Hopeful that this [illegible] elp
with these painful decisions

CHRONIC PAIN IN SMALL ANIMAL MEDICINE

Steven M Fox
MS, DVM, MBA, PhD
Surgical Specialist: New Zealand VMA
Independent Consultant, Albuquerque New Mexico, USA
Adjunct Professor, College of Veterinary Medicine, University of Illinois
Program Chairman (2000-02), President (2004), Veterinary Orthopedic Society

MANSON PUBLISHING/THE VETERINARY PRESS

ISBN: 978-1-84076-124-5

A CIP catalogue record for this book is available from the British Library.

For full details of all Manson Publishing Ltd titles please write to:
Manson Publishing Ltd, 73 Corringham Road, London NW11 7DL, UK.
Tel: +44(0)20 8905 5150
Fax: +44(0)20 8201 9233
Website: www.mansonpublishing.com

Cover illustration courtesy of Nancy Kedersha, UCLA Science Photo Library

Commissioning editor: Jill Northcott
Project manager: Kate Nardoni, cactusdesign.co.uk
Copy-editor: Joanna Brocklesby
Designer: Cathy Martin, Presspack Computing Ltd
Layout: DiacriTech, India
Colour reproduction: Tenon & Polert Colour Scanning Ltd, Hong Kong
Printed by: Grafos SA, Barcelona, Spain

CONTENTS

PREFACE

To life, which is the place of pain…

Bhagavad Gita

There is no pain pathway! Pain is the result of a complex signaling network. The cognition of pain, like cognition in general, requires sophisticated neurological hardware.

Pain has many definitions because it's an intensely subjective experience that is filtered through our emotions as well as our anatomy. It's any sensation amplified to an uncomfortable level, and it's a plethora of negative emotions called 'suffering'. No one patient feels pain the same – there is no single accepted pain experience. Like the perception of beauty, it's very real, but only in the eye of the beholder. Yet, pain is so fundamental to our well-being that it is added to heart rate, respiratory rate, temperature, and blood pressure as the 'fifth vital sign'. Without a 'pain thermometer' people in pain must rely on their language skills to describe what they are feeling. In human medicine pain is what the patient says it is, in veterinary medicine pain is what the assessor says it is! Trained as scientists, veterinarians are schooled to assess responses based on the mean ± standard deviation, yet effective pain management suggests we target the least-respondent patient within the population, so as to ensure no patient is declined the relief of pain it needs and deserves.

In its simplest sense, pain protects us from bodily harm, hence the proposal that pain is a teacher, the headmaster of nature's survival school. Dangerous things are noxious things, and pain punishes us if we take excessive risks or push ourselves beyond our physical limits. Further, pain often forces us to observe 'recovery time'. Another way of understanding pain is that any stimulus – noxious or otherwise – can become painful if the patient's ability to cope with it has been diminished.

A working definition of chronic pain is that, unlike acute pain, it lasts beyond the time necessary for healing and resists normal treatment. The primary indicator of chronic pain is not how long it persists, but whether it remains long after it should have disappeared. As the father of pain medicine, John Bonica, explains, 'Acute pain is a symptom of disease; chronic pain itself is a disease.'

The noxious stimuli that constitute pain can reconfigure the architecture of the nervous system they invade. Lasting noxious input can produce a neurobiological cycle of chemical and electrical action and reactions that becomes an automatic feedback loop: a chronic, self-perpetuating torment that persists long after the original trauma has healed.

From the human healthcare experience, pain, and in particular chronic pain, is a major problem for which current treatments are often inadequate. The tangible costs economically are in the many tens of billions of dollars, and the costs in terms of suffering are known all too well to practitioners who seek to help these patients. In veterinary medicine we are experiencing a surge of increasing focus on measuring and resolving pain and suffering, and indeed, this aspect is central to the veterinarian's oath. This focus is being supported by an increased understanding of pain neurophysiology, discovery of novel treatment targets, a greater offering of innovative pharmacologics, and consumer demand. The pharmaceutical industry has made important strides forward in bringing new therapies to address the problem of chronic pain, but to the suffering patient, this progress is glacially slow. Specific areas of exploration include peripheral nervous system targets, central nervous system targets, disease-specific targets, and development of measurement tools and applications of new technologies.

In the 1880s Friedrich Bayer and Company commercialized Bayer Aspirin®. When aspirin ('a' for acetyl, part of its chemical composition; 'spir' from a plant that contained salicin; and 'in' a popular medical suffix at the time) went over the counter in 1915, the mass production of pain alleviators for the general public was launched. Pain is the most common reason patients see a physician, while pain and pain relief are among the most robust areas of medical research.

Realistically, new discoveries and innovative drug formulations for veterinary patients will continue to lag considerably behind those for humans, despite the fact that animals are often used for the development of human therapies. This is a reality of present-day economics, appreciated as return on investment by the pharmaceutical industry. Accordingly, there are presently, and will likely in the future be, a limited number of agents and techniques actually labeled for veterinary use. It is, therefore, incumbent on the veterinarian and veterinary healthcare professional to understand both the neurobiology of chronic pain, and the mode of action of various therapies so as to determine if the therapeutic agent or technique is likely to be safe and efficacious when utilized 'off-label'. Such insights may not be readily available for the proposed target patient, but would be 'inferred' from data obtained from a different species. Herein comes the weighing of 'species specificity' vs. 'one science' in the clinical decision-making process.

This text was created for the veterinary healthcare professional seeking a greater depth of knowledge in mechanisms of pain accompanying chronic disease states, and potential targets for treatment. It aspires to go beyond the 'cookbook protocols' found in many offerings, by providing contemporary understandings of 'why and how to treat'.

Steven M. Fox

DISCLAIMER

The contents of this text are intended to further general scientific research, understanding, and discussion only and are not intended and should not be relied upon as recommending or promoting a specific method, diagnosis, or treatment by practitioners for any particular patient. The publisher and the author make no representations or warranties with respect to the accuracy or completeness of the contents of this work and specifically disclaim all warranties, including without limitation any implied warranties of fitness for a particular purpose. In view of ongoing research, equipment modifications, changes in governmental regulations, and the constant flow of information relating to the use of medicines, equipment, and devices, the reader is urged to review and evaluate the information provided in package inserts or instructions for each medicine, equipment, or device for, among other things, any changes in the instructions or indication of usage and for added warnings and precautions. Readers should consult with a specialist where appropriate. The fact that an organization or website is referred to in this work as a citation and/or a potential source of further information does not mean that the author or the publisher endorses the information the organization or website may provide or recommendations it may make. Further, readers should be aware that internet websites listed in the work may have changed or disappeared between when this work was written and when it is read. No warranty may be created or extended by any promotional statements for this work. Neither the publisher nor the author shall be liable for any damages arising from this work.

ACKNOWLEDGEMENTS

It is said that fulfillment comes from (1) having something to do, (2) having something to look forward to, and (3) having someone to love. If that is true, then I am three times blessed. I first wish to acknowledge my supportive wife Pam, who each day demonstrates compassionate care for our pets and encourages my commitment to raising the standards of pain management for veterinary patients.

I also wish to recognize the contributors to this work, who are noted international leaders in veterinary medicine. It is my good fortune to learn from their collaboration, and more importantly, to embrace them as personal friends and colleagues.

Creation of the International Veterinary Academy of Pain Management (IVAPM) and the International Association for the Study of Pain: Non-human Special Interest Group (IASP:SIG) has made a framework through which we can all collectively advance the science and practice of pain management. Congratulations to the visionaries who have invested their resources toward the creation of these organizations, and thanks to their membership who have recognized a forum for the promotion of our common interests.

Finally, I want to salute Manson Publishing for their recognition of contemporary veterinary issues, servicing their readers' interests with quality resources, and providing a congenial framework for collaboration.

The best doctor in the world is the veterinarian.
He can't ask his patients what is the matter –
he's got to just know.
Will Rogers

CONTRIBUTORS

STEVEN M. FOX MS, DVM, MBA, PhD
Surgical Specialist: New Zealand VMA
Independent Consultant, Albuquerque, New Mexico, USA
Adjunct Professor, College of Veterinary Medicine, University of Illinois
Program Chairman (2000-02), President (2004), Veterinary Orthopedic Society

SHEILAH A. ROBERTSON BVMS (Hons), PhD, DACVA, DECVA, CVA, MRCVS
Professor: Anesthesia, Pain Management and Animal Welfare
College of Veterinary Medicine
University of Florida
Gainesville, Florida

WILLIAM J. TRANQUILLI DVM, MS, DACVA
Professor Emeritus
University of Illinois
Urbana, Illinois

JAMES (JIMI) L. COOK DVM, PhD, DACVS
Associate Professor of Orthopedic Surgery and
William C. Allen Endowed Scholar for Orthopedic Research
Director: Comparative Orthopedic Laboratory
College of Veterinary Medicine
University of Missouri
Columbia, Missouri

B. DUNCAN X. LASCELLES BSc, BVSc, PhD, CertVA, DSAS(ST), DECVS, DACVS
Associate Professor: Small Animal Surgery
College of Veterinary Medicine
North Carolina State University
Raleigh, North Carolina

NICOLE EHRHART VMD, MS, DACVS
Associate Professor: Oncology
College of Veterinary Medicine
Colorado State University
Fort Collins, Colorado

ABBREVIATIONS

5-HT	5-hydroxytryptamine
AA	arachidonic acid
ACE	angiotensin converting enzyme
ADE	adverse drug event
ADP	adenosine diphosphate
ALA	alpha-linolenic acid
ALT	alanine aminotransferase
AMA	American Medical Association
AMP	adenosine monophosphate
AMPA	alpha-amino-3-hydroxy-5-methyl-4-isoxazole propionic-acid
ARS	acute radiation score
ASIC	acid-sensing ion channel
ASU	avocado/soybean unsaponifiables
ATL	aspirin triggered lipoxin
ATP	adenosine triphosphate
BDNF	brain-derived neurotrophic factor
BUN	blood urea nitrogen
cAMP	cyclic adenosine monophosphate
CCK	cholecystokinin
CCL	cranial cruciate ligament
CCLT	cranial cruciate ligament transection
CGRP	calcitonin gene-related peptide
CIPN	chemotherapy-induced peripheral neuropathy
CMPS	composite measure pain scale
CNS	central nervous system
COX	cyclo-oxygenase
CrCLD	cranial cruciate ligament deficiency
CRI	continuous rate infusion
DHA	docosahexaenoic acid
DJD	degenerative joint disease
DMOAA	disease-modifying osteoarthritic agent
DMOAD	disease modifying osteoarthritic drug
DRG	dorsal root ganglion
ELISA	enzyme-linked immunosorbent assay
eNOS	endothelian NOS
EPA	eicosapentaenoic acid
ERK	extracellular signal-regulated kinase
FDA	Food and Drug Administration
fMRI	functional magnetic resonance imaging
GABA	gamma aminobutyric acid
GAG	glycosaminoglycan
GAIT	Glucosamine/chondroitin Arthritis Intervention Trial
GCMPS	Glasgow composite measure of pain scale
GDNF	glial-derived neurotrophic factor
HA	hyaluronic acid
HCN	hyperpolarization-activated cyclic nucleotide-gated
HIV	human immunodeficiency virus
HRQL	health-related quality of life
HVA	high-voltage activated
IASP	International Association for the Study of Pain
IBS	irritable bowel syndrome
IC	interstitial cystitis
IKK	IκB kinase
IL	interleukin
iNOS	inducible NOS
KCS	keratoconjunctivitis sicca
LOX	lipoxygenase
LT	leukotriene
LVA	low-voltage activated
MFPS	multifactorial pain scales
MMP	matrix metalloproteinase
NAVNA	North American Veterinary Nutraceutical Association
NE	norepinephrine
NF-κB	nuclear factor kappaB
NGF	nerve growth factor
NMDA	N-methyl-D-aspartate
nNOS	neuronal NOS
NNT	number needed to treat

NO	nitric oxide
NOS	nitric oxide synthase
NPY	neuropeptides Y
NRS	numeric rating scales
NSAID	nonsteroidal anti-inflammatory drug
OA	osteoarthritis
OTM	oral transmucosal
P2X	ionotropic purinoceptor
P2Y	metabotropic purinoceptor
PDN	painful diabetic neuropathy
PG	prostaglandin
PHN	postherpetic neuralgia
PNS	peripheral nervous system
PSGAG	polysulfated glycosaminoglycan
SAMe	S-adenosylmethionine
SAP	serum alkaline phosphatase
SDS	simple descriptive scales
SERT	serotonin transporter
SNL	spinal nerve ligation
sP	substance P
SSRI	selective serotonin reuptake inhibitors
TENS	transcutaneous electrical nerve stimulation
TGF	transforming growth factor
TIMP	tissue inhibitor of metalloproteinase
TNF	tumor necrosis factor
TRP	transient receptor potential
TRPV	transient receptor potential vanilloid
TTX	tetrodotoxin
TX	thromboxane
VAS	visual analog scales
VDCC	voltage-dependent calcium channel
VGSC	voltage-gated sodium channel
VR	vanilloid receptor
VRS	verbal rating scales
WDR	wide dynamic range

1 PHYSIOLOGY OF PAIN

IN PERSPECTIVE

Pain management has become one of the more inspiring contemporary issues in veterinary medicine. It is an area of progressive research, revealing new understandings on an almost daily basis. Accordingly, 'current' insights to pain management is a relative term. In some respects the management of pain, especially in companion animal practice, is more thorough than in human medicine. And, although it is amusing to recognize that most pain in humans is managed based upon rodent data, considerable direction for managing pain in animals is based upon the human pain experience. This is because many physiological systems are similar across species, and large population studies often conducted in human medicine require resources prohibitive in veterinary medicine. Herein, evidence-based veterinary pain management will likely always be under some degree of scrutiny. Since our maturation of understanding the complex mechanisms of pain comes from studies in different species with many physiological processes in common, it is fitting to consider the study of pain as 'one science'.

The frontier of discovery for treating pain is founded upon an understanding of physiology and neurobiology. Physiological mechanisms underpin the evidence supporting treatment protocols and provide insights for new drug development. An overview of pain physiology is intellectually intriguing, but extensive. Therefore, the following synopsis is presented to gain an appreciation of the complex mechanisms underlying chronic pain and to encourage lateral thinking about treatment modalities. Paraphrasing Albert Einstein, 'some things can be made simple, but only so much so before they lose meaning'.

UNDERSTANDING THE PHYSIOLOGY OF PAIN

Nociception is the transduction, conduction, and central nervous system (CNS) processing of signals generated by a noxious insult. The conscious, cognitive processing of nociception results in pain, i.e. pain infers consciousness. It is reasonable to assume that a stimulus considered painful to a human, that is damaging or potentially damaging to tissues and evokes escape and behavioral responses, would also be painful to an animal because anatomical structures and neurophysiological processes leading to the perception of pain are similar across species.

The pain pathway suggests reference to the simplistic nociceptive pathway of a three-neuron chain, with the first-order neuron originating in the periphery and projecting to the spinal cord, the second-order neuron ascending the spinal cord, and the third-order neuron projecting into the cerebral cortex and other supraspinal structures (**1**).

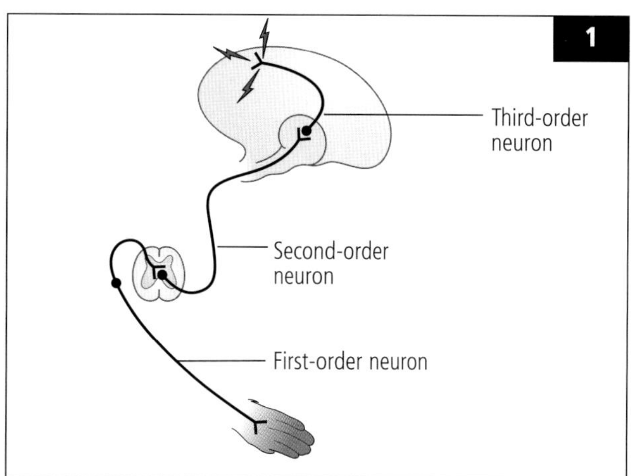

1 The Pain Pathway infers a three-neuron chain. The first-order neuron originates in the periphery and projects to the spinal cord. The second-order neuron ascends the spinal cord and the third-order neuron projects into the cerebral cortex and other supraspinal structures. (Adapted from: Tranquilli WJ, *et al.* Pain Management for the Small Animal Practitioner. Teton NewMedia 2004, 2nd edition (with permission)).

'For every complex issue, there is an answer that is simple, neat...and wrong!' There are no 'pain fibers' in nerves and no 'pain pathways' in the brain. Pain is not a stimulus. The experience of pain is the final product of a complex information-processing network.

AFFERENT RECEPTORS

Peripheral sensory receptors are specialized terminations of afferent nerve fibers exposed to the tissue environment, even when the fiber is myelinated more centrally. Such receptors are plentiful in the epidermis/dermis and display differentiated functions (2):

- Low-threshold mechanoreceptors: Aα, Aβ in humans; Aα, Aβ, Aδ, and C in animals.
- Displacement: Ruffini endings–stretch; hair follicle with palisade endings of 10–15 different nerve fibers each.

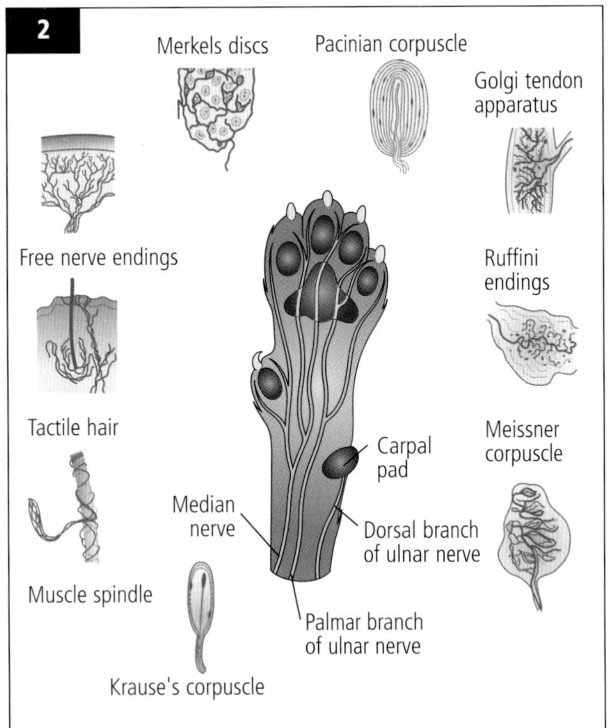

2 Afferent receptors are widely dispersed and serve different functions, allowing the animal to sense its environment. (Adapted from: Tranquilli WJ, *et al.* Pain Management for the Small Animal Practitioner. Teton NewMedia 2004, 2nd edition (with permission)).

- Velocity: Meissner corpuscle.
- Vibration: Pacinian corpuscle, fluid environment with onion-like lamellae acting as high-pass filter.
- Thermal receptors.
  - Cold: discriminates 0.5°C, 100 μm diameter field, Aδ.
  - Warm: mostly C fibers.
- Nociceptors:
  - Myelinated: Aδ, most conduct in 5–25 m/s range, 50–180 μm field, 10–250 receptors/mm^2.
  - C polymodal nociceptors; pain.

As terminations of afferent nerve fibers, peripheral sensory receptors allow the receptor to transduce or translate specific kinds of energy into action potentials. Most peripheral receptors act either by direct coupling of physical energy to cause changes in ion channel permeability or by activation of second messenger cascades. Chemoreceptors detect products of tissue damage or inflammation that initiate receptor excitation. Free nerve endings are also in close proximity to mast cells and small blood vessels. Contents of ruptured cells or plasma contents, together with neurotransmitters released from activated nerve terminals, create a milieu of proteins, allowing the free nerve endings, capillaries, and mast cells to act together as an evil triumvirate to increase pain (3).

Although there are no pain fibers or pain pathways, there are anatomically and physiologically specialized peripheral sensory neurons–nociceptors–which respond to noxious stimuli, but not to weak stimuli (*Table 1*). These are mostly thinly myelinated Aδ and unmyelinated C afferents, and they end as free, unencapsulated peripheral nerve endings in most tissues of the body including skin, deep somatic tissues like muscles and joints, and viscera. (The brain itself is not served by these sensory fibers, which is why cutting brain tissue does not hurt.) Thickly myelinated Aβ afferents typically respond to light tactile stimuli. They also respond to noxious stimuli, but they do not increase their response when the stimulus changes from moderate to strong, i.e. they do not encode stimuli in the noxious range. Although Aβ afferents do respond to painful stimuli, electrical stimulation, even at high frequency, normally produces a sensation not of pain, but of nonpainful pressure. Convergence of large- and small-diameter afferents of various sorts at the level of the dorsal horn, with further processing in the brain, gives rise to a variety of everyday sensations.

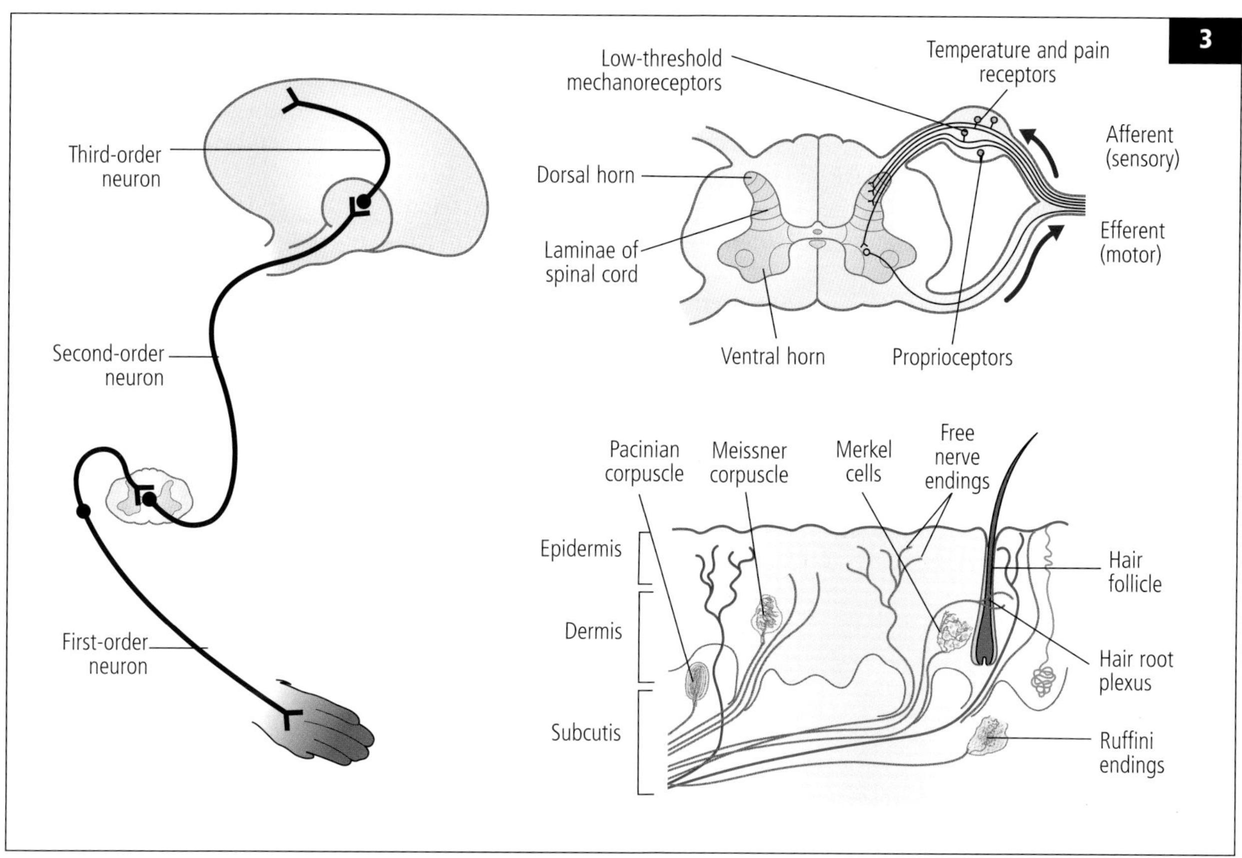

3 A milieu of inflammatory mediators results in receptor excitation that transduce or translate specific forms of energy into action potentials. Such action potentials become the nociceptive messengers for pain.

Table 1 Nociceptors and fiber types.

Nociceptors	Fiber type and response
Aδ	Small myelinated fibers; slowest conducting are nociceptors
AMH type I (A mechano-heat)	Respond to mechanical stimuli; have heat threshold of 53°C, but sensitize rapidly to heat; most common
AMH type II	Respond to mechanical stimuli; threshold 47°C, also respond to noxious cold
AM	Respond only to noxious mechanical stimulation
CMH	Most common C (polymodal nociceptor); responds to mechanical stimuli; thermal threshold 45–49°C; noxious cold ≤4°C
CH	Responds to heat only; thermal threshold 45–49°C
CMC	Like CMH, responds to noxious cold instead of heat
CC	Responds to noxious cold only
Silent nociceptors	Do not fire in absence of tissue injury

A change in temperature or an agonist binding to a membrane may cause a conformational change in the shape of a receptor protein allowing influx of ions or triggering second messenger pathways (**4**). When transient receptor potential (TRP) (vanilloid or capsaicin) receptors are activated, they directly allow calcium ion cell influx, which can be sufficient to initiate neurotransmitter release.

Primary afferents will fire action potentials at different adaptive rates. For example, touch receptors or vibration detectors and hair follicle afferents fire at the beginning and sometimes at the end of a maintained stimulus–they respond to the change (delta) of a stimulus. In contrast, nociceptors never fully adapt and stop firing in the presence of a stimulus. They are difficult to turn off once they are activated.

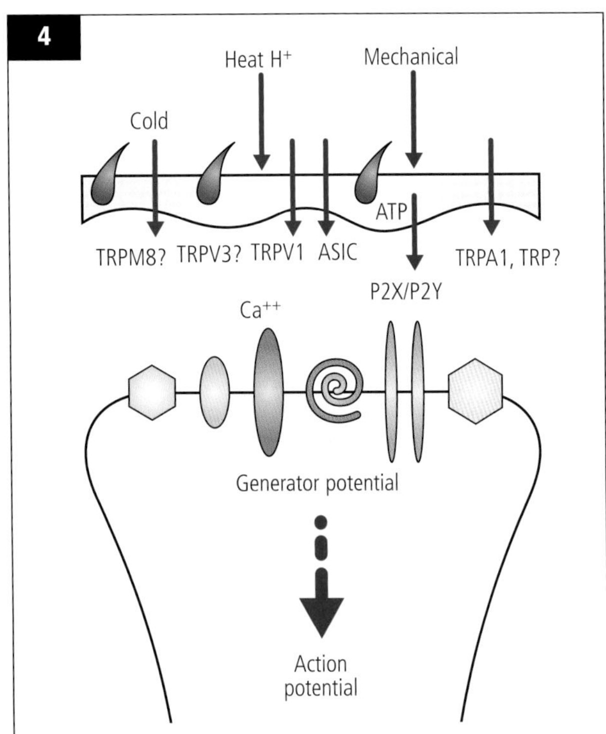

4 Receptor activation may allow ion influx or trigger a second messenger pathway that initiates an action potential.

The term *vanilloid* refers to a group of substances related structurally and pharmacologically to capsaicin, the pungent ingredient of chili peppers. The principal action of capsaicin and other vanilloids on the sensory neuron membrane is to produce a nonselective increase in cation (+) permeability, associated with the opening of a distinct type of cation channel. The inward current responsible for depolarization and excitation of the neurons is carried mainly by sodium ions, but the channel is also permeable to divalent cations, including calcium. The vanilloid receptor VR1 (also called TRPV1) shows a remarkable characteristic of heat sensitivity (and also acidic pH), with robust channel opening in response to increases in ambient temperature. The physiological effects of capsaicin are numerous:

- Immediate pain.
- Various autonomic effects caused by peripheral release of substance P (sP) and calcitonin gene-related peptide (CGRP), inducing profound vasodilatation, while release of sP promotes vascular leakage and protein extravasation; components of the neurogenic inflammatory response: rubor (redness), calor (heat), and tumor (swelling).
- An antinociceptive effect of varying duration, associated with desensitizative effect of capsaicin on the peripheral terminals of C fibers. The cellular mechanisms underlying the neurodegenerative consequences of capsaicin likely involve both necrotic and apoptotic cell death.
- A fall in body temperature: a reflex response generated by thermosensitive neurons in the hypothalamus following capsaicin activation of primary afferent fibers.

Capsaicin acts on nonmyelinated peripheral afferent fibers to deplete sP and other transmitter peptides; the net effect is first to stimulate and then to destroy C fibers.[1]

A number of receptor systems reportedly play a role in the peripheral modulation of nociceptor responsiveness. The vanilloid receptor, TRPV1, is present on a subpopulation of primary afferent fibers and is activated by capsaicin, heat and protons. Following inflammation, axonal transport of TRPV1 mRNA is induced, with the proportion of TRPV1-labeled unmyelinated axons in the periphery being increased by almost 100%.[2] The inflammatory mediator bradykinin lowers the threshold of TRPV1-mediated heat-induced currents in dorsal root ganglion (DRG) neurons, and increases the proportion of DRG cells that respond to capsaicin.[3]

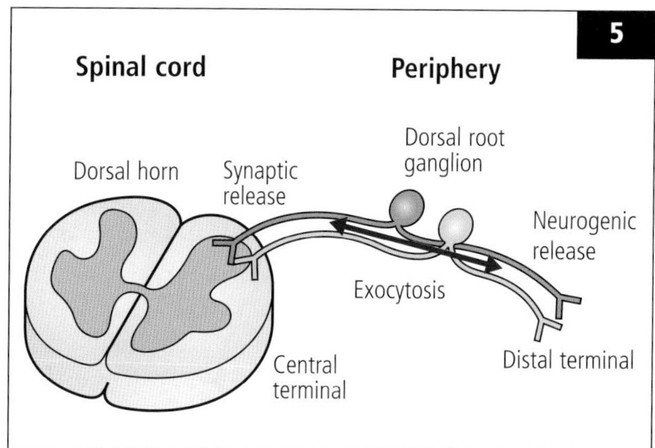

5 Neurotransmitters and modulators are transported from the DRG both centrally and peripherally.

In addition, there is a synergism between an acid pH and the capsaicin (VR1) receptor, such that transmembrane current is significantly increased from the inflammatory environment.[4] To date, strong evidence exists showing that nociceptor firing and human perception of pain are correlated (the animal corollary is not yet validated).

Cell bodies manufacture neurotransmitters and modulators of all kinds, as well as receptors and ion channels. These are transported from the DRG both centrally and peripherally (**5**). Glutamate is the major excitatory neurotransmitter of nociceptors. sP and CGRP are peptide transmitters of nociceptors. Ion channels exist along the length of the primary afferent fibers and functional receptors, while mechanisms to release at least some neurotransmitters also prevail along the length of the axon. Several neurotransmitters can exist in a single neuron.

Depolarization induces the release of neurotransmitters (**6**), and excesses of released neurotransmitters (e.g. glutamate) are recycled by the presynaptic terminal. Further, it has been shown that calcium flow through transient receptor potential (TRV) receptors along the course of the axon is sufficient to cause release of neurotransmitters, independent of axon depolarization.[5] This implies that inflammatory mediators, heat, or changes in pH can cause release of potentially pain-producing substances along the entire length of a nerve. However, the patient will sense the pain emanating from the peripheral terminations. It is also noted that the release of some neurotransmitters cannot be evoked by individual inflammatory mediators, such as prostaglandin (PG) E_2; however, together with bradykinin, PGE_2 can enhance neurotransmitter release.

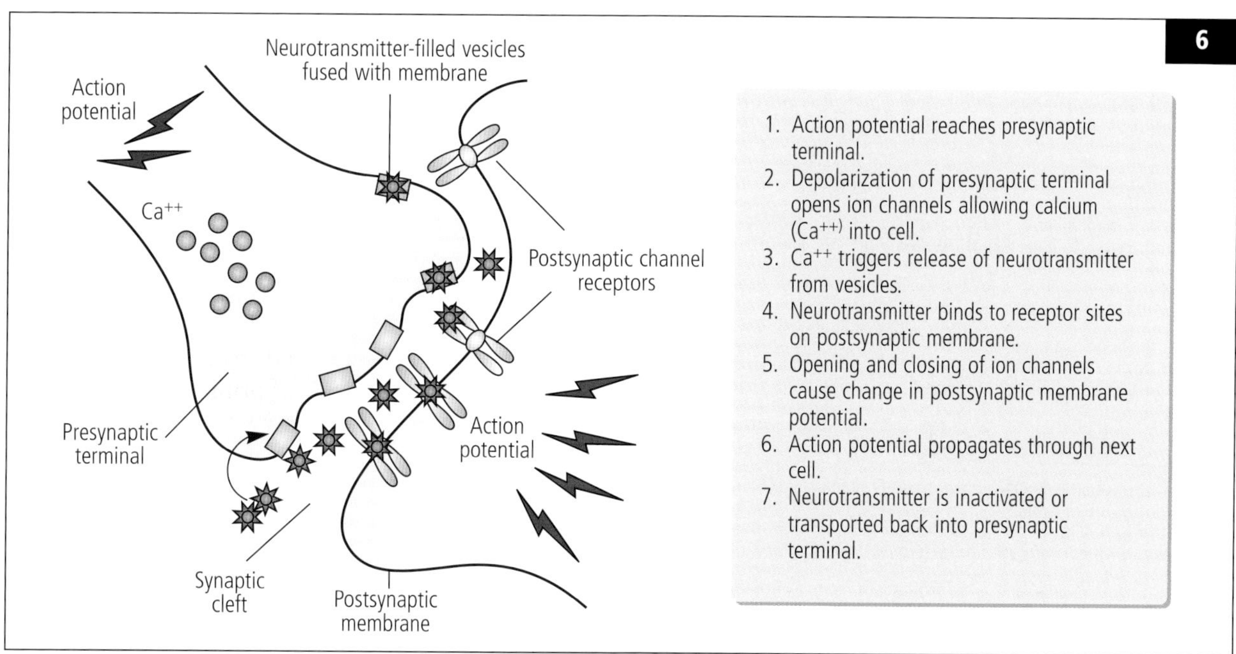

6 At the synapse, there is a chemical transmission of the nerve impulse.

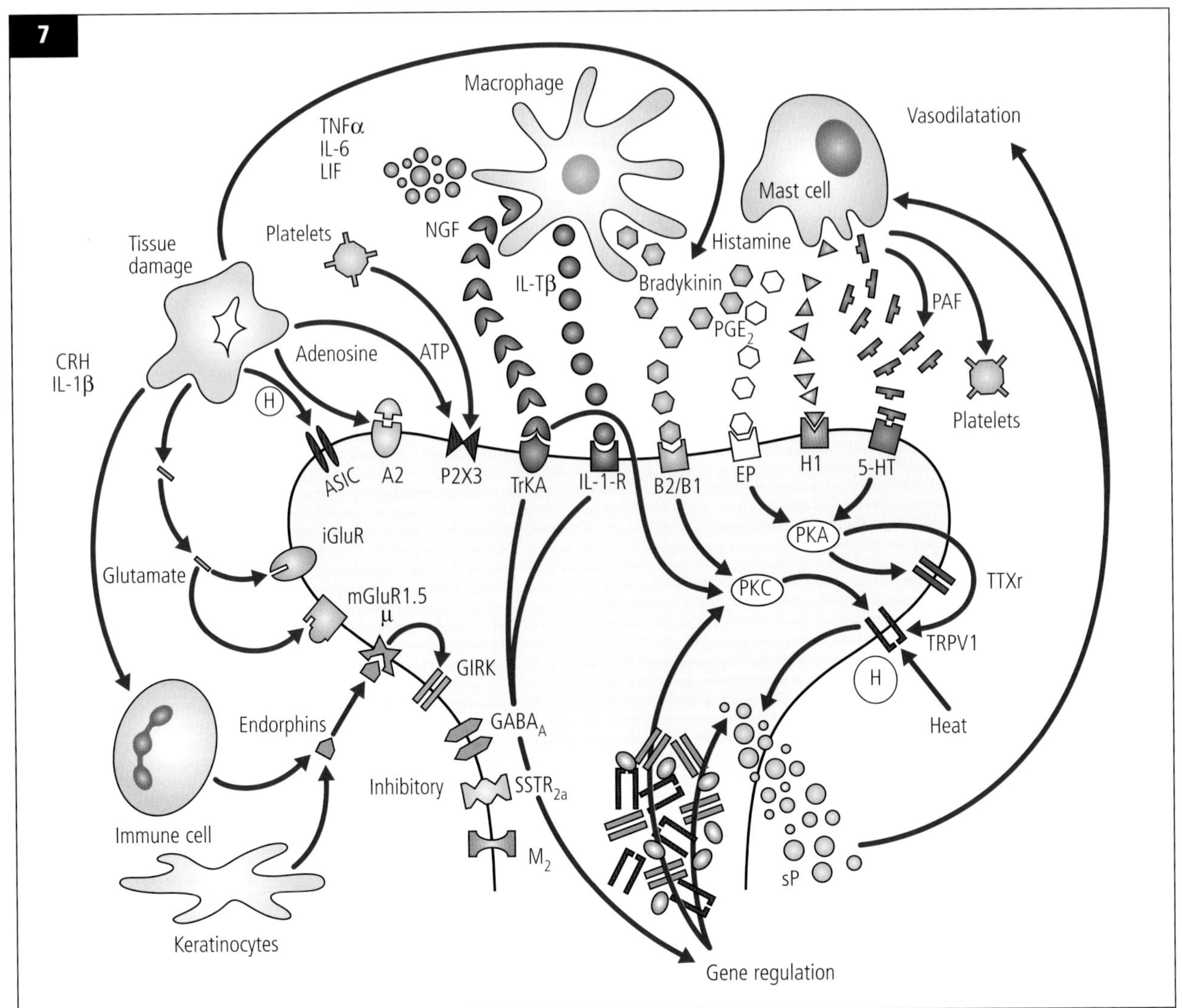

7 Many different types of receptors may reside on primary afferent terminals. (Adapted from Woolf CJ, Costigan M. Transcriptional and posttranslational plasticity and the generation of inflammatory pain. *Proc Natl Acad Sci* 1999; **96**: 7723–7730).

Neurotransmitters are noted as such only if they have a receptor for binding. Other criteria include: (1) synthesis in the neuron DRG, (2) seen in presynaptic terminal (central or peripheral) and released in sufficient quantities to exert a defined action on the postsynaptic neuron or tissue, (3) exogenous administration mimics endogenously released neurotransmitter, (4) a mechanism exists for its removal, and (5) it is released by neuronal depolarization in a Ca^{++}-dependent fashion. Many different neurotransmitters exist, most notably glutamate, sP, and CGRP. Glutamate is the most prevalent neurotransmitter in the CNS, and is synthesized not only in the cell body, but also in the terminals.

Several receptors reside on primary afferent terminals, which regulate terminal excitability: serotonin, somatostatin, interleukin, tyrosine kinase, ionotropic glutamate, etc. (7).

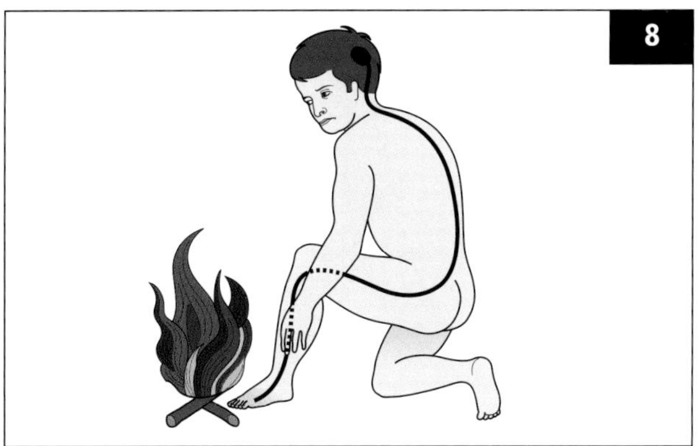

8 In the seventeenth century, René Descartes proposed that pain was transmitted through tubes of transfer.

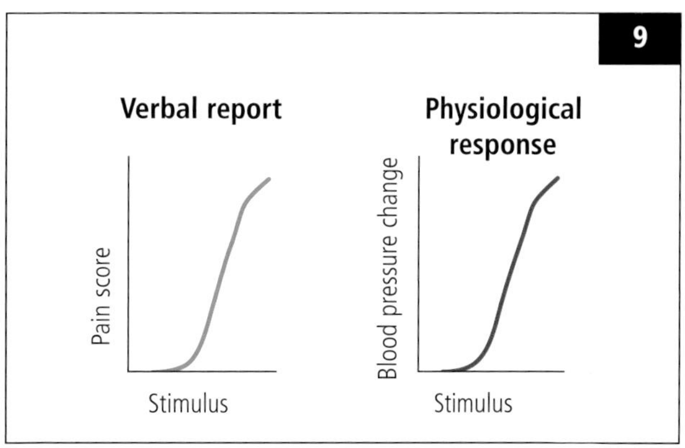

9 Cartesian model: psychophysical experience (pain report) = *f* (stimulus intensity).

MEDIATORS OF PAIN

PGs are not the only chemical mediators of inflammation and hypersensitivity. The acidity and heat of injured, inflamed tissue enhances pain and hypersensitivity through response of the capsaicin/vanilloid receptor (TRPV1). sP and CGRP can be released from the peripheral terminals of activated C fibers and contribute to neurogenic inflammation by causing vasodilatation. Affected tissues are subsequently in a state of *peripheral sensitization*. sP is an 11-amino-acid peptide neurotransmitter, often co-occurring with CGRP, which, when released in the spinal dorsal horn, activates second-order transmission neurons that send a nociceptive ('pain') signal to the brain.

PLASTICITY ENCODING

René Descartes (1596–1650) proposed that 'pain' was transmitted from the periphery to a higher center through tubes of transfer (**8**). From the concept of Descartes came the Cartesian model: a fixed relationship between the magnitude of stimulus and subsequent sensation (**9**).

The Cartesian model has evolved over the centuries through the contributions of many, including C.S. Sherrington (1852–1952), who coined the term 'nociception', stating that a nociceptive stimulus will evoke a constellation of responses which define the pain state. Nociception, *per se*, separates the detection of the event (noxious stimulus) from the production of a psychological or other type of response (pain). In a simple example, injury in the legs of a paraplegic produces nociception from impulses in nociceptors, exactly as in a normal subject, but there is no pain perceived. A common clinical example is routine surgery, where neurobiolgical data confirms nociception (response to the noxious stimulus), but pain is not experienced while the patient is at an appropriate stage of anesthesia, i.e. there is no cognitive processing of the nociception.

The classic Cartesian view of pain stemmed from René Descartes' 'bell ringer' model of pain in which pain, as a purely quantitative phenomenon, is designed to alert us to physical injury. Studying World War II injuries, Henry Beecher observed that some soldiers with horrendous injuries often felt no pain, while soldiers with minor injuries sometimes had severe pain. Beecher concluded that Descartes' theory was all wrong: there is no linear relationship between injury and the perception of pain.

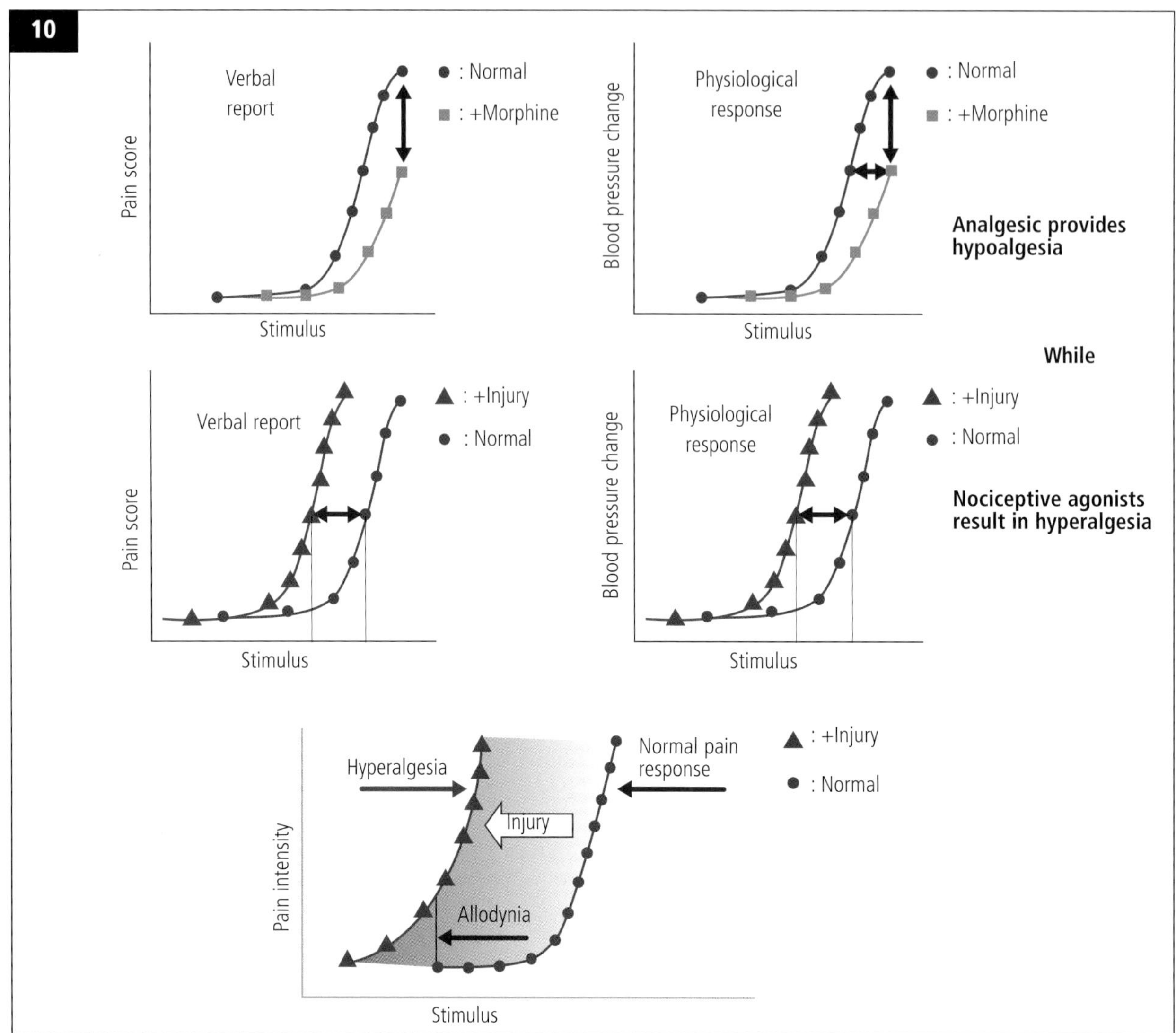

10 Pain encoding is dynamic. An analgesic can provide hypoalgesia, while complementary nociceptive agonists can result in hyperalgesia. A left shift in the stimulus–response curve can result in allodynia, i.e. a normally non-noxious stimulus becomes noxious.

It is now appreciated that there exists a plasticity of pain encoding. A diminished response (as with the analgesic morphine) to a given noxious stimulus can give rise to hypoalgesia/analgesia. On the other hand, local injury can shift the stimulus–response curve to the left, giving rise to the same pain report with a lower stimulus: hyperalgesia. If the curve is shifted such that a non-noxious stimulus becomes noxious, the state is referred to as allodynia (**10**).

Hyperalgesia to both heat and mechanical stimulus that occurs at the site of an injury is due to sensitization of primary afferent nociceptors.[6,7] Mechanisms of the phenomenon have been studied in various tissues, including the joint, cornea, testicle, gastrointestinal tract, and bladder. Hyperalgesia at the site of injury is termed *primary hyperalgesia*, while hyperalgesia in the uninjured tissue surrounding the injury is termed *secondary hyperalgesia*.

GATE THEORY

The existence of a specific pain modulatory system was first clearly articulated in 1965 by Melzack and Wall[8] in the gate control theory of pain. This was the first theory to propose that the CNS controls nociception. The basic premises of the gate control theory of pain are that activity in large (non-nociceptive) fibers can inhibit the perception of activity in small (nociceptive) fibers and that descending activity from the brain also can inhibit that perception, i.e. interneurons of the substantia gelatinosa regulate the input of large and small fibers to lamina V cells, serving as a gating mechanism. Most simplistically: fast moving action potentials in myelinated fibers activate inhibitor neurons that shut down second-order neurons before slower arriving signals reach the inhibitor neurons via nonmyelinated fibers (**11**). These signals from unmyelinated fibers would normally shut down inhibitor neurons, thereby allowing further transmission through second-order neurons. With the gate theory, Melzack and Wall formalized observations that encoding of high-intensity afferent input was subject to modulation. Although their concept was accurate, details of their explanation have since been more accurately modified.

As an example, transcutaneous electrical nerve stimulation (TENS) therapy is a clinical implementation of the gate theory. TENS is thought to act by preferential stimulation of peripheral somatosensory fibers, which conduct more rapidly than nociceptive fibers. This results in a stimulation of inhibitory interneurons in the second lamina of the posterior horn (substantia gelatinosa) that effectively blocks nociception at the spinal cord level. Further, the gate theory may explain why some people feel a decrease in pain intensity when skin near the pain region is rubbed with a hand ('rubbing it better'), and how a local area is 'desensitized' by rubbing prior to insertion of a needle. An additional example would be the shaking of a burned hand, an action that predominantly activates large nerve fibers.

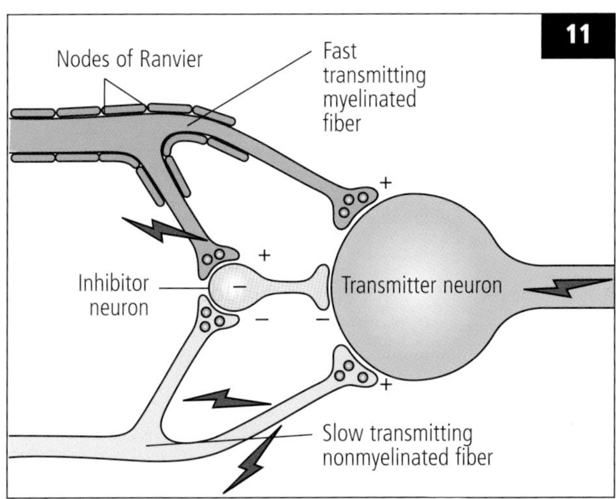

11 Melzack and Wall's gate control theory of pain; the first theory proposing that nociception was under modulation by the CNS.

ACTIVITY OF NOCICEPTORS

Injured nerve fibers develop ectopic sensitivity. A substantial proportion of C fiber afferents are nociceptors, and abnormal spontaneous activity has been observed in A fibers and C fibers originating from neuronal-resultant nerve transections. In patients with hyperalgesic neuromas, locally anesthetizing the neuroma often eliminates the pain.[9]

Nociceptor activity induces increased sympathetic discharge. In certain painful patients, nocipeptors acquire sensitivity to norepinephrine (NE; noradrenalin) released by sympathetic efferents. Pain caused by activity in the sympathetic nervous system is referred to as *sympathetically maintained pain*. In human studies of stump neuromas and skin,[10] it is concluded that apparently sympathetically maintained pain does not arise from too much epinephrine (adrenalin), but rather from the presence of adrenergic receptors that are coupled to nociceptors. In sympathetically maintained pain, nociceptors develop α-adrenergic sensitivity such that the release of NE by the sympathetic nervous system produces spontaneous activity in the nociceptors. This spontaneous activity maintains the CNS in a sensitized state. Therefore, in sympathetically maintained pain, NE that normally is released from the sympathetic terminals acquires the capacity to evoke pain. In the presence of a sensitized central pain-signaling neuron (second order), pain in response to light touch is induced by activity in low-threshold mechanoreceptors–allodynia. In this circumstance, α_1-adrenergic antagonists lessen nociceptor activity and the resultant hyperalgesia or allodynia.

VOLTAGE-GATED ION CHANNELS

Following thermal, mechanical or chemical stimulation of primary afferents, the excitatory event must initiate a regenerative action potential involving voltage-gated sodium, calcium or potassium channels culminating in neurotransmitter release, if sensory information is to be conveyed from the periphery to the second-order afferent neuron located in the spinal cord dorsal horn.

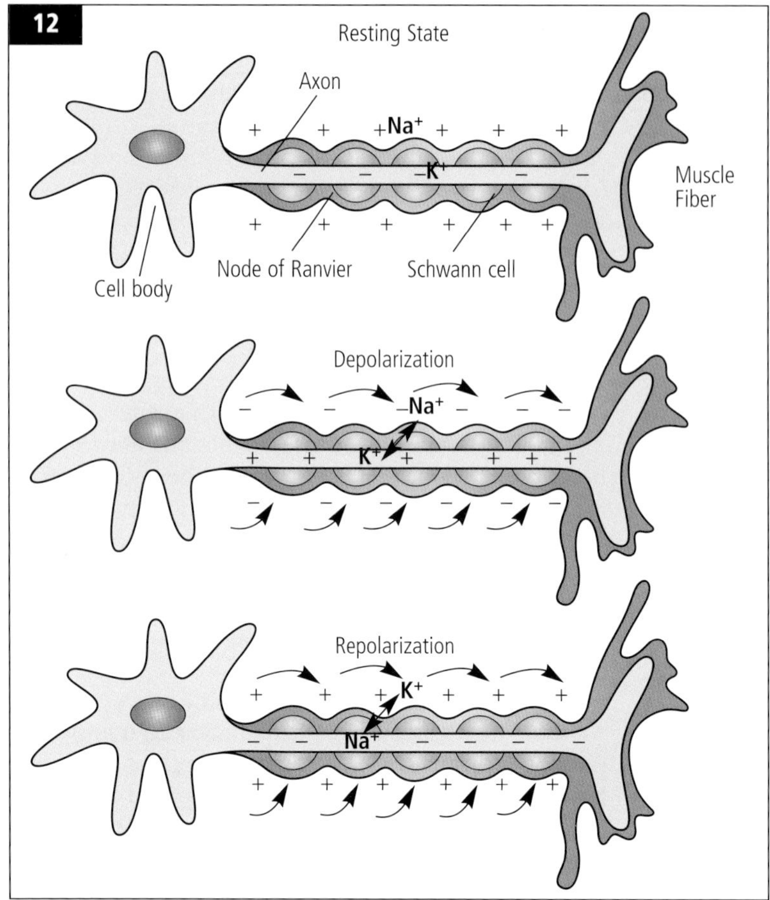

12 Sequential events during the action potential showing the normal resting potential, development of a reversal potential during depolarization, and re-establishment of the normal resting potential during repolarization.

Within the dorsal horn, the CNS 'decides' if the message lives or dies. The hypersensitization of *windup* is testimonial that the CNS dorsal horn is dynamic, and the important role of these voltage-gated ion channels makes them attractive targets for novel and selective analgesics. Voltage-gated calcium channels open when the membrane potential depolarizes and they cause intracellular calcium concentration to rise. The calcium then causes contraction of muscle and secretion of neurotransmitters and hormones from nerves. There are at least nine different types of voltage-gated sodium channel (VGSC) genes expressed in mammals[11] and three calcium channel gene families.[12] In the field of pain, calcium channel diversity is meaningful because N-type channels (from subtypes L, N, P, R and T) are critical for neurotransmission in sensory neurons, but relatively less important for excitatory transmission in the CNS. Therefore, it is important that the most effective analgesics, opiates, act upon sensory neurons by inhibiting their N-type calcium channels. Voltage-gated potassium channels are not essential for the action potential, but influence the shape of action potentials and tune their firing time. When open, they steer the membrane potential toward the potassium equilibrium potential, thereby decreasing the excitability of a cell. This makes them prime molecular targets for suppressing hyperactive neurons and suppressing hyperalgesia.

Excitability of a neuron can be changed by channels as well as receptors:

- Na^+: increased excitability with increased permeability.
- K^+: increased excitability with decreased permeability, and *vice versa*.
- Ca^{++}: increased neurotransmitter release; increased second messenger action.
- Cl^-: variable, depending on chloride equilibrium potential.

VGSC are complex, transmembrane proteins that have a role in governing electrical activity in excitable tissue. The sodium channel is activated in response to depolarization of the cell membrane that causes a voltage-dependent conformational change in the channel from a resting, closed conformation to an active conformation, the result of which increases the membrane permeability to sodium ions (**12**). Based on the sensitivity to a toxin derived from puffer fish, tetrodotoxin (TTX), sodium currents can be subdivided as being either TTX-sensitive (TTXs: $Na_v1.7$ channel, plentiful in the DRG) or TTX-resistant (TTXr: $Na_v1.8$ and $Na_v1.9$, which are exclusively expressed in cells of the DRG, and predominantly in nociceptors). Loss of function mutation of the gene that encodes $Na_v1.7$ is associated with the condition of insensitivity or indifference to pain, e.g. hot-ember barefoot walkers. In contrast, a gain of function mutation is the major cause of erythromelalgia–a condition of heat allodynia in the extremities of humans.

Accumulating evidence shows that upregulation of subtyes of sodium channels takes place in both neuropathic and inflammatory models of pain.[13] Many drugs used clinically to treat human peripheral neuropathies, including some local anesthetics (e.g. lidocaine), antiarrhythmics (e.g. mexiletine), and anticonvulsants (e.g. phenytoin and carbamazepine) are VGSC blockers.

In contrast to VGSCs, voltage-gated potassium channels act as brakes in the system, repolarizing active neurons to restore baseline membrane potentials. The hyperpolarization-activated cyclic nucleotide-gated (HCN) channel is structurally homologous to the potassium channel, prevails in cardiac tissue and DRG neurons, and modulates rhythm and waveform of action potentials–thereby also contributing to resting membrane potentials.[14]

Calcium ions play an important role in neurotransmission, being essential for transmitter release from terminals (**13**). They also play a key role in neurons, linking receptors and enzymes, acting as intracellular signals, forming a channel-gating mechanism, and contributing to the degree of depolarization of the cell. The means by which calcium enters the neuron and terminal is via calcium channels, making calcium channels targets for a variety of neurotransmitters, neuromodulators, and drugs. Two families of voltage-dependent calcium channels (VDCC) exist:

- Low threshold, rapidly activating, slowly deactivating channels (low-voltage activated (LVA) also referred to as T-type).
- High-threshold, slowly activating, fast-deactivating channels (high-voltage activated (HVA)). Zicnotide (a synthetic version of a ω-conotoxin found in the venoms of predatory marine snails) blocks depolarization-induced calcium influx through VDCC binding.

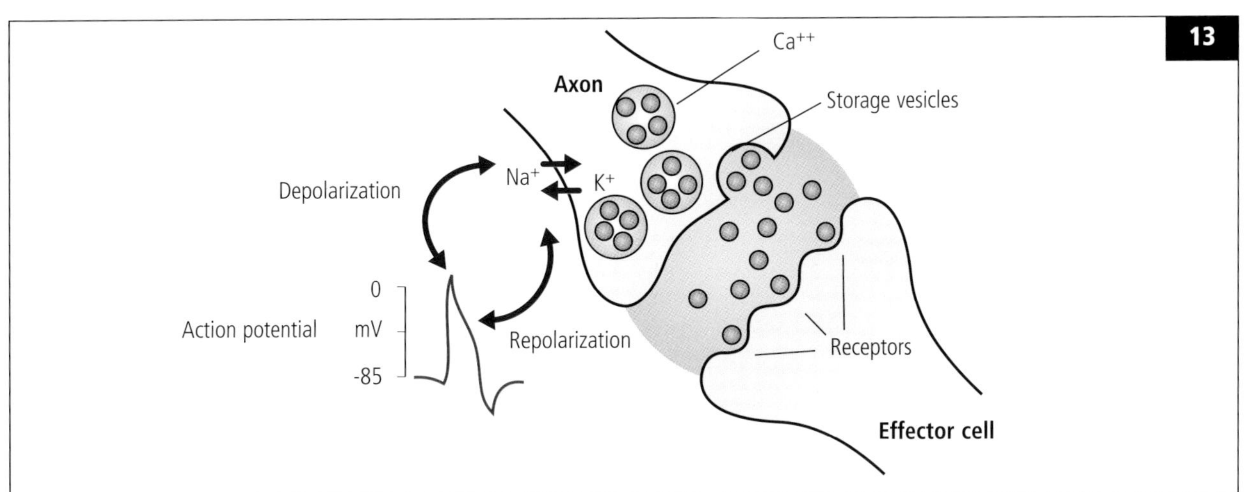

13 Neurohumoral transmission. The axonal action potential expresses a depolarization–repolarization of the axon, characterized by an influx of sodium and efflux of potassium. Arriving at the nerve terminal, the action potential facilitates an inward movement of calcium, which triggers the discharge of neurotransmitters from storage vesicles into the junctional cleft. The neurotransmitters react with specialized receptors on the postjunctional membranes and initiate physiological responses in the effector cell.

Calcium channels include receptor-operated channels, stretch-operated channels, calcium channels operated by second messengers, and voltage-sensitive channels (*Table* 2). The only channels that are responsive to the current calcium channel blockers are L-type calcium channels.[15]

The role of nitric oxide (NO) in nociception is unclear, although it appears to function both centrally and peripherally. Nitric oxide is synthesized from L-arginine by the enzyme nitric oxide synthase (NOS), of which three isoforms are known to exist: endothelian NOS (eNOS), neuronal NOS (nNOS), and inducible NOS (iNOS). Of these isoforms, eNOS and nNOS are constitutively expressed, whereas the expression of iNOS is induced in a wide cell range by immune or inflammatory stimuli. nNOS is not confined to the CNS, but is the predominant form in the CNS. NO may influence nociceptive processing at many levels, and may potentially have different effects, depending on the site and concentration of NO.[16] NO itself is a very short-lived molecule (half-life of milliseconds to seconds); however, models of its diffusional spread suggest that a point source synthesizing NO for 1–10 seconds would lead to a 200 μm sphere of influence: in the brain this volume could encompass 2 million synapses.[17] The main role of spinal NO appears to be in mediating hyperalgesia. In the periphery, the antinociceptive actions of opioids are mediated by NO and the analgesic actions of endogenous opioids, acetylcholine, and α_2-adrenoreceptor agonists may all involve NO in an antinociceptive role. There also appears to be a link between NO and the prostanoid pathway. Interleukin-1β (IL-1β) can induce both NOS and cyclo-oxygenase (COX) expression, and NO can increase the synthesis and release of prostanoids.[18]

Within the body, the endogenous nucleotide adenosine performs multiple functions. It can be progressively phosphorylated to generate the high-energy molecules adenosine mono-, di-, and triphosphate (AMP, ADP, and ATP), and from ATP, may be further modified to generate the intracellular second-messenger cyclic-AMP (cAMP). Generally its effects are inhibitory, and it acts as a depressant in the CNS. Equilibrative transporters facilitate adenosine release across cell membranes into the extracellular space, to the extent that under severe hypoxic conditions the concentration of adenosine may rise 100-fold.[19] Species differences exist in adenosine receptor pharmacology, but early studies suggest adenosine agonists were effective in antinociceptive tests mainly by acting as general CNS depressant agents.

ATP can have diverse origins from which to activate sensory nerve terminals. ATP can be co-released with NE following sympathetic stimulation, possibly underlying the maintenance of 'sympathetic pain', as well as by antidromic stimulation of sensory nerves. Painful stimulation can also be associated with sympathetic activity–proposed as a contributor to arthritic pain. Purinoceptors for ATP fall into two broad groups: ionotropic receptors, which are termed

Table 2 Types of calcium channel.

Types of calcium channel	Activity stimulus
Receptor-operated channels	Binding of a specific ligand, such as a neurohormone, to receptors within the channel
Stretch-operated channels	Vascular stretch
Second messenger-operated channels	Intracellular second messengers, such as inositol phosphate
Voltage-sensitive calcium channels	Voltage change across the membrane, such as depolarization
Neuronal (N-type)	Are involved with transmitter release at synaptic junctions (as well as P/Q channels)
Transient (T-type)	Low-voltage activated channels that permit calcium flux at resting membrane potentials, hence their role in pacemaking, neuronal bursting, and synaptic signal boosting
Long lasting (L-type)	Key determinants of membrane excitability. (The only channels affected by calcium channel blocking agents)

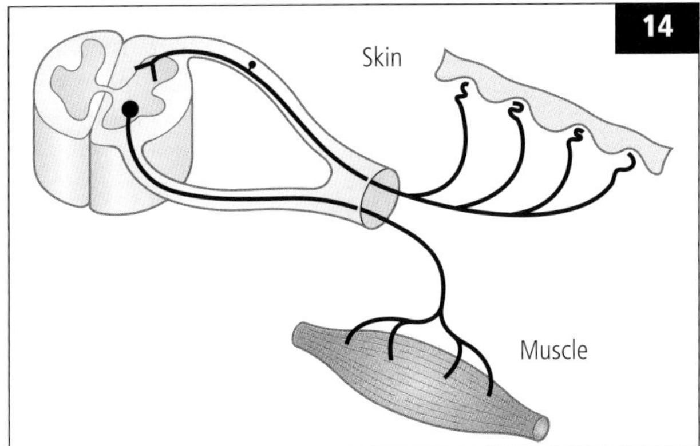

14 Nociception is initially influenced by first-order neurons in the PNS, prior to reaching the dorsal horn of the spinal cord.

P2X, and metabotropic receptors, termed P2Y. P2X receptors appear to be localized to nociceptive nerve endings in the joint capsule.[20] Support for the role of P2Y receptors in pain is weak. There is, however, strong evidence that the ultimate breakdown product of ATP, adenosine, plays a role in nociceptive processing,[21] and it may be that P2X and adenosine (P_1) receptors act together as physiological regulators of nociceptive traffic. Accordingly, the P2X receptor would be considered a candidate for pharmacological intervention in treating nociceptive pain.

ATP is also sourced from damaged cells, which could underlie the pain associated with tissue trauma. Vascular endothelial cells also appear to release ATP readily, without any concomitant cellular lysis.[22]

Adenosine receptor agonists can be highly effective antinociceptive agents, where their activity is similar to, but not identical with, that of opioids. Both classes of compounds are effective against thermal nociceptive stimuli; opioids tend to be more efficacious against mechanical nociception, whereas adenosine agonists are more efficacious against inflammatory and neuropathic pain. Their therapeutic window is small, however.[23]

PERIPHERAL NERVOUS SYSTEM AND DORSAL ROOT GANGLION

The peripheral nervous system (PNS) comprises nervous tissue outside the spinal canal and brain. Nociception first undergoes change in the PNS, followed by dynamic changes in the dorsal horn of the spinal cord (**14**). Peripheral receptors (specialized axon terminals in skin) transduce nociceptive and proprioceptive events for processing by first-order sensory neurons in the ipsilateral, segmental DRG, whose extension terminates in the dorsal horn (substantia gelatinosa) of the spinal cord.

The PNS includes cranial nerves, spinal nerves with their roots and rami, peripheral components of the autonomic nervous system, and peripheral nerves whose primary sensory neurons are located in the associated DRG, also a part of the PNS. Axons are extensions of the cell body and contain a continuous channel of neuronal cytoplasm.

As a theory of electrical engineering, there is a relationship between fiber size and conduction velocity (*Table 3*); however, conduction velocity may be enhanced by Schwann cell activity or reduced by pathology.

Nearly all large-diameter myelinated Aβ fibers normally conduct non-noxious stimuli applied to the skin, joints, and muscles, and thus these large sensory neurons usually do not conduct noxious stimuli.[24] In contrast, most small-diameter sensory fibers–unmyelinated C fibers and finely myelinated A-fibers–are specialized sensory neurons known as nociceptors, whose major function is to detect environmental stimuli that are perceived as harmful and convert them into electrochemical signals that are then transmitted to the CNS.

The term 'nerve fiber' refers to the combination of the axon and Schwann cell as a functional unit. The Schwann cell (the oligodendrocyte is the corresponding CNS cell) significantly accelerates the speed of action potential propagation and acts as a first-line phagocyte. It also plays a major role in nerve regeneration and axonal maintenance. All peripheral nerve axons are surrounded by segmental Schwann cells, although only some Schwann cells produce myelin–a lipid-rich insulating covering.

Table 3 Relationship between fiber size and conduction velocity.

Cutaneous nerve	Muscle nerve	Conduction velocity in cat (m/s)	Diameter (μm)
	Group I	72–130	12–22
Aαβ		35–108	6–18
	Group II	36–72	6–12
Aδ	Group III	3–30	3–7
C	Group IV	0.2–2	0.25–1.35

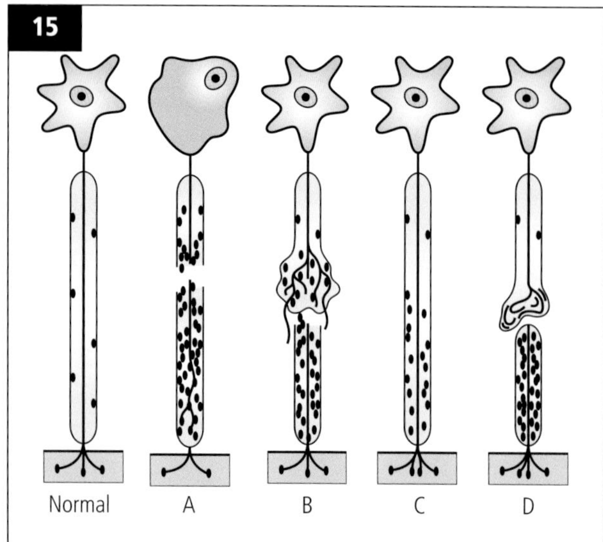

15 Wallerian degeneration includes: (A) transection injury and degeneration in the distal segment of nerve (minimal degeneration proximally), (B) regeneration following degeneration, as injured axons form many small sprouts that are guided by trophic factors to target tissue (often following remnant basal lamina of Schwann cells that have themselves degenerated), (C) axon size then increases, as the axon develops and remyelinates, (D) occasionally a very painful neuroma forms when regeneration lacks a terminal target.

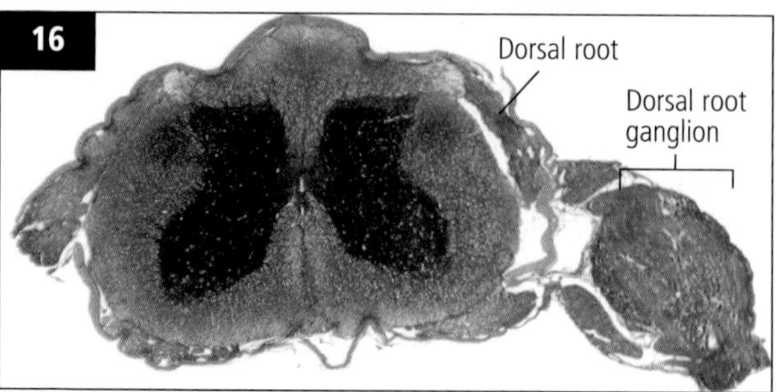

16 DRG neurons are first-order sensory neurons with axons branching both centrally and peripherally.

Myelin is formed by serial wrapping of Schwann cell cytoplasm around an axon, and sequential myelinated Schwann cells are separated by nodes of Ranvier, a location of high sodium channel concentration. Nodes of Ranvier provide rapid axon saltatory conduction. After nerve injury, new axonal sprouts arise from a node of Ranvier. In the perinodal region of the axon high concentrations of potassium channels are exposed during early phases of demyelination.

The most common cause of neuropathy following axonal injury is associated with Wallerian degeneration, named after Augustus Waller, who in 1850 described a pathological process following nerve transection that included an initial reaction at the injury site, then degeneration and phagocytosis of myelin and axons distal to the injury (**15**). Wallerian degeneration occurs after axonal injury of any type, including crush and severe ischemia.

The anatomy of nerve circulation influences its homeostasis. Surface circulation of a peripheral nerve is sinusoidal in its longitudinal course. This allows the nerve to stretch approximately 10% without injury, and this compensatory design can be compromised by scar formation within adjacent tissue. Endoneurial vessels are free of innervation, and blood flow is not modulated by sympathetic activity, but by local perfusion pressure and vessel caliber. Since the endoneurial space can expand by edema or by the influx of hematological or neuronal cells, the perineurium can expand, pinching transperineurial

Table 4 Classification of axoplasmic proteins by transport rate.

Group	Velocity (mm/day)	Substances
I	>240	Membrane constituents, transmitter vesicles, glycoproteins, glycolipids, lipids, cholesterol, acetylcholine, norepinephrine, serotonin, sP, other putative transmitters, associated enzymes
II	40	Mitochondrial components, fodrin
III–IV	2–8	Actin, myosin-like proteins, glycolytic enzymes, calmodulin, clathrin, some additional fodrin
V	1	Cytoskeleton proteins, neurofilament proteins

vessels closed. At 50% compromise to blood flow, neurological consequences can become apparent.

DRG neurons are the first-order sensory neurons, with their distal axons connected to sensory receptors or their free ends localized in tissue space (**16**). DRG axons leave the cell body and then bifurcate into a central and peripheral process.

Axonal cell bodies 'sense' their environment, which provides a 'backflow' to alter cell transcription and axonal protein flow (*Table 4*). Normally, the transcription machinery is devoted primarily to making neurotransmitters, but following peripheral nerve injury, the DRG senses the requirement for skeletal proteins for regeneration and shifts its production for that purpose. The process of axonal transport is functional in all viable axons, both myelinated and unmyelinated.

There are other support cells in the PNS including mast cells, fibroblasts, endothelial cells, and resident macrophages.

THE DORSAL HORN ACTS AS A 'GEAR BOX' IN PAIN TRANSMISSION

In the early 1960s it became clear that pain manifests several distinct perceptual components. There is clearly a sensory–discriminative feature that signals the intensity, localization and modality of the nociception, e.g. 'I have a pain of seven, on a scale of one to ten, in my right index finger'. There is also, clearly, an affective–motivational component reflecting stimulus context and a variety of higher order functions such as memory and emotion, e.g. 'The pain in my finger makes life miserable–impacting everything I do'. These different components are highly integrated, involving distinct anatomical systems.

Complex networks of pathways from various sites in the brain integrate together to modulate the spinal processing of sensory information in a top-down manner. Higher-order cognitive and emotional processes, such as anxiety, mood, and attention, can influence the perception of pain through convergence of somatic and limbic systems into a so-called descending modulatory system, providing a neural substrate through which the brain can control pain (**17**). The pharmacology of the descending systems is complex, but broadly, the two major defined transmitters in the pathways from brain to spinal cord are the monoamines, NE and 5-hydroxytryptamine (5-HT).

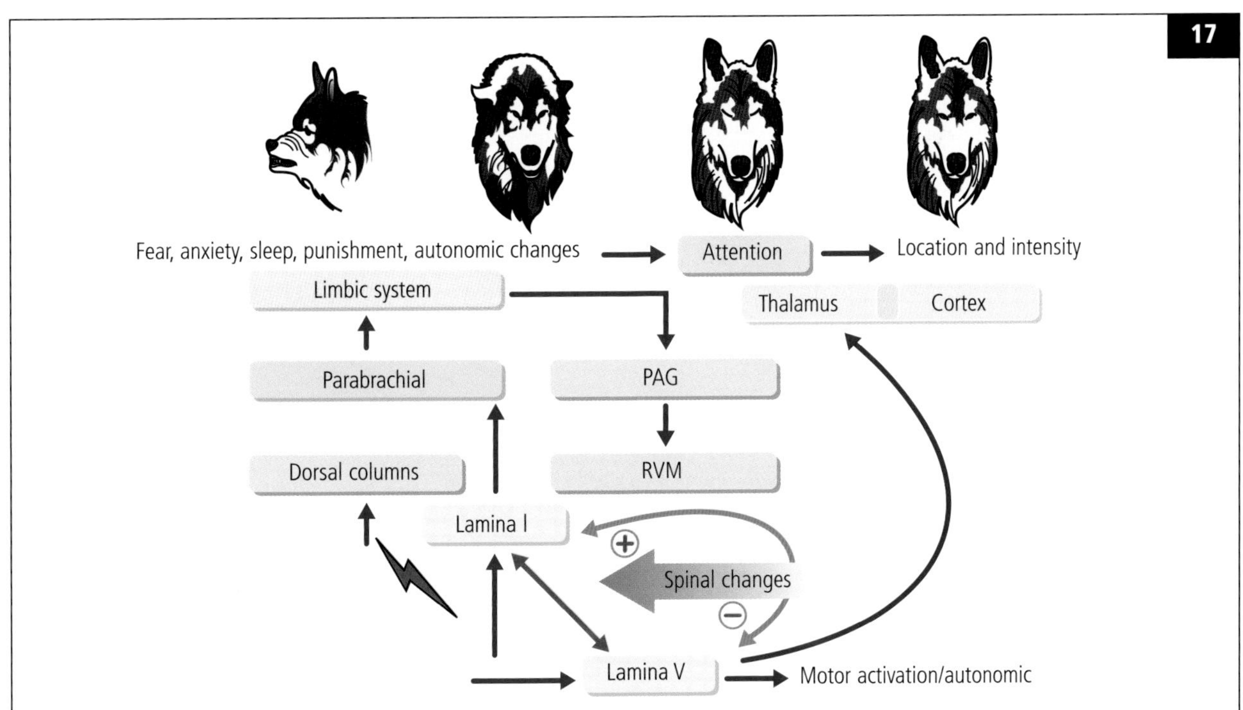

17 The brain and spinal cord are able to 'talk to one another'. The emotional center of the brain is a series of nerves and tissue called the limbic system, which creates a rainbow of emotions. The limbic system not only influences pain signals, but also adds emotional texture to them. (RVM = rostral ventromedial medulla; PAG = periaqueductal gray)

An important tenet underlies enhanced response of the CNS to mechanical stimuli of cutaneous injury: 'the peripheral signal for pain does not reside exclusively with nociceptors; under pathological circumstances, other receptor types, which are normally associated with the sensation of touch, acquire the capacity to evoke pain'.[25] This principle applies to secondary hyperalgesia, as well as to neuropathic pain states in general. *Central sensitization* is the term denoting augmentation of responsiveness of central pain-signaling neurons to input from low-threshold mechanoreceptors. It is central sensitization that plays the major role in secondary hyperalgesia, not peripheral sensitization. This underlies the value of local anesthetic blocks: when the CNS is spared the input from nociceptors at the time of the acute insult, hyperalgesia does not develop.[26]

The predominant neurotransmitter used by all primary afferent fibers is glutamate, although other excitatory transmitters, notably ATP, act to depolarize dorsal horn neurons directly or on presynaptic autoreceptors to enhance glutamate release during action potential firing.[27] Primary afferents, unique in their capacity to release neurotransmitters peripherally, and so underlie neurogenic inflammation, convey information to the CNS. In the dorsal horn, peptides such as sP impact postsynaptic dorsal horn neurons–setting the gain or magnitude of the nociceptive response.[28]

The dorsal horn of the spinal cord is organized into lamellae comprised of dorsal horn neurons and the inhibitory and excitatory synaptic connections they receive and make. Non-neural glial cells–the oligodendrocytes, astrocytes, and microglia–modulate the operation of these neuronal circuits. A key feature of the somatosensory system, modifiability or *plasticity*, resides in the dorsal horn.[29] Neuronal information processing is not fixed, but is instead dynamic, changing in a manner that is dependent on levels of neuronal excitability and synaptic strength, profoundly diversifying for either a short period (seconds) or prolonged periods (days), or perhaps indefinitely.

In 1954 Rexed demonstrated that the gray matter of the spinal cord can be divided into cytoarchitecturally distinct laminae or layers (**18**). Physiological studies have since demonstrated an analogous, functional laminar organization. Lamina I (marginal layer) is comprised of cells that respond primarily, and in some cases exclusively, to noxious stimuli. Some also respond to innocuous, i.e. noninjurious stimulation, including moderate temperatures. Many lamina I cells contribute axons to the spinothalamic tract. Lamina II (substantia gelatinosa) contains small interneurons, many responding to noxious inputs. Lamina II neurons modulate cells of laminae I and V. Laminae I and II receive direct primary afferent input only from small-diameter fibers. Laminae III and IV cells respond to innocuous stimuli, hair brush and tactile skin stimulation, and do not increase their response when noxious stimuli are presented. Lamina V cells respond to noxious and non-noxious stimulus–they are wide

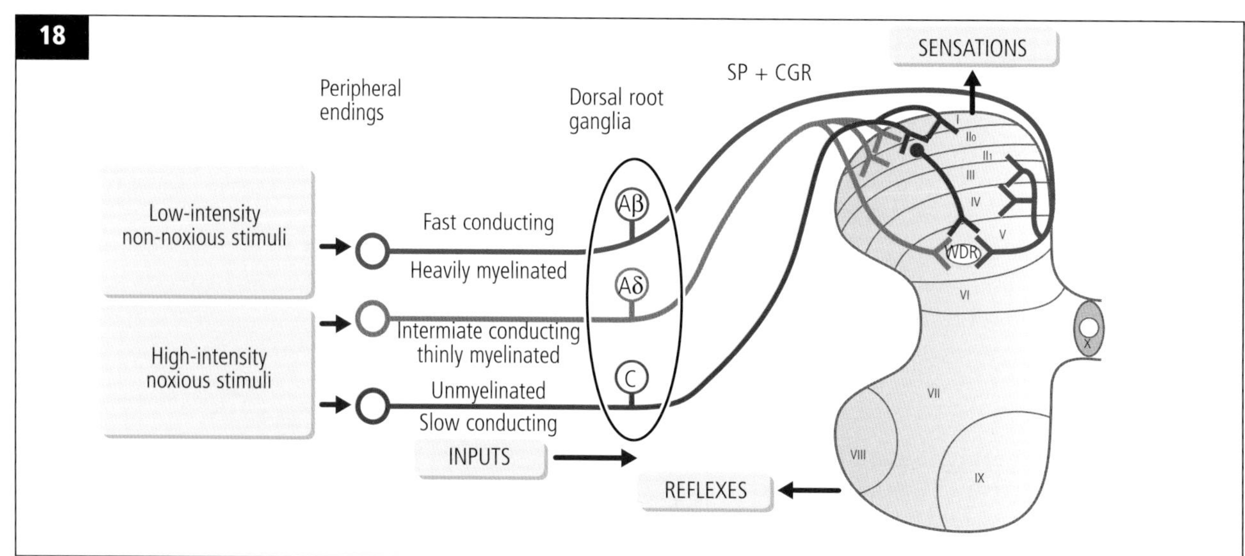

18 The dorsal horn of the spinal cord is comprised of lamellae, with characteristic afferents and efferents.

dynamic range (WDR) cells. They also respond to noxious visceral stimuli.

Spinal cord transmissions work as a binary response: low-intensity stimuli interpreted as innocuous or nonpainful, such as touch, vibration or hair movement, versus high-threshold stimuli producing pain. Different perceptions are elicited depending upon whether low- or high-threshold afferents have been activated, because of the different central circuits engaged.

Dorsal horn neurons consist primarily of projecting neurons, propriospinal neurons, and local interneurons (**19**). Their distribution as well as dendritic arborization determine which and how many inputs each receives. *Projection neurons* transfer sensory information to higher CNS levels and are also involved in the activation of descending control systems. *Propriospinal neurons* transfer inputs from one segment of the spinal cord to another, and local *interneurons*, comprising the majority of intrinsic dorsal horn neurons, serve as short-distance excitatory and inhibitory interneurons. Most inhibitory interneurons contain gamma aminobutyric acid (GABA) and/or glycine as neurotransmitters, and synapse both presynaptically on primary afferent endings and postsynaptically on dorsal horn neurons.[30] Presynaptic inhibition decreases transmitter release from primary afferent terminals, while postsynaptic inhibition hyperpolarizes postsynaptic membranes. Many inhibitory interneurons are spontaneously active, maintaining an ongoing tonic inhibitory control within the dorsal horn.

Contributing to CNS plasticity is neuronal capacity for structural reorganization of synaptic circuitry. Schwann cells accrue and promote neuronal redevelopment, resulting in deafferentation of injured and uninjured fibers. Resultant collateral branching can lead to misdirected targeting of fibers and inappropriate peripheral innervation, so that cutaneous areas once occupied by the lesioned nerve

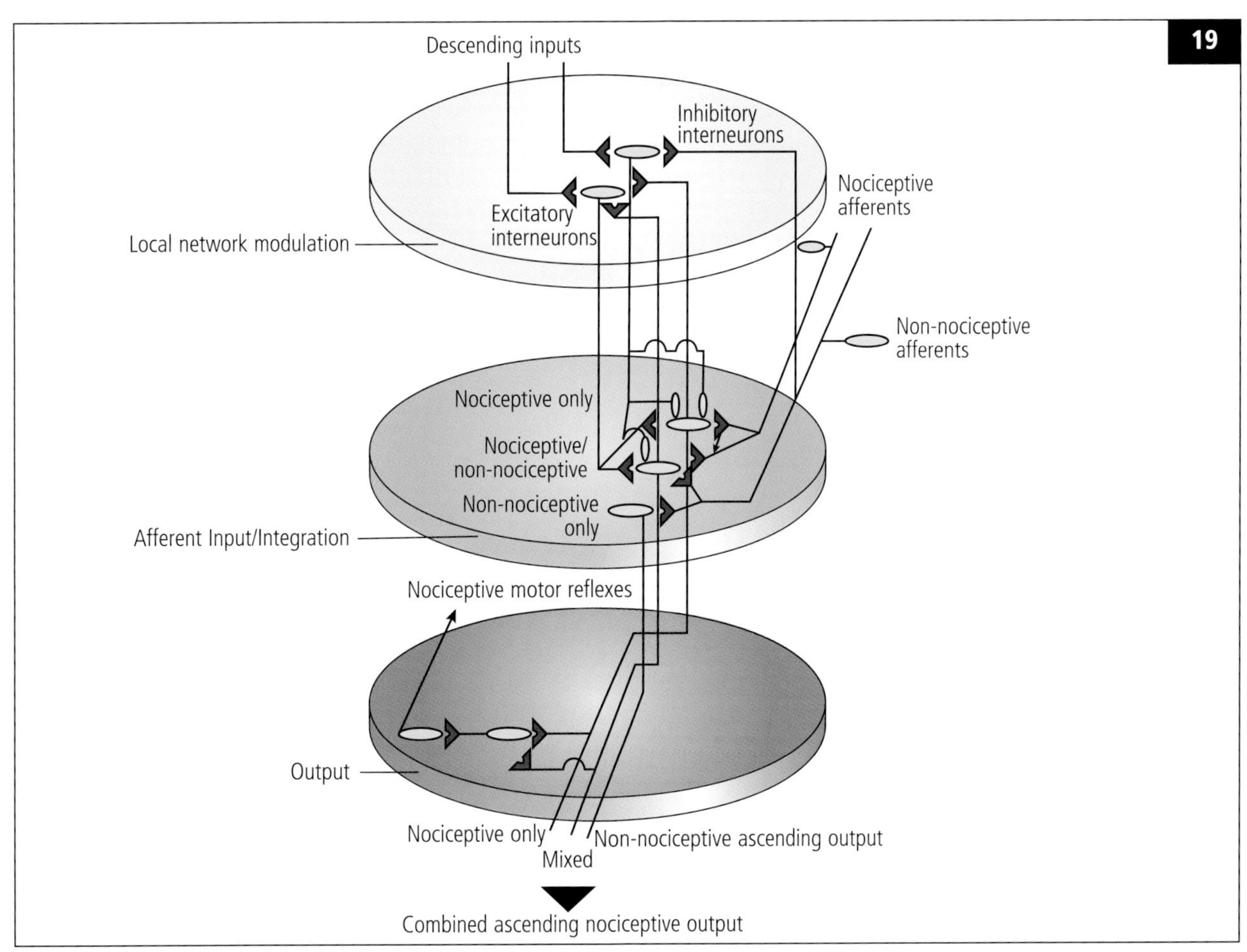

19 Dorsal horn neurons consist of projecting neurons, propriospinal neurons, and local interneurons.

become hyperinnervated by low- and high-threshold fibers. Neurons may die, axon terminals may degenerate or atrophy, new axon terminals may appear, and the structural contact between cells at the synapses may be modified. This can result in the loss of normal connections, formation of novel abnormal connections and an alteration in the normal balance between excitation and inhibition.[31] Structural reorganization and its functional sequelae can result in changed sensory processing long after the initial injury has healed.

WHAT MAKES THE CNS SO DYNAMIC?

AFFERENT SIGNAL SUPPRESSION

Spinal cord sensory transmissions can be endogenously suppressed, as might be necessary for survival value, enabling, for example, flight or fight reactions in the presence of substantial injury. Inhibitory mechanisms can be activated by peripheral inputs of TENS, acupuncture, placebo, suggestion (in humans), distraction, and cognition. Further, endogenous inhibitory mechanisms can be mimicked pharmacologically with agents such as opiates, GABA-mimetics, and α-adrenergic agonists.

GABA exerts a powerful inhibitory tone within the spinal cord dorsal horn mediated by both $GABA_A$ receptors (pre- and postsynaptic on primary afferents) and $GABA_B$ receptors located principally on presynaptic sites. Although GABAergic inhibition may be upregulated during peripheral inflammatory states, GABAergic interneurons are subject to excitotoxic or apoptotic death following nerve injury, resulting in a loss of inhibitory tone, which, in turn, may contribute to hyperalgesia and allodynia.[32]

WINDUP

Windup is a form of activity-dependent plasticity characterized by a progressive increase in action potential output from dorsal horn neurons elicited during the course of a train of repeated low-frequency C fiber or nociceptor stimuli.[33] Repetitive discharge of primary afferent nociceptors results in co-release of neuromodulators such as sP and CGRP, together with glutamate (the main neurotransmitter used by nociceptors synapsing with the dorsal horn) from nociceptor central terminals. These neuropeptides activate postsynaptic G-protein-coupled receptors, which lead to slow postsynaptic depolarizations lasting tens of seconds.[34] Resultant cumulative depolarization is boosted by recruitment of NMDA (N-methyl-D-aspartate) receptor current through inhibition of magnesium channel suppression.

NMDA receptor and windup

The most involved receptor in the sensation of acute pain, AMPA (alpha-amino-3-hydroxy-5-methyl-4-isoxazole propionic-acid), is always exposed on afferent nerve terminals. In contrast, those most involved in the sensation of chronic pain, NMDA receptors, are not functional unless there has been a persistent or large-scale release of glutamate (**20**).

Repeated activation of AMPA receptors dislodges magnesium ions that act like stoppers in transmembrane sodium and calcium channels of the NMDA receptor complex. Calcium flowing into the cell activates protein kinase C, the enzyme needed for NOS production of NO. NO diffuses through the dorsal cell membrane and synaptic cleft into the nociceptor and stimulates guanyl synthase-induced closure of potassium channels. Since endorphins and enkephalins inhibit pain by opening these channels, closure induces opiate resistance. NO also stimulates the release of sP, which by binding to NK-1 receptors in the dorsal horn membrane, triggers *c-fos* gene expression and promotes neural remodeling and hypersensitization. Accompanying this windup, less glutamate is required to transmit the pain signal and more antinociceptive input is required for analgesia. Endorphins cannot keep up with their demand and essentially lose their effectiveness. The clinical implications are under-appreciated: *inadequately treated pain is a much more important cause of opioid tolerance than use of opioids themselves.* NMDA activation can also cause neural cells to sprout new connective endings.[35]

Calcium entry by NMDA receptor activation activates the neuronal isoform of NOS (nNOS) localized within both primary afferent nociceptors in the DRG and neurons of the spinal cord dorsal horn (primarily laminae I–II and X).[36] NO, acting as a retrograde transmitter within the dorsal horn, thereby potentiates excitatory amino acid and neurokinin release, contributing to central sensitization, and plays a key role in nociceptive processing.

It is important to note that NMDA-associated windup is a process where 'normal' underlying nociceptive signaling (much of which occurs in the spinothalamic tract) is *facilitated* by activity of the NMDA receptor. When this facilitation is blocked by an NMDA antagonist, the underlying nociception signaling remains, which must be treated with other analgesics. For this reason, NMDA antagonists serve best as adjuncts in a multimodal analgesic protocol (**21**).

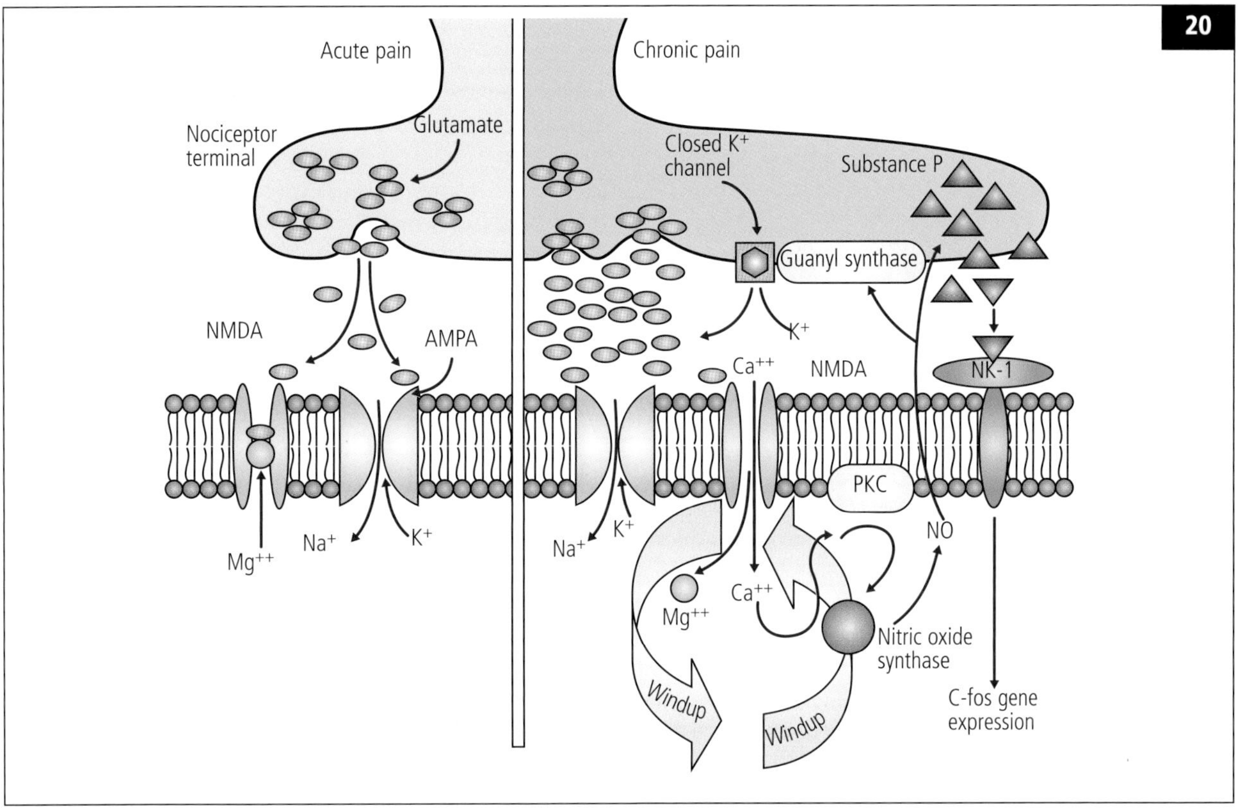

20
Acute pain
Chronic pain
Nociceptor terminal
Glutamate
Closed K+ channel
Substance P
Guanyl synthase
NMDA
AMPA
Ca++
NMDA
K+
NK-1
PKC
Mg++
Na+
K+
Na+
K+
NO
Mg++
Ca++
Nitric oxide synthase
Windup
Windup
C-fos gene expression

20 CNS windup involves the NMDA receptor.

21
Dorsal horn neuron
CGRP
sP
Glu
Nociception
Primary afferent neuron
CGRP
NK-1
AMPA
Spinothalamic tract
Activate
NMDA
facilitate
Hypersensitivity
Opioid
Inhibition
Hyperalgesia
Windup

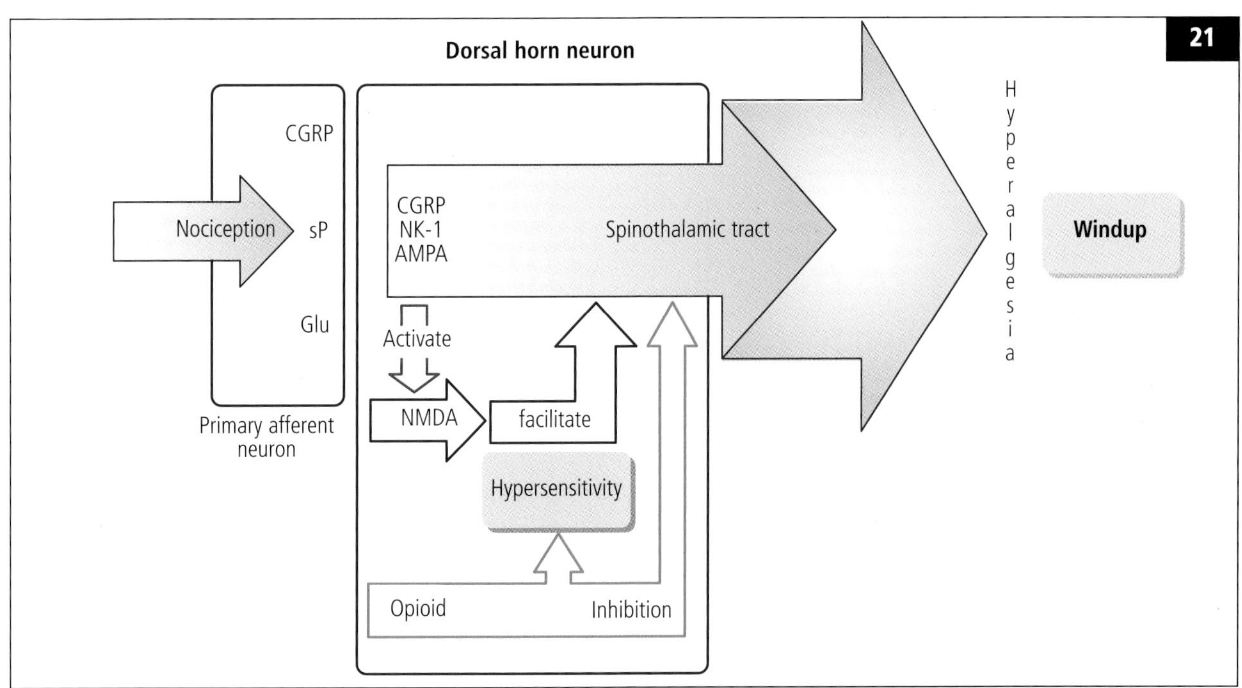

21 NMDA-mediated windup facilitates the underlying nociceptive signaling, resulting in a state of hyperalgesia. Therefore, NMDA-antagonists are administered as 'adjuncts' to a baseline protocol for optimal results.

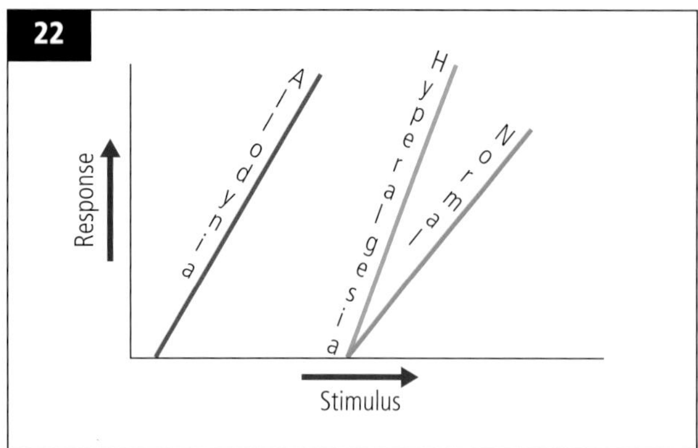

22 Stimulus–response curve of noxious insult.

Pain memories imprinted within the CNS, mediated by NMDA receptors, produce hyperalgesia and contribute to allodynia (**22**). In several animal experiments, *c-fos* expression (the *c-fos* gene serves as a marker for cellular activation, i.e. nociception), central sensitization, and windup do not occur if nociceptive blockade is applied prior to the nociceptive event. Such findings suggest that presurgical blockade of nociception may prevent postsurgical wound pain or pain hypersensitivity following surgery, i.e. pre-emptive analgesia, as advocated by the eminent pain physiologist, Patrick Wall.[37] Successful pre-emptive analgesia must meet three criteria: (1) intense enough to block all nociception, (2) wide enough to cover the entire surgical area, and (3) prolonged enough to last throughout surgery and even into the postoperative period.

It is important to note that adequate levels of general anesthesia with a volatile drug such as isoflurane do *not* prevent central sensitization. The potential for central sensitization exists even in unconscious patients who are unresponsive to surgical stimuli. This has been somewhat validated in the dog,[38,39] where ('pain-induced distress') cortisol spikes in response to noxious stimuli of ovariohysterectomy during the anesthetic period suggest a link between surgical stimulus and neural responsiveness during anesthetic-induced unconsciousness (**23**).

As indicated by the expression of *c-fos* (early genomic expression), noxious stimuli still enter the spinal cord during apparently adequate anesthesia.[40]

In 1988, Professor Patrick Wall introduced the

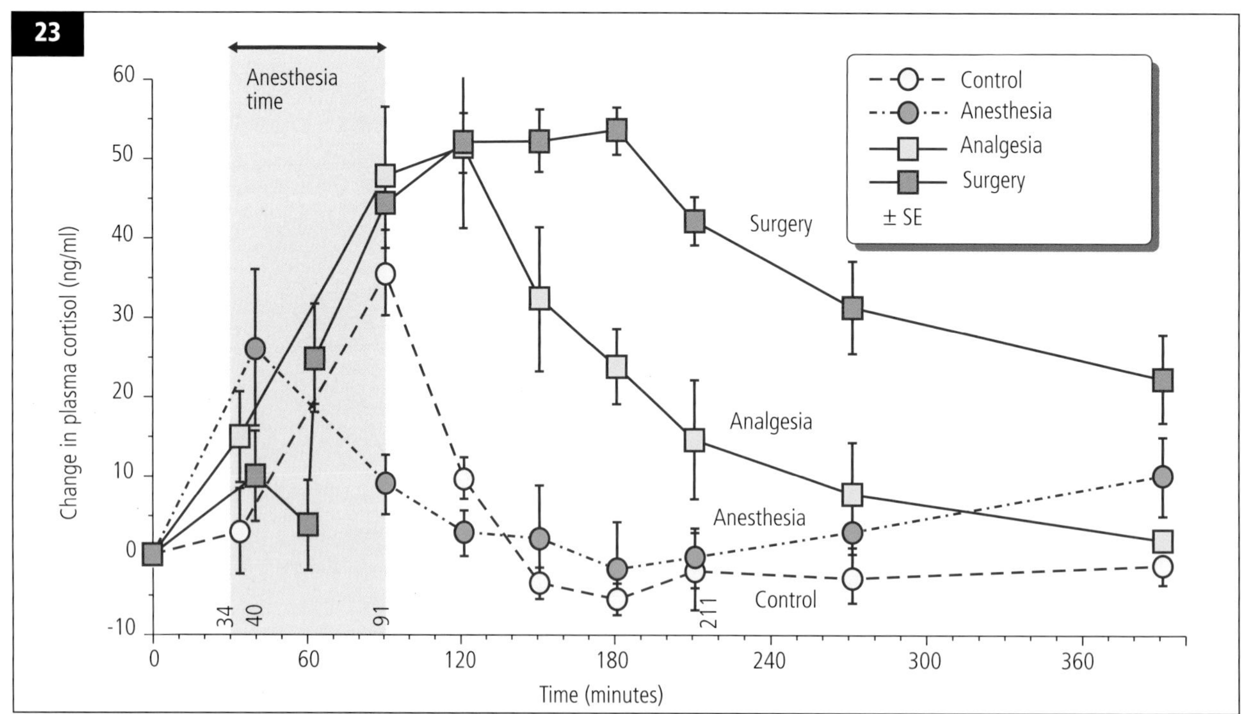

23 Changes in plasma cortisol concentrations from pretreatment values for control, anesthesia, analgesia, and surgery treatments; the curves demonstrate that although canine patients were under the appropriate stage of gaseous anesthesia, nociception was apparent. Technically, these dogs were not painful, because the nociception was not being cognitively processed.[38]

concept of pre-emptive analgesia to clinicians with his editorial in the journal *Pain*.[41] The emphasis of pre-emptive analgesia is to prevent sensitization of the nervous system throughout the perioperative period. Pain is to be expected from an initial surgery and the hypersensitivity that subsequently develops. Analgesia administered after sensitization may decrease pain somewhat, but has little long-term benefit in addressing the pain resultant from postsurgical inflammation. Analgesia administered before surgery limits inflammatory pain and decreases subsequent hypersensitivity. The most effective pre-emptive analgesic regimen occurs when initiated before surgery and continued throughout the postoperative period (**24**).

A review of pre-emptive analgesia, with inclusion of suggested drugs (available in 2001) and dosage has been provided elsewhere.[42] A logical pre-emptive drug protocol would include an opioid, alpha-2 agonist, ±NMDA antagonist,[43] and a nonsteroidal anti-inflammatory drug (NSAID).[44] The implementation of perioperative NSAIDs is controversial based upon their antiprostaglandin effect, which in the face of hypotension, might enhance the potential for acute renal failure. This is why perioperative fluid support is such an important consideration. However, anti-inflammatory drugs play a substantial role in perioperative pain management[45] because surgery cannot be performed without subsequent inflammation. Reducing the inflammatory response in the periphery, and thereby decreasing sensitization of the peripheral nociceptors, should attenuate central sensitization.[46] It has also been recognized for some time that NSAIDs synergistically interact with both μ-opioid and α_2-adrenoceptor agonists.[47–50] In human medicine, the use of perioperative NSAIDs has reduced the use of patient-controlled analgesic morphine by 40–60%.[51,52]

GLIAL CELLS

By the early 1990s, a large body of literature had accumulated with evidence that CNS proinflammatory cytokines (tumor necrosis factor (TNF), IL-1, and IL-6) were critically involved in the generation of every sickness response studied.[53] Further, glia were recognized as a major source of these proinflammatory substances. This built on the 1970s data that CNS microglia and astrocytes became activated following trauma to peripheral nerves.[54] Further, the drug MK801, which blocks neuropathic pain behaviors, was demonstrated to block glial activation as well, hence correlating neuropathic pain and glial activation. Although microglia and astrocytes have become attractive treatment targets for neuropathic pain, proinflammatory cytokines, for example, can also be produced by fibroblasts, endothelial cells, and other types of glia and some neurons.[55]

The term 'glia' means glue, and the CNS contains three types of glial cells: astrocytes, oligodendrocytes, and microglia. Microglia are the resident tissue macrophages of the CNS and, as such, are thought to be the first line of defense against injury or infection.[56] Microglia cells, which outnumber neurons by 10 to 1 in the CNS, play a central role in the pathophysiology of neuropathic pain. Activated microglia release chemical mediators that can act on neurons to alter their function: expression and release of cytotoxic or inflammatory mediators, including IL-1β, IL-6, TNF-α, proteases, and reactive oxygen intermediates, including NO.[57]

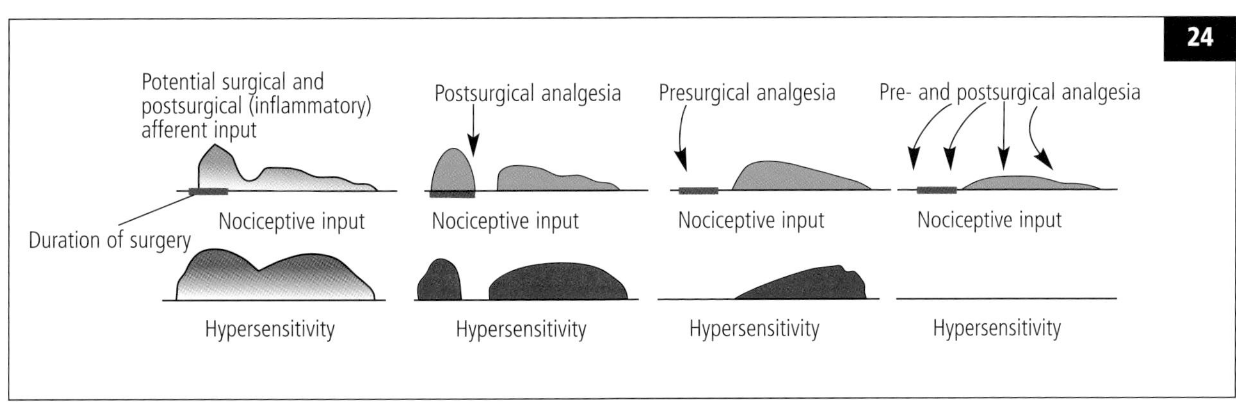

24 The most effective pre-emptive analgesia is initiated before surgery and continued throughout the postoperative period.

Normally, microglia are quiescent, having no known basal function other than surveillance for debris, pathogens, and CNS 'clutter'. Astrocytes, on the other hand, regulate extracellular ions, sequester extracellular neurotransmitters, and perform other homeostatic functions. Astrocytes encapsulate synapses and actively participate in synaptic communication by responding to synaptically released neurotransmitters by releasing glial substances into the synapse as well.[58] As such, astrocytes are 'active', but not 'activated'.

Activation is a fundamentally different phenomenon in neurons compared with that in glia. For neurons, activation is unidimensional, i.e. it relates to the production of action potentials. In contrast, activation of glia is multidimensional because glia perform numerous functions. Responding to different activational states, substances released by activated glia include proinflammatory cytokines (TNF, IL-1, IL-6), NO, reactive oxygen species, PGs, excitatory amino acids, and ATP.[59] Microglia and astrocytes can synergize in their functions, and so products released by one cell type can stimulate the release of proinflammatory substances from the other. A shift from the basal state to activation can occur quite rapidly, as microglia are extremely sensitive to changes in their microenvironment. Stimuli that trigger microglial activation include CNS trauma, ischemia, tumors, neurodegeneration, and immune stimuli such as bacteria or viruses.

It is noteworthy that glia do not have axons. They cannot relay sensory information from the spinal cord to the brain. Accordingly, their role is indirect. Conceptually, glia can be recognized as 'volume controls', where substances released by activated glia cause incoming sensory afferents to increase their release of neurotransmitter, thereby amplifying their 'pain' message. It follows that preventing such glial alterations in the functioning of the 'pain pathway' can be conceptualized as 'turning down the gain on pain'.[60]

The origin of microglia is uncertain, however evidence suggests that microglia arise from mesodermal cells, probably of hematopoietic lineage.[61] After development, microglia can arise from two primary sources. First, resident microglial cells undergo mitosis and therefore replenish their numbers throughout life. Secondly, peripheral blood monocytes migrate into the CNS through the intact blood–brain barrier, and these cells subsequently transform into resident microglia. In response to CNS immune challenge or trauma, microglia are stimulated to actively proliferate.[62] Further, CNS trauma and ischemia can lead to site-specific recruitment of peripheral blood monocytes. Such monocytes can again mature into macrophages within the CNS that, over time, become morphologically identical to microglia. After microglia maturation through three stages and clearance of immune challenges, microglia reverse their maturation toward the basal condition where they remain in a 'primed' state from which they can respond more rapidly as in an anamnestic response. Microglia appear to be required for the development of neuropathic pain, but not its maintenance.

Astrocytes appear to arise from dorsal regions of the neural tube, comprise 40–50% of all glial cells, and outnumber neurons. Multipotential neuroepithelial stem cells are thought to give rise to astrocytes, as well as to neurons and oligodendrocytes.[63] Astrocytes have been divided into two groups: protoplasmic astrocytes are predominant in gray matter, while fibrous astrocytes are primarily found within white matter.

Astrocytes are closely apposed to neurons. They enwrap the majority of synapses in the CNS, and also ensheath nonsynaptic sites (neuronal cell bodies, dendrites, nodes of Ranvier). In contrast to microglia, the basal state of astrocytes is not quiescent, as they perform a wide array of functions in the normal CNS. Astrocytes provide neurons with energy sources and neurotransmitter precursors.[64] They also play an important role in trophic support via the release of growth factors, regulation of extracellular ions and neurotransmitters, neuronal survival and differentiation, neurite outgrowth and axon guidance, and formation of synapses.[65] The concept of the 'tripartite synapse' (instead of the traditional two elements) is now widely accepted: the presynaptic terminal, the postsynaptic terminal, and the surrounding astrocytes (**25**).[66]

Synaptic activation of low frequency or intensity elicits no response by astrocytes. In contrast, axonal activity of high frequency or intensity activates astrocytes and induces oscillatory changes in intracellular calcium: activation. Elevations in intracellular calcium in astrocytes lead to glial release of various substances, including glutamate, PGE_2, and proinflammatory cytokines.[67] These, in turn, increase the synaptic strength of excitatory synapses, increase the expression of AMPA receptors by neurons, and induce an increase in intracellular calcium and action potential frequency in nearby neurons,[68] at least in part via glutamate-mediated activation of extrasynaptic NMDA receptors.

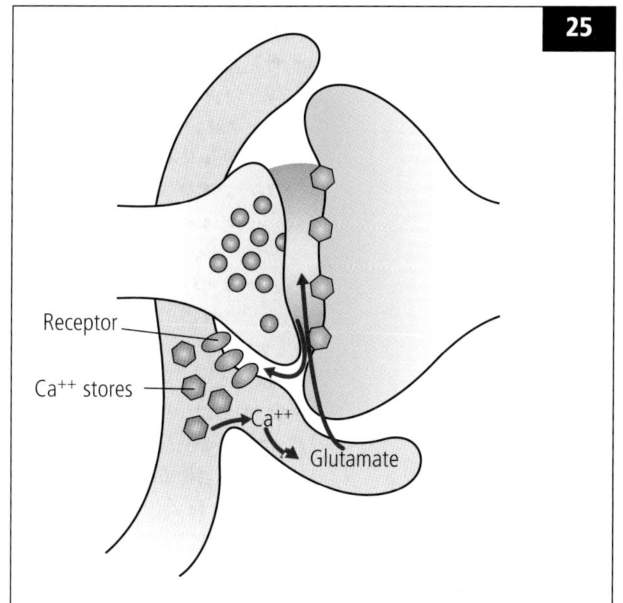

25 Representation of a tripartite synapse in which the process of an astrocyte (gray) wraps around a synaptic connection. Synaptic activity elicits postsynaptic potentials while GABA or glutamate can act on astrocytic receptors and trigger calcium release from internal stores to increase astrocytic calcium levels. Elevated astrocytic calcium evokes the local release of the chemical transmitter glutamate, which can modulate the synapse.

The following summarizes mechanisms by which proinflammatory cytokines alter neuronal excitability. Neurons, including those in the spinal cord dorsal horn, express receptors for proinflammatory cytokines. Neuronal excitability in the dorsal horn and trigeminal nucleus increases rapidly in response to these glial products, suggestive of a direct effect on neurons. IL-1 has been demonstrated to enhance neuronal NMDA conductance, including within the spinal cord dorsal horn. TNF rapidly upregulates membrane expression of neuronal AMPA receptors and also increases AMPA conductance. TNF also enhances neuroexcitability in response to glutamate, and IL-1 induces the release of the neuroexcitant ATP via an NMDA-mediated mechanism. Additionally, proinflammatory cytokines can induce the production of a variety of neuroexcitatory substances, including NO, PGs, and reactive oxygen species. Accordingly, proinflammatory cytokines exert multiple effects, each of which would be predicted to increase neuronal excitation and each of which would serve as a future target for analgesic drug development.

Astrocytes also communicate among themselves. They do not generate action potentials, but create calcium waves wherein intracellular calcium elevations are propagated in a nondecremental fashion from astrocyte to astrocyte. Calcium waves, by leading to the activation of distant astrocytes, result in the release of glial products at distant sites (**26**).[66] Glial gap junctions may also be involved in the spread of pain to distant sites.[68]

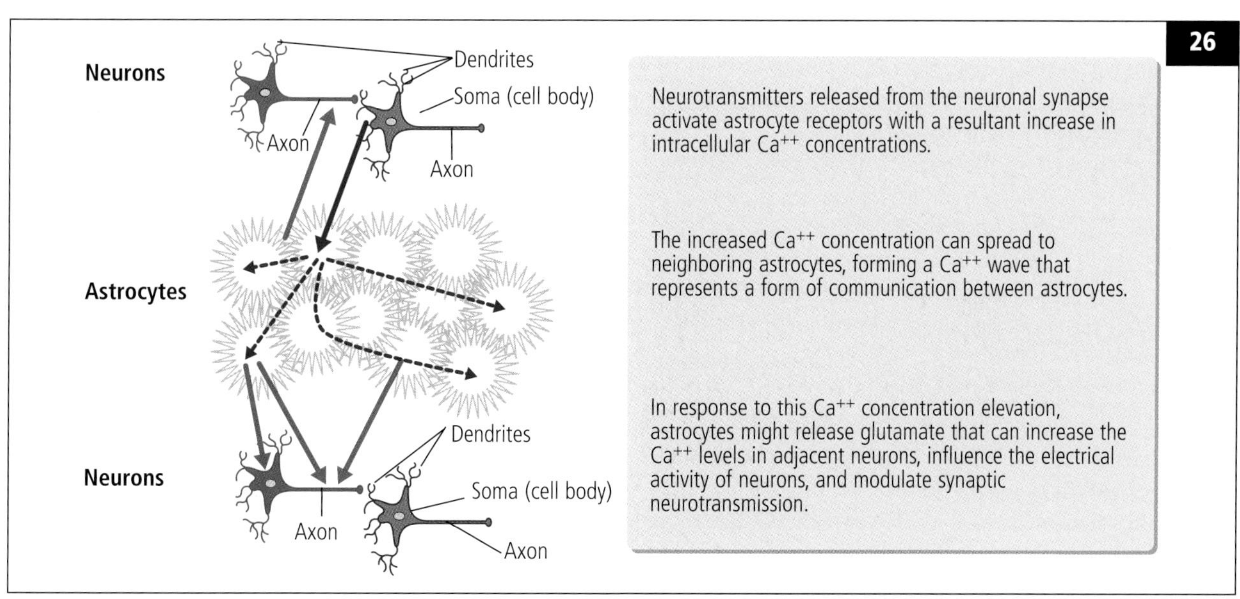

26 Calcium waves within astrocytes provide bi-directional communication between astrocytes and neurons.

Two interrelated points are worth noting: (1) the actions of glial products can synergize and (2) substances released by activated microglia can, in turn, activate astrocytes, and *vice versa*.

Fractalkine is a neuron-to-glia signal[69] that can trigger release of neurostimulating agents such as NO, ATP, excitatory amino acids, and classical immune mediators, inducing spinal nociceptive facilitation.[70] Considering that glial cells are not normally involved in pain processing and are only activated during excessive nervous system activity, agents targeting these cells, or their neuroactive

Table 5 Different strategies targeting glial activity.

Strategy	Pros	Cons	Developments
Disrupt glial activation	If basal homeostatic functions of glia are left intact, could be promising	Disrupting basal glial intracellular functions is not acceptable. Drugs targeting microglia alone may not be clinically effective in reversing established pain	Minocycline is being explored as a microglia-selective inhibitor in animal models
Block proinflammatory cytokine actions	Proinflammatory cytokines are involved in the initiation and maintenance of pain facilitation. This strategy is effective for blocking as well as reversing pain facilitation	Proinflammatory cytokines are redundant as unblocked cytokines may take over their function: thus, blocking a single cytokine is unlikely to be clinically effective. Current compounds do not cross the blood–brain barrier	Antagonists of TNF, IL-1, and IL-6 are being assessed in animal models
Inhibit proinflammatory cytokine synthesis	If synthesis of all proinflammatory cytokines could be blocked, pain problems are predicted to be resolved	No apparent disadvantage as long as treatment is reversible/controllable to allow expression of cytokines under conditions where they would be beneficial	Some thalidomide derivatives cross the blood–brain barrier and might be worth assessing for potential effects on glial function
Disrupt cytokine signaling and synthesis	Broad-spectrum approaches to shut down creation or effectiveness of key mediators of pain facilitation. Some p38 MAP kinase inhibitors are orally active and cross the blood–brain barrier. Intrathecal nonviral gene therapy (controllable by insertion of appropriate control sequences) reversibly generates IL-10 site-specifically, using a safe and reliable outpatient delivery system	P38 MAP kinase is not the only cascade involved; it may be only transiently involved and not restricted to glia (expressed by neurons); effect of inhibiting neuronal signaling is unknown. IL-10 gene therapy involves an invasive procedure (lumbar puncture)	Efficacy of both p38 MAP kinase inhibitors and IL-10 nonviral gene therapy is being assessed in animal models

Ref: 2008 IASP meeting, Glasgow UK

Note: IL-10 is an anti-inflammatory cytokine, does not cross the blood–brain barrier, and is effective in reversing pain facilitation; however, it is very short-acting.

Note: these pursuits and other clinical trials can be sourced at: http://clinicaltrials.gov

products, hold analgesic hope for the future (*Table 5*). Modulation of the immune system is becoming the 'new approach' to managing neuropathic pain.

Under the influence of ATP activation, $P2X_4$ is upregulated with a time course that parallels that of the development of allodynia.[71] $P2X_4$ receptors are nonspecific cation channels that are permeable to calcium ions. Apparently, ATP stimulation of these receptors leads to calcium influx that activates signaling proteins leading to the release of factor(s) that enhance transmission in spinal pain transmission neurons. This could occur through enhanced glutamatergic synaptic transmission or through *reversal of GABA/glycinergic inhibition*.[72] In the rat peripheral nerve compression model, Coull *et al.*[72] observed that reversing the direction of anionic flux in lamina I neurons reverses the effect of GABA and glycine. It is believed that increased cellular calcium impacts the capacity of neurons to pump chloride out of the cytoplasm through the potassium chloride cotransporter, KCC-2. Opening anion channels in the setting of intracellular chloride accumulation results in chloride efflux instead of influx. Reversing the direction of anionic flux reverses the effect of GABA and glycine, changing inhibition to excitation (**27**). Microglial activation occurs only following C fiber neuropathic injury and is not typically seen following peripheral inflammation.

DYNAMIC TRAFFICKING

A variety of pathological processes affecting peripheral nerves, sensory ganglia, spinal roots, and CNS structures can induce neuropathic pain. When an axon is severed, the proximal stump (attached to the cell body) seals off, forming a terminal swelling 'endbulb'. Within a day or two, numerous fine processes ('sprouts') start to grow out from the endbulb. Regenerating sprouts may elongate within their original endoneurial tube, reforming connections, or they may become misdirected, forming a variety of different types of neuromas (**15**). Various neuroma endings have been identified to give rise to 'ectopic' activity, which originates in axonal endbulbs, sprouts, patches of dysmyelination, and in the cell soma, rather than at the usual location, the peripheral sensory ending.[73]

Axotomy experiments have revealed that there are high levels of *ectopic discharge* in dorsal roots following peripheral axotomy, with activity apparently originating in the DRG.[74] When axons are cut close to the DRG, 75% of ectopic afferent activity originates in the DRG, and 25% in the neuroma.[75] When the nerve is injured further distally, the neuroma makes a relatively greater contribution. DRG ectopia may be important in herniated intervertebral disk in which the DRG is directly impacted by the disease. A direct relationship exists between ectopic afferent firing and allodynia in neuropathic pain. Preventing the generation of ectopia, or blocking its access to the CNS, suppresses the allodynia, while enhancing ectopia accentuates allodynia. The most convincing specific sign of spontaneous neuropathic pain in animals (rodents to primates) is 'autotomy', their tendency to lick, scratch and bite numb (but presumably painful) denervated body parts.[76]

Other mechanisms, such as *ephaptic cross-talk*, distort sensory signals in neuropathy. Each sensory neuron normally constitutes an independent signal conduction channel, however excitatory interactions can develop among neighboring neurons, amplifying sensory signals and causing sensation spread.

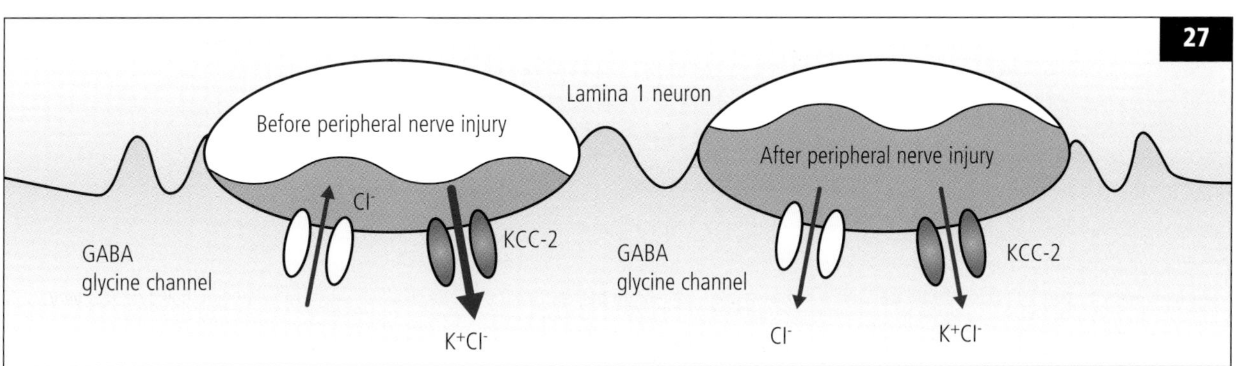

27 Paradoxically, GABA/glycinergic inhibition can be reversed to a state of excitation.

Herein, cross-excitation in the PNS may contribute to windup. Ephaptic (electrical) cross-talk occurs when there is a sufficient surface area of close membrane apposition between adjacent neurons in the absence of the normal glial insulation.[77] Different types of fibers are frequently coupled.

Membrane remodeling also impacts afferent hyperexcitability in neuropathy. Membrane proteins responsible for transduction and encoding are synthesized on ribosomes in the DRG cell soma. Thereafter, they are inserted into the local membrane in a process called 'vesicle exocytosis', after being loaded into the membrane of intracytoplasmic transport vesicles and vectorially transported down the axon. Dynamic 'trafficking' in normal neurons is closely regulated to ensure molecules arrive at their correct destination in appropriate numbers. For example, the turnover half-life of sodium channels is thought to be only 1–3 days.[78] Various ion channels, transducer molecules, and receptors are synthesized in the cell soma, transported along the axon, and incorporated in excess into the axon membrane of endbulbs and sprouts associated with injured afferent neurons (**28**).[79] This remodeling appears to be a causative factor in altered axonal excitability in some patients.

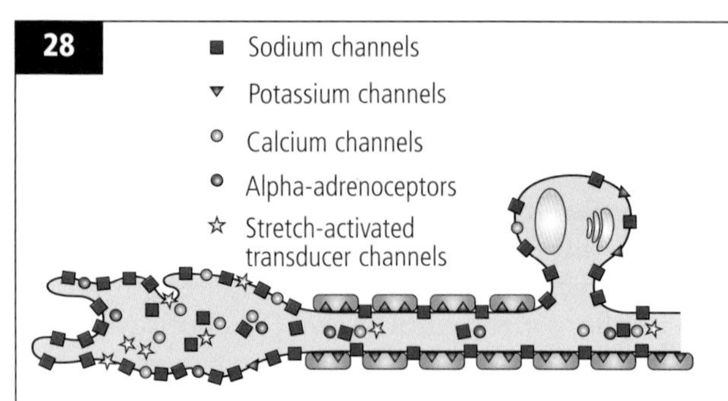

28 Injured afferent neurons can express an increased state of hyperexcitability. The cell stoma synthesizes various ion channels, transducer molecules, and receptors that are transported along the axon and incorporated in excess into the axon membrane of the endbulbs and sprouts associated with the injury. (Adapted from Devor M. Nerve pathophysiology and mechanisms of pain in causalgia. *J Auton Nerv Syst* 1983; **7**: 371–384).

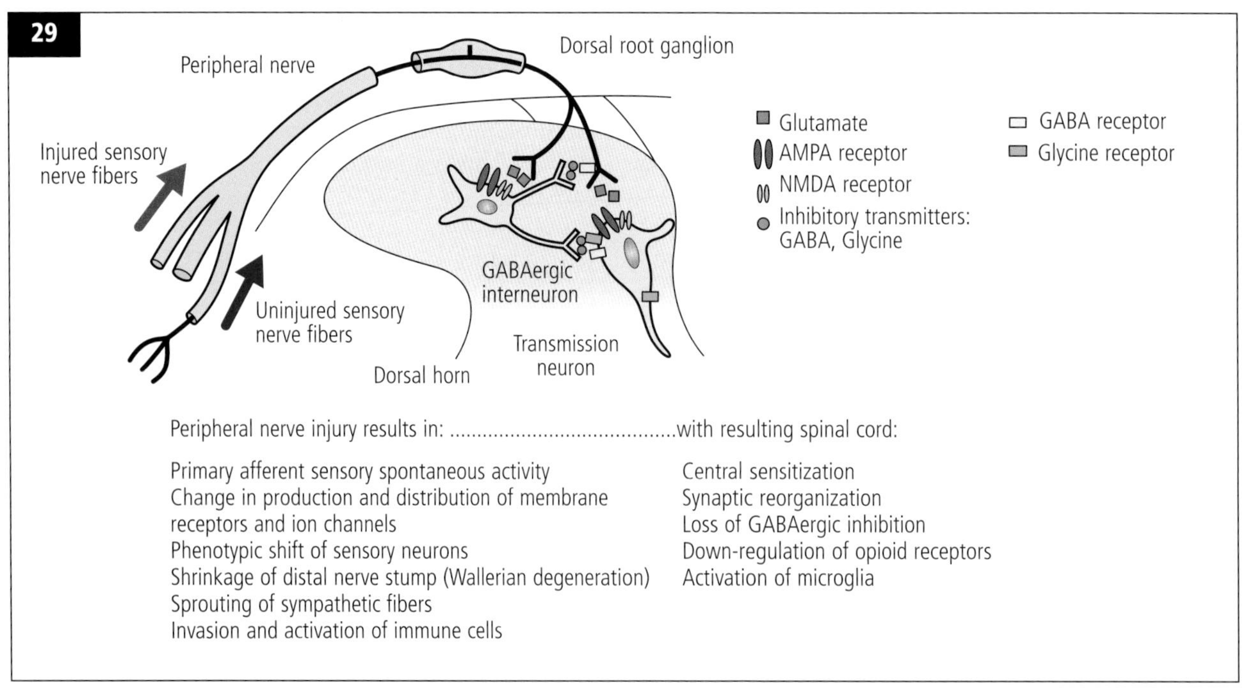

29 Relationships between peripheral nerve injury and spinal cord responses.

Neuronal hyperexcitability may also be dependent upon *intrinsic kinetic properties* of the ion channel. For example, cAMP-dependent phosphorylation or dephosphorylation of the sodium channel molecule regulates sodium ion current. Certain hormones, trophic factors, neuromodulatory peptides, and inflammatory mediators (notably PGs) can activate dephosphorylating enzymes that are positioned to affect afferent excitability by this mechanism. That is to say, some diffusible mediators change sodium and potassium current density, regulating neuronal firing without necessarily changing membrane potential.[80] In the understanding of neuropathic pain, it is important to differentiate excitation from excitability. *Excitation* refers to the transduction process, the ability of a stimulus to depolarize a sensory neuron, creating a generator potential. *Excitability* refers to the translation of the generator potential into an impulse train, where sodium and potassium channels play a major role. This distinction has medical treatment implications. Neuronal excitation can result from a large number of physical and chemical stimuli. Eliminate one, and many others are still at play. In contrast, if excitability is suppressed, the cell loses its ability to respond to all stimuli. See **29**.

ACUTE PAIN

Everyday acute pain, or 'nociceptive pain', occurs when a strong noxious stimulus (mechanical, thermal or chemical) impacts the skin or deep tissue. Nociceptors, a special class of primary sensory nerve fibers, fire impulses in response to these stimuli which travel along the peripheral nerves, past the sensory cell bodies in the DRG, along the dorsal roots, and into the spinal cord (or brainstem). Thereafter, the conscious brain interprets these transmissions from populations of second- and third-order neurons of the CNS. Acute pain is purposeful. It protects us from potentially severe tissue injury of noxious insults from everyday activities (**30**). Acute pain is also short-acting, and relatively easy to treat.

Physiological pain, a term synonymous with nociceptive pain, occurs after most types of noxious stimulus, and is usually protective. This type of pain plays an adaptive role as part of the body's normal defensive mechanisms, warning of contact with potentially damaging environmental insults and it initiates responses of avoidance. Dr. Frank Vertosick states, 'Pain is a teacher, the headmaster of nature's survival school.'[81] This protective system relies on a sophisticated network of nociceptors and sensory neurons that encode for insult intensity, duration, quality, and location. Physiological pain is rarely a clinical entity for treatment, but rather a state to avoid. *Pathological pain*, inferring that tissue damage is present, is not transient, and may be associated with significant tissue inflammation and nerve injury. It is often further classified into inflammatory pain or neuropathic pain. From a temporal perspective, recent pathological pain can be considered a symptom, whereas chronic pain can be considered a disease.

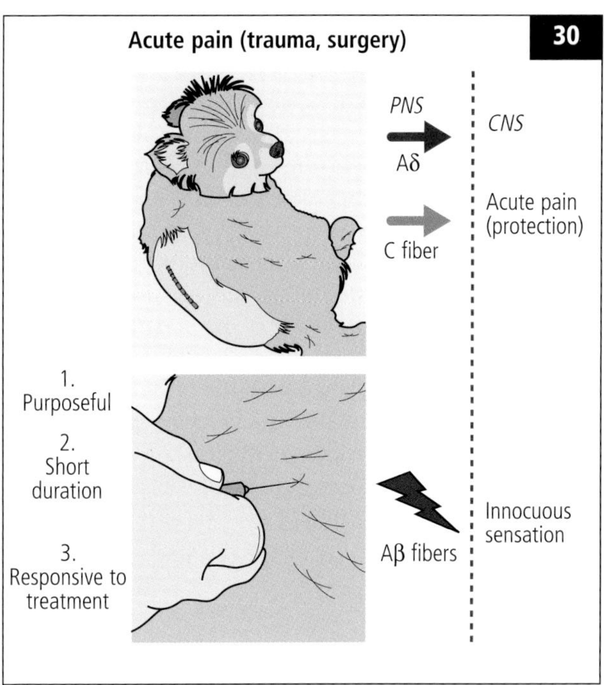

30 Acute pain is a signal of life. It is purposeful, of short duration, and most often responsive to treatment.

INFLAMMATORY PAIN

Inflammatory pain, often categorized along with acute pain as 'nociceptive', refers to pain and tenderness felt when the skin or other tissue is inflamed, hot, red, and swollen (**31**).

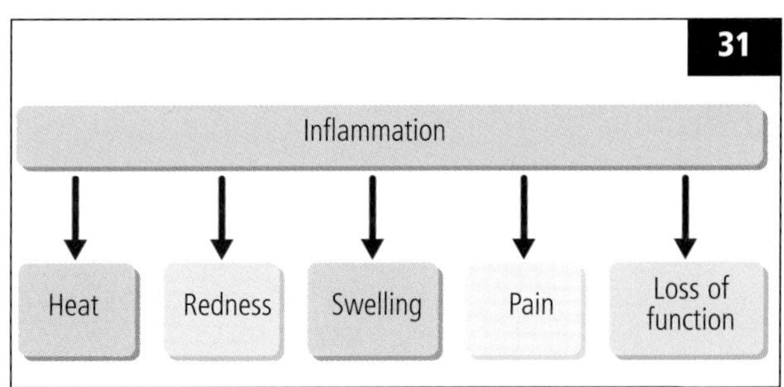

31 Inflammatory pain is associated with heat, redness, swelling, and loss of function.

The inflammatory process is mediated and facilitated by the local release of numerous chemicals, including bradykinin, PGs, leukotrienes (LTs), serotonin, histamine, sP, thromboxanes, platelet-activating factor, adenosine and ATP, protons and free radicals. Cytokines, such as ILs and TNF, and neurotropins, especially nerve growth factor (NGF), are also generated during inflammation (**32**).

When there is tissue injury and inflammation, the firing threshold of the Aδ and C nociceptive afferents in response to heating of the skin is lowered into the non-noxious range. This is a result of PG production from COX activity in the arachidonic acid cascade, which acts directly on the peripheral terminals of the Aδ and C fibers, lowering their threshold to thermal (but not electrical) stimuli.

INCISIONAL PAIN

Postoperative, incisional pain is a specific and common form of acute pain. Studies in rodents have characterized the primary hyperalgesia to mechanical and thermal stimuli.[82] Primary hyperalgesia to mechanical stimuli lasts for 2–3 days, while hyperalgesia to heat lasts longer–6 or 7 days (after plantar incision). The secondary hyperalgesia is present only to mechanical, not thermal, stimuli.[83] Conversion of mechanically insensitive silent nociceptors to mechanically responsive fibers is thought to play an important role in the maintenance of primary mechanical hyperalgesia, while release of ATP from injured cells is considered to play an important role in the induction of mechanical allodynia following skin incision.[84] The incision-induced spontaneous activity in primary afferent fibers helps to maintain the sensitized state of WDR neurons of the dorsal horn, in contrast to other forms of cutaneous injury (e.g. burns), where hyperalgesia is NMDA dependent.

VISCERAL PAIN

Healthy viscera are insensate or, at best, minimally sensate. Such observation dates back to 1628 when Sir William Harvey exposed the heart of a patient, and with pinching and pricking determined that the patient could not reliably identify the stimulus.[85] This is in contrast to the body surface which is always sensate. Injury to the surface of the body initiates the reflex response of fight or flight, whereas visceral pain tends to invoke immobility. In general, there is a poor correlation between the amount of visceral pathology and intensity of visceral pain. Clinical lore has it that: (1) viscera are minimally sensate, whereas

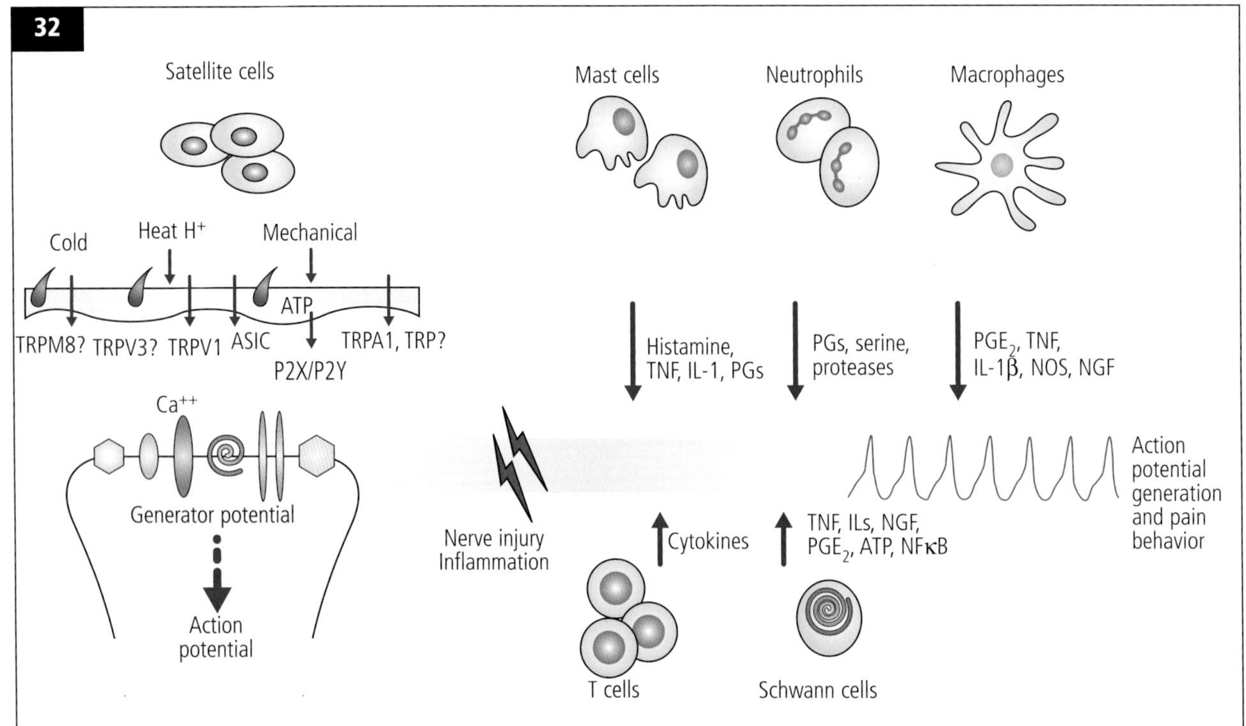

32 Many different cell types and neuromodulators contribute to the pain associated with inflammation.

body surfaces are always highly sensate, (2) visceral pain has poorer localization than superficial pain, and (3) visceral pain is more strongly linked to emotion than superficial pain.

A separate pathway for transmitting visceral input from the site of origin to the brain does not exist. Every cell that has visceral input has somatic input: visceral–somatic convergence. There are cells that receive somatic input only, but there are no cells that receive visceral input only. During normal activities, information is conducted from somatic origin, such as skin through the spinothalamic tract, to CNS areas of interpretation for nociception. With myocardial infarct/angina, for example, the same spinothalamic tract cells are activated, and theory has it that the spinothalamic tract may have become 'conditioned' to the everyday somatic responses; so it now 'presumes' it is sensing a somatic input rather than visceral nociception (**33**).

A suggested mechanism for referred pain is that visceral and somatic primary neurons converge on to common spinal neurons (**34**). This is the *convergence–projection* theory, which has considerable supporting experimental evidence.[86]

To better explain 'referred pain with somatic hyperalgesia', two theories have been proposed. The *convergence–facilitation* theory proposes that abnormal visceral input would produce an irritable focus in the relative spinal cord segment, thus facilitating messages from somatic structures. The second postulates that the *visceral afferent barrage* induces the activation of a reflex arc, the afferent branch of which is presented by visceral afferent fibers and the efferent branch by somatic efferents and sympathetic efferents toward the somatic structures (muscle, subcutis, and skin). The efferent impulses toward the periphery would then sensitize nociceptors in the parietal tissues of the referred area, thus resulting in the phenomenon of somatic hyperalgesia.

Visceral pain is also processed differently. Although primary afferents subserving visceral, cutaneous, and muscle pain are mostly distinct, at the dorsal horn there is considerable convergence of these pathways so that spinothalamic, spinoreticular, and spinomesencephalic tracts all contain neurons that respond to both somatic and visceral stimuli.[87] Functional magnetic resonance imaging (fMRI) reveals a common cortical network subserving cutaneous and visceral pain that could underlie similarities in the pain experience. However, differential activation patterns within insular, primary somatosensory, motor, and prefrontal cortices of the brain have been identified that may account for the ability to distinguish visceral and cutaneous pain as well as the differential emotional, autonomic, and motor responses associated with different sensations.[88]

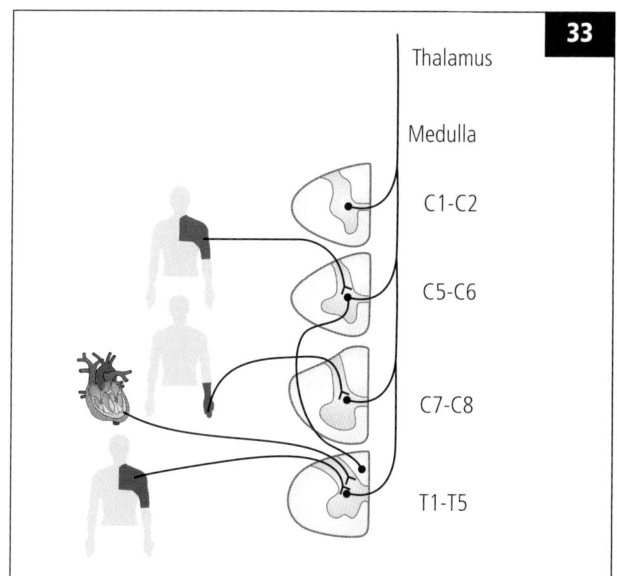

33 Neural mechanism underlying angina pectoris. The same spinothalamic cells are activated as by skin, and the 'default' source is considered to be peripheral.

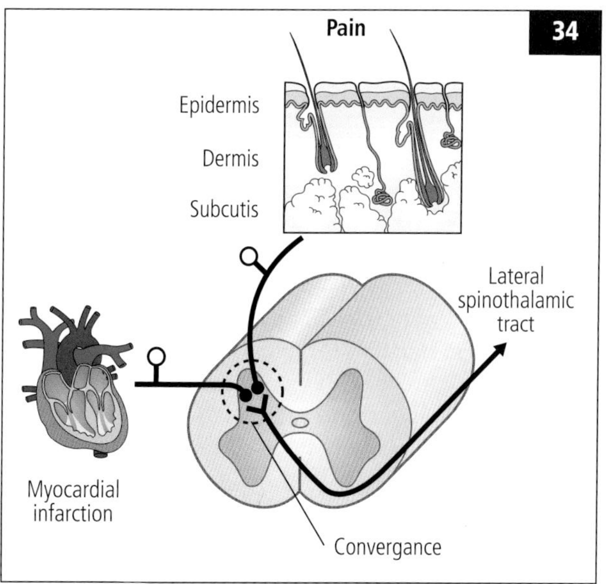

34 Convergence–projection theory: visceral and somatic primary neurons converge on to common spinal neurons.

GENDER AND VISCERAL PAIN

A review of the human literature[89] demonstrates that women are more likely than men to experience a variety of recurrent and visceral pains. Generally, women report more severe levels of pain, more frequent pain, and pain of longer duration than do men. Reports of visceral pain in veterinary patients is sparse. A report of veterinary outpatients visiting the Ohio State University showed that in the year 2002 1,153 dogs and 652 cats were presented.[90] Twenty percent of the dogs and 14% of the cats were diagnosed as painful, with approximately half of each species being diagnosed with visceral pain. No differences were noted related to gender; however, most animals presented were neutered or spayed. Studies in rats show that visceral hypersensitivity varies over the estrous cycle, where rats are more sensitive during proestrus, and proestrous rats are more hypersensitive than male rats.[91] Kamp *et al.* have shown that female mice are more sensitive to visceral pain than males in a colorectal distention model, but have also shown that response varies with the strain of mouse.[92] There is a stunning over-representation of male subjects in the study of pain (approximately 20:1),[93] perhaps reflecting the concern of experimental variability with female subjects, supporting the case for inclusion of more female subjects in basic science studies of pain.

VISCERAL PAIN MODELS

A number of visceral pain models exist. Distention of hollow organs is a common model. More often distension of the distal gastrointestinal tract (colon, rectum) has been used to evoke respiratory, cardiovascular, visceromotor, behavioral, and neurophysiological responses in multiple species including horse, dog, cat, rabbit, and rat. Contemporary thinking is that viscera are not insensate, but are minimally sensate in the healthy state and can become very sensitive following pathology that upregulates sensation from a subconscious state to the conscious state.

Strigo *et al.* have used psychophysical measures to directly compare visceral and cutaneous pain and sensitivity.[94] Healthy human subjects evaluated perceptions evoked by balloon distention of the distal esophagus and contact heat on the upper chest. For esophageal distention, the threshold for pain intensity was higher than that observed for unpleasantness, whereas for contact heat, pain and unpleasantness thresholds did not differ for either phasic or tonic stimulus application. Results support that visceral pain is more unpleasant, diffuse, and variable than cutaneous pain of similar intensity, independent of the duration of the presented stimuli (35).

VISCERAL STIMULI

A lack of sensitivity in viscera at baseline may relate to the sparse population of visceral afferents themselves, which are quantitatively fewer per unit area than similar measures of cutaneous afferents. This may suggest that increased activity is required to cross a threshold for perception. The large proportion of silent afferents in viscera also help explain the variation of sensitization. Silent afferents have been frequently noted in visceral structures to form up to 50% of the neuronal sample.[95]

The mucosa, muscle, and serosa of hollow organs as well as the mesentery, but not the parenchyma of solid organs, contain visceral receptors.[96] Inflammation will lower nociceptor firing thresholds, resulting in a more broad recognition of pain experienced at lower distension pressures. As previously mentioned, inflammation also recruits 'silent' nociceptors, which fire at lower thresholds or become sensitized by hypoxemia and ischemia.[97] Acute pain is the sum of high-threshold nociceptors activated at high pressures, where chronic noxious stimuli recruit previously unresponsive or silent nociceptors through hypoxemia or inflammation. Pain sensations correlate with generated intracolonic or small bowel pressures and increased wall tension rather than intraluminal volume.[98] Accordingly, patients may have ileus without pain.

Stimulated visceral nociceptors release both sP and CGRP within synapses of the dorsal horn. Activation of visceral afferents also results in upregulation of NOS in the spinal cord dorsal horn and causes expression of the oncogene *c-fos*.[99] Kappa receptor agonists bind to peripheral visceral afferents suppressing the release of sP and expression of *c-fos* in the dorsal horn.[100]

Peripheral reduction in nociceptive thresholds leads to primary visceral hypersensitivity. Secondary hypersensitivity is a central neuroplastic reaction to activated C-fibers and convergence. Visceral central hypersensitivity is maintained by glutamate release that binds to NMDA receptors, the activation of which leads to NOS expression, NO production, and PG production.[101]

POOR LOCALIZATION OF VISCERAL PAIN

Much of our knowledge surrounding the poor localization of visceral pain comes from clinical practice in humans. Visceral pain is not normally perceived as localized to a given organ, but to somatic

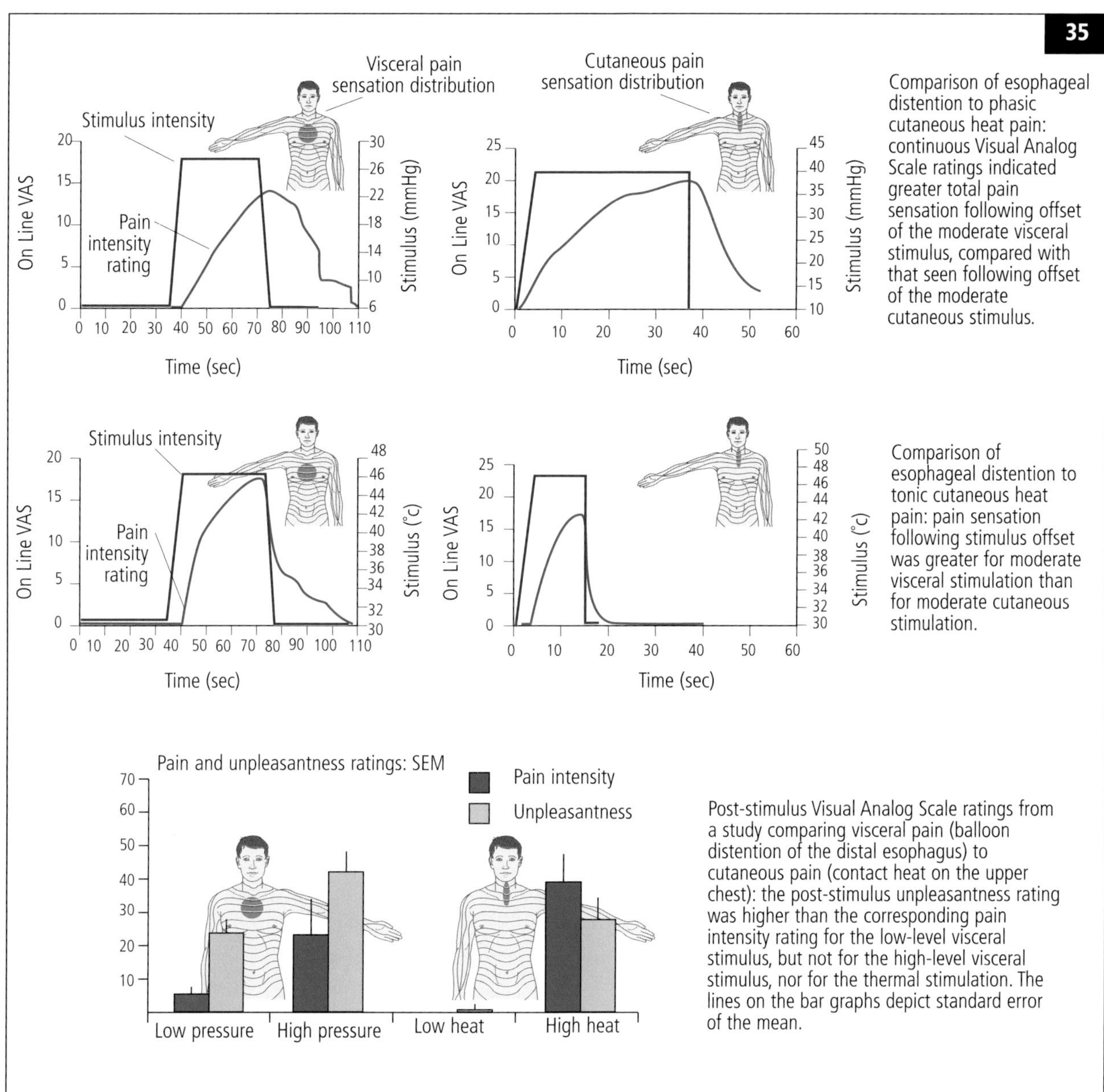

35 In human studies, visceral pain is more unpleasant, diffuse and variable than cutaneous pain of similar intensity.

structures that receive afferent inputs at the same spinal segments as visceral afferent entry. The actual source of the visceral pain may only be localized when manipulation or physical examination might stimulate the painful organ. Classically, visceral pain is considered either as wholly unlocalized pain or as referred pain, with two separate components: (1) the diseased viscera sensation is transferred to another site (e.g. ischemic myocardium felt in the neck and arm) or (2) hypersensitivity at other sites from inputs directly applied to those other sites (e.g. flank muscle becoming sensitive to palpation concurrent with urolithiasis)–a phenomenon called *secondary somatic hyperalgesia.*

The very neuroanatomy of viscera suggests their unique pain response (**36**). The pattern of distribution for visceral primary afferents differs markedly from that of cutaneous primary afferents. Visceral sensory pathways tend to follow perivascular routes that are diffuse in nature. Visceral afferent pathways have peripheral sites of neuronal synaptic contact that occur with the cell bodies of prevertebral ganglia such as the celiac ganglion, mesenteric ganglion, and pelvic ganglion. This architecture can lead to alterations in local visceral function outside central control. The gut is probably an extreme example, where it functions by its own 'independent brain' that regulates the complex activities of digestion and absorption.

DRG neurons innervating the viscera tend to follow the original location of structural precursors of the viscera during embryological development. Afferents of a given viscus may have cell bodies in the dorsal root ganglia of 10 or more spinal levels, bilaterally distributed. Further, individual visceroceptive afferent fibers branch once they enter the spinal cord and may spread over a dozen or more spinal segments, interacting with neurons in at least five different dorsal horn laminae located bilaterally in the spinal cord.[102] Upon further examination, spinal dorsal horn neurons with visceral inputs have multiple inputs, from the viscera, joints, muscle, and cutaneous structures (**37**).

Collectively, there is an imprecise and diffuse organization of visceral primary inputs appearing consistent with an imprecise and diffuse localization by the CNS.

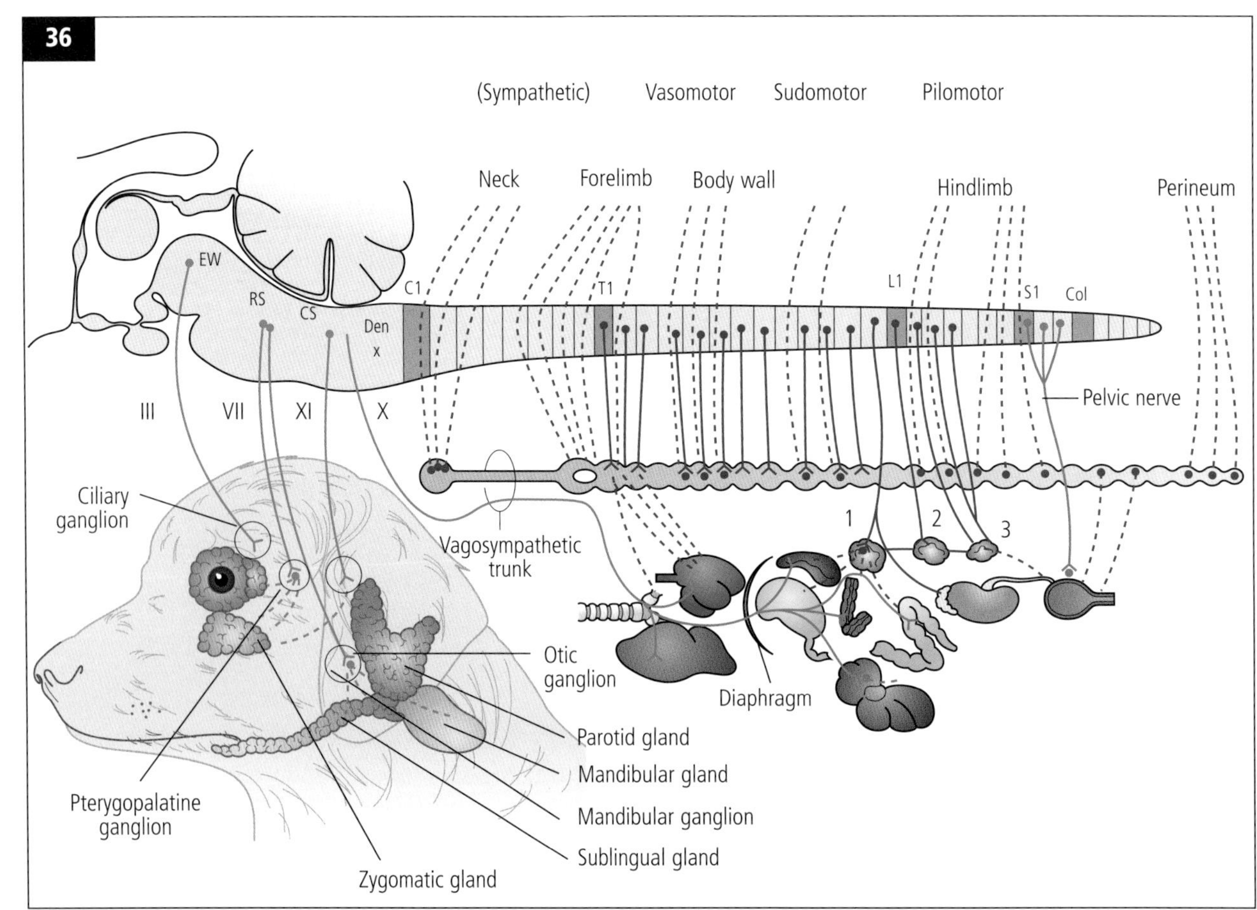

36 The neuroanatomy of canine viscera suggests their unique pain response.

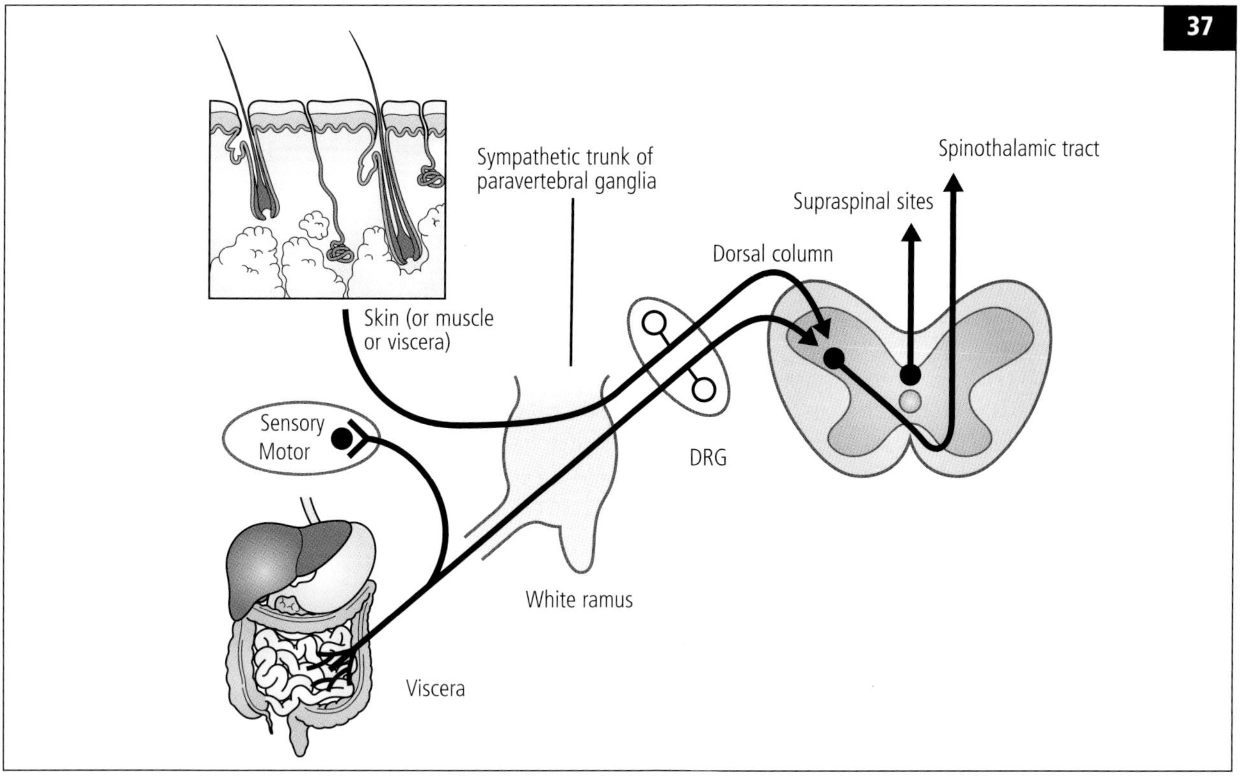

37

Sympathetic trunk of paravertebral ganglia
Spinothalamic tract
Supraspinal sites
Dorsal column
Skin (or muscle or viscera)
Sensory
Motor
DRG
White ramus
Viscera

37 Spinal dorsal horn neurons with visceral inputs have multiple inputs from the viscera, joints, muscle and cutaneous structures.

VISCERAL HYPERSENSITIZATION

The bladder is one of the few viscera that have recognized sensation when healthy and when diseased. As with irritable bowel syndrome (IBS), hypersensitivity to somatic stimuli is noted in people with interstitial cystitis (IC). Subjects with IC are significantly more sensitive to deep tissue measures of sensation related to pressure, ischemia, and bladder stretch than healthy subjects, showing an upward and left shift of reported discomfort with bladder filling (**38**).[103]

Cross-organ communication: visceral organs

As many as 40–60% of human patients diagnosed with IBS also exhibit symptoms and fulfill diagnostic criteria for IC; correspondingly, 38% of patients diagnosed with IC also have symptoms and fulfill diagnostic criteria for IBS.[104,105] Because neural cross-talk exists under normal conditions, alterations in neural pathways by disease or injury may play a role in development of overlapping chronic pelvic pain disorders and pelvic organ cross-sensitization.

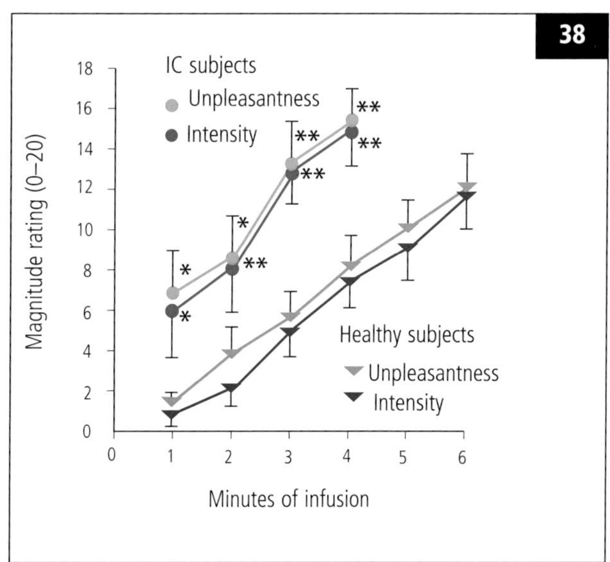

38 Human subjects with interstitial cystitis (IC) show an upward and left shift of discomfort with bladder filling compared to normal, healthy subjects. Single asterisk indicates significantly different in subjects with IC vs. healthy subjects ($p < 0.05$). Double asterisks indicate significantly different in subjects with IC vs. healthy subjects ($p < 0.01$).[103]

Pezzone *et al.*[106] have developed a rodent model for studying pelvic organ reflexes, pelvic organ cross-talk, and associated striated sphincter activity that has shown (1) colonic afferent sensitization occurs following the induction of acute cystitis and (2) urinary bladder sensitization occurs following the induction of acute colitis. A possible explanation might be that the inflamed colon and urinary bladder have a common afferent axon that enters the spinal cord, resulting in the observed effect (**39**).

In the rat, approximately 14% of superficial and 29% deeper L6–S2 spinal neurons receive convergent inputs from both urinary bladder and colon.[107] In cats, approximately 30% of the sacral and thoracolumbar compound spinal interneurons have convergent inputs from both the urinary bladder and colon, and both of these visceral organs either excite or inhibit approximately 50% of the neurons.[108] These facts suggest that pelvic pain conditions and disorders might be a result of the interaction between algogenic conditions of more than one visceral organ (**40**).

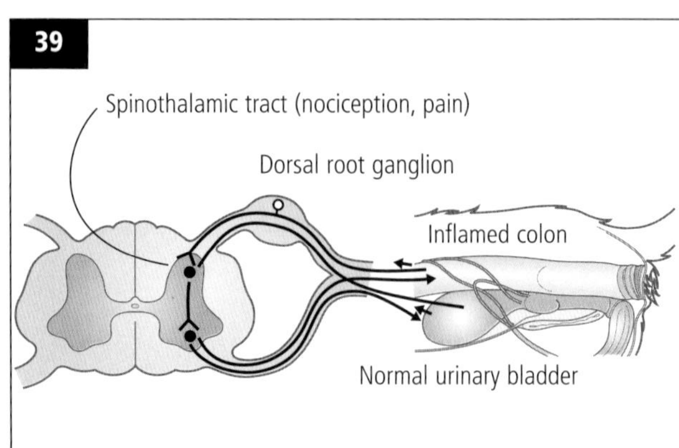

39 Cross-organ convergence: convergence of colonic and urinary bladder afferent fibers onto a spinothalamic tract cell.

VISCERAL PAIN AND EMOTION

Human studies, as well as animal models, have demonstrated that visceral pain is strongly linked to emotion. The emotional state frequently alters function of the viscera,[109] and the reverse is true – far more pronounced than with equal intensity of superficial pain. This tends to evoke an unending cycle of feedback between visceral pain and anxiety. Therefore, it would appear appropriate to include an anxiolytic in a pharmacotherapeutic regimen targeting chronic visceral pain syndromes.

VISCERAL PAIN SUMMARY

Visceral pain is unique for several reasons:

- There is a poor correlation between the amount of tissue injury and visceral pain.
- Patterns of referred pain are a result of convergence of somatic and visceral afferents on the same dorsal horn neurons within the spinal cord.
- Clinical visceral pain is poorly localized (in humans), midline, and perceived as deep because, in part, of poor representation within the primary somatosensory cortex.
- More so than in somatic pain, visceral pain is accompanied by autonomic responses.
- Only a minority of visceral afferents are sensory, most relate to motor or reflex responses, and few have specialized sensory terminals.
- Pain severity is transmitted by the sum of activity from nonspecific sensory receptors within mucosa, smooth muscle, and serosa.

See *Table 6*.

Anatomical differences influencing visceral pain, where perception and psychological processing are different from somatic pain, include:

- A low number of visceral nociceptors compared with somatic nociceptors.
- Lack of specialization.
- Visceral polymodal nociceptors.
- Convergence with somatic afferents on dorsal horn laminae resulting in referred pain.
- Hypersensitivity that is both peripherally and centrally mediated, but not by windup characteristic of somatic pain.
- Unique ascending tracts through the dorsal column, low and poor representation with primary somatosensory cortex, rich input through the medial thalamus to the limbic cortex, amygdala, anterior cingulate, and insular cortices.
- Close association with autonomic nerves.

Visceral sensitization mechanisms are:

- Ongoing pain sensation.
- Enhanced response to given stimulation.

Peripheral mechanisms are:

- Activation of visceral afferent fibers.

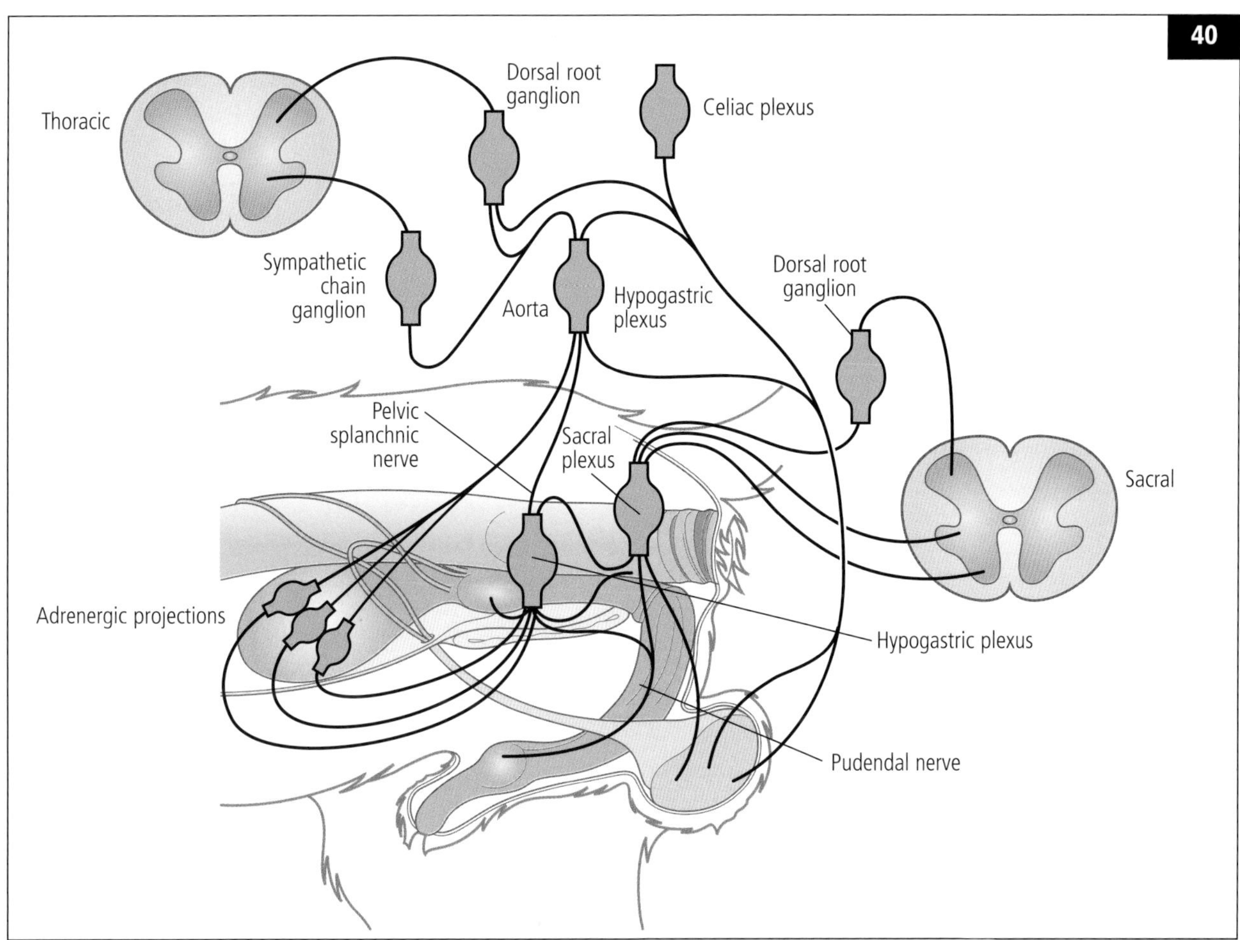

40 Pelvic pain severity is transmitted by the sum of activity from nonspecific sensory receptors within mucosa, smooth muscle, and serosa. Further, convergence makes it difficult to identify a single focus of input.

Table 6 Differences between visceral and somatic pain processing.

	Visceral pain	Superficial pain
Innervation	Spinal + vagal	Spinal
Injury	No	Yes
Noxious	Stretch Inflammation Ischemia	Damage Threat of damage
Localization	Poor	Excellent
Referred pain	The rule	The exception
Pathology	Not related to intensity	Related to intensity

- Sensitization of mechano-/chemosensitive terminals.
- Continuous afferent input to the spinal cord.
- Activation of silent mechanosensitive afferent fibers.

Spinal mechanisms are:

- Sensitization of spinal neurons.
- Expanded spatially distributed spinal input.

See *Table 7*.

NEUROGENIC INFLAMMATION

Release of sP and NGF into the periphery causes a tissue reaction termed *neurogenic inflammation*. Neurogenic inflammation is driven by events in the CNS and does not depend on granulocytes or lymphocytes as with the classic inflammatory response to tissue trauma or immune-mediated cell damage. Cells in the dorsal horn release chemicals that cause action potentials to fire backwards down the nociceptors. The result of this dorsal root reflex is that nociceptive dendrites release sP and CGRP into peripheral tissues, causing degranulation of mast cells and changing vascular endothelial cell characteristics. The resultant outpouring of potent inflammatory and vasodilatating agents causes edema and potentiates transmission of nociceptive signals from the periphery (**41**).

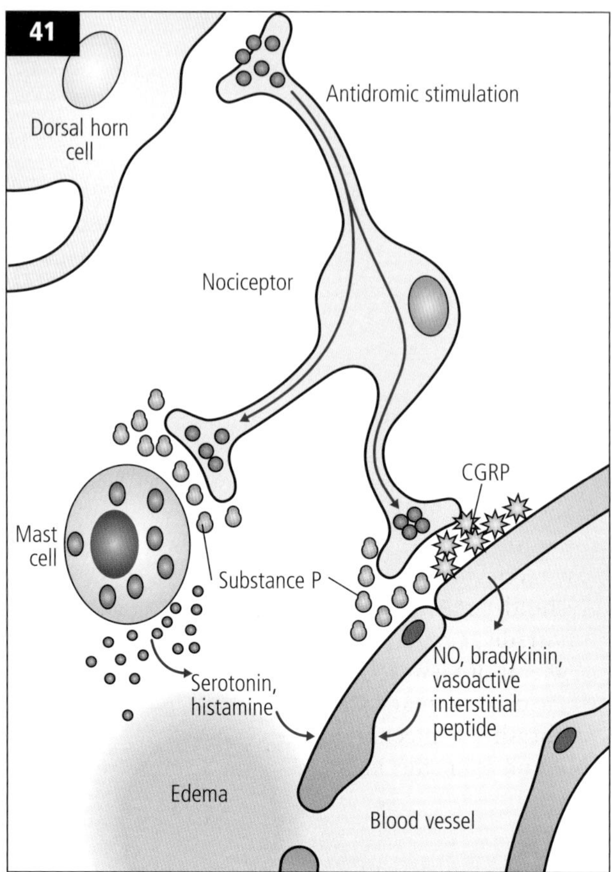

41 Neurogenic inflammation varies from the classic inflammatory response, as it is driven by events in the CNS.

Table 7 Potentially useful agents in the management of visceral pain.

Agent	Mode of action
Kappa opioid agonist	Peripheral kappa receptor agonists on visceral afferents reduce sP and CRGP
Mu and delta opioids	Central mu and delta receptors reduce primary nociceptor activity and central hypersensitivity through periaqueductal gray activity
NSAIDs	Block spinal cord and peripheral PG and central hypersensitivity
Ketamine, methadone, amantadine	Block dorsal horn NMDA receptors
Corticosteroids	Block expression of spinal cord NOS and reduce hypersensitivity
Gabapentin	Reduces central glutamate levels and NMDA binding for hypersensitivity
Alpha-2-adrenoreceptor agonists	Facilitate descending inhibitory tracts through the periaqueductal gray
Tricyclic antidepressants	Facilitate descending inhibitory tracts in periaqueductal gray
Anticholinergics	Reduce colic and intestinal secretion
Somatostatin	Inhibits vasointestinal peptide and decreases colic and intestinal secretion Reduces central hypersensitivity

TACTILE ALLODYNIA

Tactile allodynia appears to be a sensory response to impulse activity in low-threshold mechanosensitive Aβ afferents, abnormally 'amplified' by central sensitization. Aβ afferents normally signal touch and vibration, but in neuropathy (and inflammation) they evoke pain. 'Aβ' pain has opened new insights into the understanding of pain systems, displacing Aδ and C fibers as the exclusive, and perhaps even the most important, primary afferent signaling channel for pathophysiological pain.

Cervero and Laird[110] proposed a model for the phenomenon of touch-evoked pain (allodynia), expanding on the gate theory and neurogenic inflammation (axon reflexes). Their model is based on the notion that Aβ mechanoreceptors can gain access to nociceptive neurons by means of a presynaptic link, at the central level, between low-threshold mechanoreceptors and nociceptors. Purportedly, excitation of nociceptors provoked by a peripheral injury activates the spinal interneurons that mediate primary afferent depolarization between low-threshold mechanoreceptors and nociceptors. Resultant from the increased and persistent barrage driving these neurons, their excitability is increased such that, when activated by low-threshold mechanoreceptors from areas surrounding the injury site, they produce a very intense primary afferent depolarization in the nociceptive afferents, capable of generating spike activity. Such activation is conducted antidromically in the form of dorsal root reflexes, but would also be conducted forward, activating the second-order neurons normally driven by nociceptors. The sensory consequence of this mechanism is pain evoked by the activation of low-threshold mechanoreceptors from an area surrounding an injury site (allodynia).

CHRONIC PAIN

In contrast to acute pain, where the pain stops quickly after the noxious stimulus has been removed, the pain and tenderness of inflammation may last for hours, days, months, and years. Recognition of the potential peripheral mediators of peripheral sensitization after inflammation gives insight as to the complexity of this process. Persistent, or chronic, pain is often *neuropathic pain*, which arises from injury to the PNS or CNS (*Table 8*).

Table 8 Human conditions in which neuropathic/neurogenic pain may appear.

Peripheral

Traumatic (including iatrogenic) nerve injury
Ischemic neuropathy
Nerve compression/entrapment
Polyneuropathy (hereditary, metabolic, toxic, inflammatory, infection, paraneoplastic, nutritional or in amyloids or vasculitis)
Plexus injury
Root compression
Stump and phantom pain after amputation
Postherpetic neuralgia
Trigeminal and glossopharyngeal neuralgia
Cancer-related neuropathy (i.e. due to neural invasion of the tumor, surgical nerve damage, radiation-induced nerve damage, or chemotherapy-induced neuropathy)
Scar pain

Central

Stroke (infarct or hemorrhage)
Multiple sclerosis
Spinal cord injury
Syringomyelia/syringobulbia

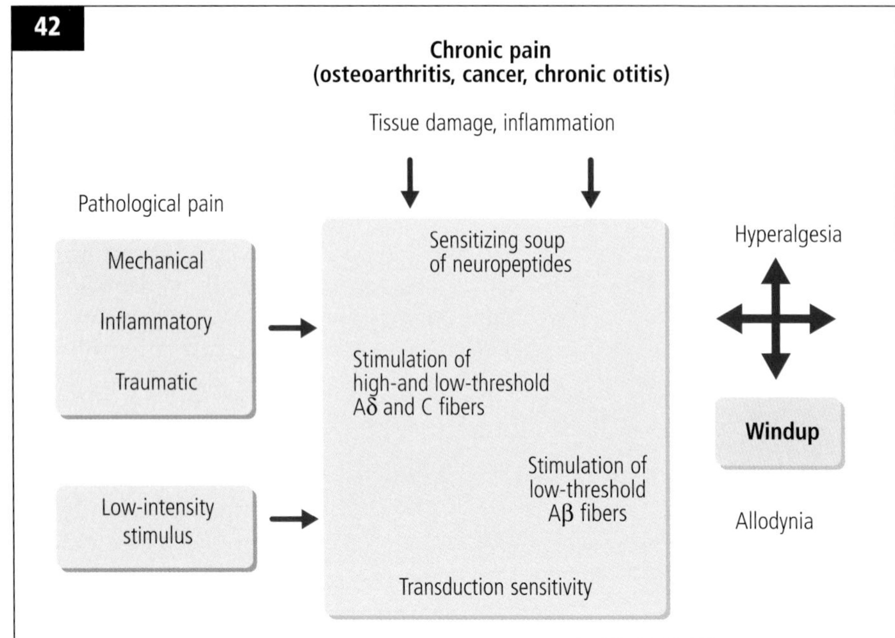

42 Chronic pain appears to have no purpose, lasts beyond an expected normal physiological response to the noxious insult, and is often difficult to treat.

Chronic pain appears to have no purpose, is characterized by extended duration, and is frequently difficult to treat (**42**), but may respond to certain anticonvulsants, tricyclic antidepressants (TCAs), and antiarrhythmics (*Table 9*). Local anesthetics applied systemically, topically, or to block nerves may also be effective. The separation between inflammatory and neuropathic pain does not exclude inflammatory components in neuropathic pain or neuropathic components in inflammatory pain. There are no systematic studies in neuropathic pain patients on the correlation between the intensity of the symptoms and the nature and severity of the nerve injury.

Chronic pain can result from sustained noxious stimuli such as ongoing inflammation or it may be independent of the inciting cause. Regardless of its etiology, chronic pain is maladaptive and offers no useful biological function or survival advantage. The nervous system itself actually becomes the focus of the pathology and contributes to patient morbidity. Effective treatment for chronic pain can be an enigma. Several studies have shown that the longer a pain lingers, the harder it is to eradicate. This is because pain can reconfigure the architecture of the nervous system it invades.

Chronic pain was traditionally defined as pain lasting more than 3 or 6 months, depending on the source of the definition.[111,112] More recently, chronic pain has been defined as 'pain that extends beyond the period of tissue healing and/or with low levels of identified pathology that are insufficient to explain the presence and /or extent of pain'.[113] There is no general consensus on the definition of chronic pain. In clinical practice it is often difficult to determine when acute pain has become chronic.

ACUTE TO CHRONIC PAIN

Normally, a steady state is maintained in which there is a close correlation between injury and pain. Yet, long-lasting or very intense nociceptive input or the removal of a portion of the normal input can distort the nociceptive system to such an extent that the close correlation between injury and pain can be lost. A progression from acute to chronic pain might be considered as three major stages or phases of pain, proposing that different neurophysiological mechanisms are involved, depending on the nature and time course of the originating stimulus.[114]

These three phases include: (1) the processing of a brief noxious stimulus, (2) the consequences of prolonged noxious stimulation, leading to tissue damage and peripheral inflammation, and (3) the consequences of neurological damage, including peripheral neuropathies and central pain states (**43**).

Table 9 Mechanisms of neuropathic pain with corresponding drug targets.

Mechanism	Target	Drug (human use)
Peripheral sensitization	TRPV1 receptors	Capsaicin
Altered expression, distribution, and function of ion channels	Voltage-gated K^+ channels	-
	Voltage-gated Na^+ channels	Local anesthetics, e.g. lidocaine; antiepileptics, e.g. carbamazepine, lacosamide, lamotrigine; antiarrhythmic agents, e.g. mexiletine
	HCN channels	-
	P2X-receptor-gated channels	-
	Voltage-gated Ca^{2+} channels	Ziconotide, gabapentin, pregabalin
Increased central excitation	NMDA receptors	Ketamine, ifenprodil
	NK1 receptors	-
Reduced spinal inhibition	Opioid receptors	Morphine, oxycodone, tramadol
	GABA receptors	Baclofen
	Glycine receptors	-
Deregulated supraspinal control	Monoamines	Tricyclic antidepressants, e.g. amitryptiline, nortriptyline; serotonin and norepinephrine reuptake inhibitors, e.g. duloxetine, tramadol
Immune system involvement	Cytokines	NSAIDs
	TNF-α	-
	Microglia	-
Schwann cell dedifferentiation	Growth factors	-

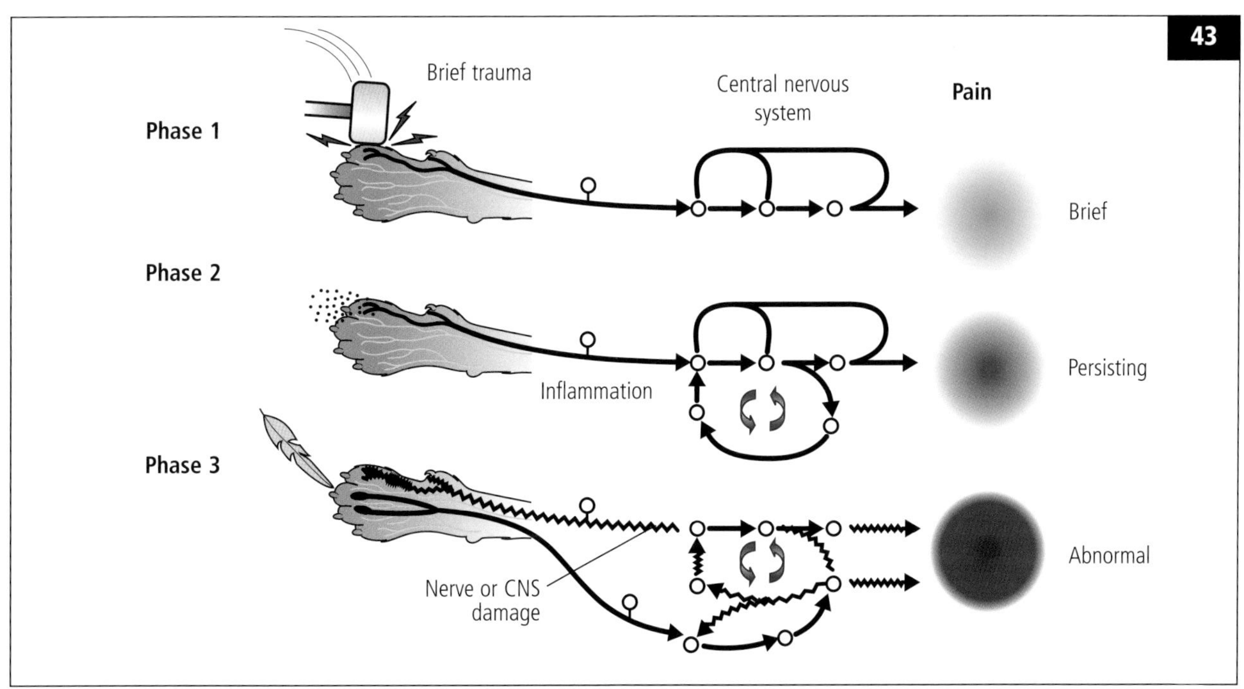

43 Progression of acute to chronic pain can be considered as phases of pain: brief (acute nociceptive), persisting (inflammatory), and abnormal (neuropathic).

- Phase 1: acute nociceptive pain (physiological pain). Mechanisms underlying the processing of brief noxious stimuli are fairly simple, with a direct route of transmission centrally toward the thalamus and cortex resulting in the conscious perception of pain, with the possibility for modulation occurring at synaptic relays along the way. It is reasonably easy to construct plausible and detailed neuronal circuits to explain the features of phase 1 pain.
- Phase 2: inflammatory pain. If a noxious stimulus is very intense, or prolonged, leading to tissue damage and inflammation, it might be considered phase 2 pain, as influenced by response properties of various components of the nociceptive system changing. These changes note that the CNS has moved to a new, more excitable state as a result of the noxious input generated by tissue injury and inflammation. Phase 2 is characterized by its central drive, a drive that is triggered and maintained by peripheral inputs. Patients experience spontaneous pain and sensation changes evoked by stimulation of the injured and surrounding area. Such change is known as hyperalgesia – a leftward shift of the stimulus–response curve. Hyperalgesia in the area of injury is termed primary hyperalgesia, and in the areas of normal tissue surrounding the injury site, as secondary hyperalgesia.
- Phase 3: neuropathic pain. Phase 3 pain is abnormal pain, generally the consequence of either damage or altered neuroprocessing within peripheral nerves or within the CNS itself, characterized by a lack of correlation between injury and pain. Clinically, phase 1 and 2 pains are symptoms of peripheral injury, whereas phase 3 pain is a symptom of neurological disease. These pains are spontaneous, triggered by innocuous stimuli, or are exaggerated responses to minor noxious stimuli. A particular combination of mechanisms responsible for each of the pain states is likely unique to the individual disease, or to a particular subgroup of patients. Phase 3 pain may involve genetic, cognitive, or thalamic processing that has yet to be identified. Activation of these mechanisms may be abnormally prolonged or intense due to abnormal input from damaged neurons, or simply because the regenerative properties of neurons are very poor or 'misdirected'. Healing may never occur. Finally, there are many mixed nociceptive–neuropathic pains, not only in malignant disease, but also in conditions such as herniated intervertebral disk and postamputation (phantom) limb pain.

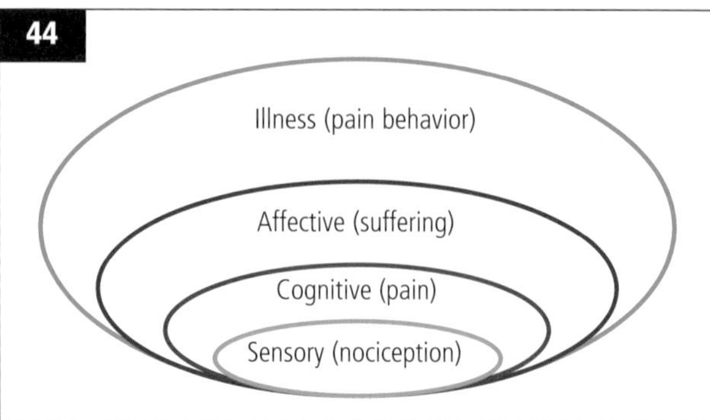

44 Integration of the physical dimensions of pain with the psychological factors, which are closely linked, gives insight to the complexity of managing pain-induced distress (suffering).

Consideration of chronic pain as a disease per se, rather than a symptom, enables the fundamental importance of the nonphysical elements of pain to be considered. Integration of the physical dimensions of pain with the psychological and social factors, which are closely linked together, allows a significant and deliberate move away from traditional Cartesian dogma (**44**).

As a result, treatment of one dimension alone may not result in improvement at other levels, and the complexity of suffering (pain-induced distress) (particularly in humans) is a challenge mandating a multifaceted approach.

NEUROPATHIC PAIN

Primary sensory neurons are able to signal specific sensory experiences because they respond with electrical impulses to specific types of stimuli (touch, pinch, heat, cold, vibration, etc.), and because they communicate with second-order sensory neurons in the spinal cord via specific synaptic connectivity using specific neurotransmitters. Maintaining these settings requires a complex biological process. If there has been nerve injury, the electrical properties, neurochemistry, and central connectivity of these neurons can change, bringing havoc on normal sensory processing, and sometimes inducing severe chronic neuropathic pain.

The International Association for the Study of Pain[115] defines neurogenic pain as 'pain initiated or caused by a primary lesion or dysfunction or transitory perturbation in the peripheral or central nervous system'. Due to potential vagaries within this definition, simplistically, neuropathic pain can be identified as pain due to a primary lesion or malfunction of the PNS or CNS. Neuropathic pain is divided between diseases with demonstrable neural lesions in the PNS and CNS and those conditions with no tangible lesion of major nerves and CNS. Therefore, there are ambiguities in identifying neuropathic diseases and currently no tests are available that can unequivocally diagnose neuropathic pain. Nevertheless, a large body of evidence validates the theory of the physiological process underlying neuropathic pain.

Many kinds of nerve inury can induce electrical changes: trauma, viral or bacterial infection, poor nutrition, toxins, autoimmune events, etc. Axon and myelin damage are known to cause a number of key changes in the functioning ('phenotype') of sensory neurons, some of which lead to ectopic spontaneous discharge.

The relative role of peripheral and central mechanisms in neuropathic pain is not well understood and likely reflects different disease states and genetic differences; however, the abnormal input of neural activity from nociceptor afferents plays a dynamic and ongoing role in maintaining the pain state. Two key concepts are critical to an understanding of neuropathic pain: (1) inappropriate activity in nociceptive fibers (injured and uninjured) and (2) central changes occur in sensory processing that arise from these abnormalities.

Neuropathic pain is caused by pathological change or dysfunction in either the PNS or CNS (**45**). Neurogenic pain, deafferentation pain, and dysesthetic pain are all terms used to describe this entity.

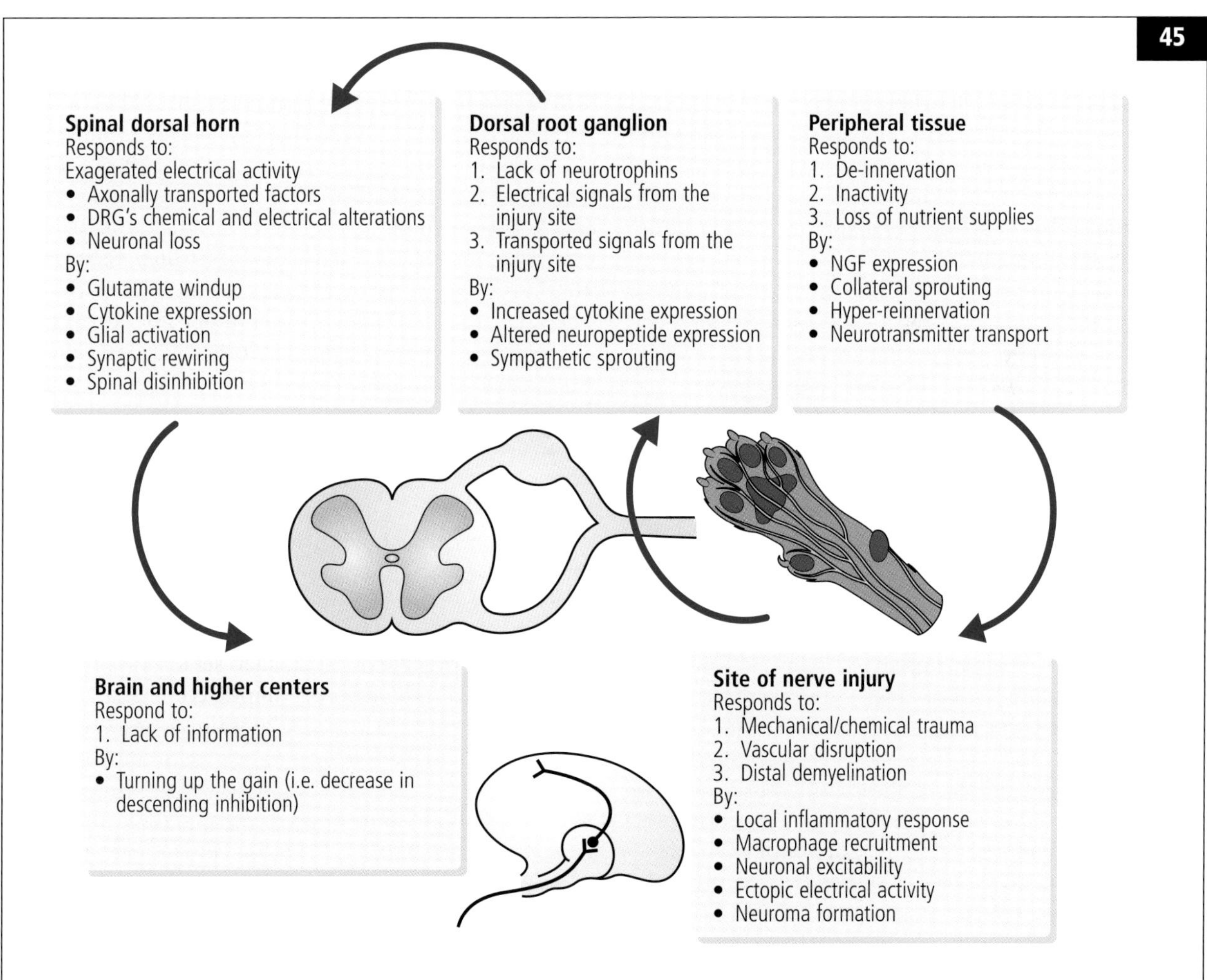

45 Possible sites for neuropathic pain generation.

The word 'neuropathic' is preferred because it encompasses changes in function as well as damage to a nerve as possible causes of pain.

Two major consequences for pain in neuropathy result from central sensitization. Input from residual uninjured Aβ touch afferents is rendered painful. More than amplification, this is a change in modality, from touch to pain. Secondly, central sensitization may render spontaneous ectopic Aβ fiber activity painful.

An understanding of neuropathic pain is increasing with the realization that the nervous system is not a 'hard-wired, line-labeled system', but one that demonstrates 'plasticity', in that the function and structure of the system alter with continuing development, experience, or consequences of injury. The nervous system appears to retain a 'memory of pain', explained, perhaps, by induction of the *c-fos* gene from prolonged peripheral input leading to structural change.

CONTRIBUTION OF SCHWANN CELLS, GROWTH FACTORS, AND PHENOTYPIC SWITCHES TO NEUROPATHIC PAIN

The degree of primary afferent fiber myelination is dependent on the integrity of enveloping Schwann cells that control sensory neuron development and function. Nerve injury can result in Schwann cell dedifferentiation and a consequent switch from normal myelin production to the deregulated synthesis of neurotrophic factors. Excessive growth factors in the neuronal environment for a prolonged time can adversely affect neighboring intact and injured neurons, contributing to the pain phenomenon.[116]

Constitutive availability of growth factors in peripheral sensory neurons maintains the normal neuronal phenotype. For example, NGF is taken up by free sensory nerve endings and transported retrograde to the cell body, where it controls the expression of genes that are crucial for homeostatic sensory function. Such genes include those encoding neurotransmitters, receptors, and ion channels. One consequence of this disruption, as from nerve injury, is a downregulation of sP and CGRP in peptidergic fibers, with a concomitant upregulation of the usually quiescent sP in Aβ fibers.[117] Tissue NGF can additionally drive peripheral and central sensitization by upregulating neuronal content of brain-derived neurotrophic factor (BDNF). Surrogate sources of BDNF have potent neuroprotective effects on axotomized sensory neurons, and can reverse some of the changes in sodium channel expression that are consequent to Schwann cell disorganization and neuropathic pain.[118]

MODELS OF NEUROPATHIC PAIN

Neuropathic pain can be broadly divided into central and peripheral neuropathic pain, depending on whether the primary lesion or dysfunction is situated in the CNS or PNS, and may be due to mechanical trauma, ischemia, degeneration, or inflammation. A broad range of pathologies may result including transient ischemia, giving rise to a selective loss of specific neuronal type, or perhaps complete denervation.

Animal models of neuropathic pain have largely focused on peripheral nerve injury: trigeminal neuralgia,[119] diabetic neuropathy,[120] and vincristine neuropathy,[121] and can be broadly divided into peripheral mononeuropathic, peripheral polyneuropathic, and central neuropathic pain, in line with the human conditions. The spinal nerve ligation (SNL) model of peripheral mononeuropathy, where the L5 and L6 spinal nerves are unilaterally ligated close to their respective ganglia to produce a restricted partial denervation of the hindlimb, is favored by many investigators.

In 1979, Wall *et al.*[76] introduced a neuroma model, where the sciatic and saphenous nerves of rats were transected and removed, thereby assessing pain that occurs following complete nerve transection. From this model it is unclear if resultant autotomy (self-mutilation of the limb) is due to spontaneous pain or complete absence of sensation. Further, many pain conditions seen following nerve injury are due to partial, rather than complete, nerve injury. Accordingly, several models of partial nerve injury have been developed, including chronic constriction injury,[122] partial nerve ligation,[123] spinal nerve transection[124] or ligation,[125] cryoneurolysis,[126] and sciatic nerve ischemia.[127] In these models input is preserved, allowing analysis of changes in mechanical and thermal thresholds in addition to the guarding and autotomy that are believed to be signs of spontaneous pain. Animal models are most useful in gaining an understanding of the physiological processes involved in the development and maintenance of chronic pain, in exploring and developing new treatments, and providing insights into clinical presentations; however, it is extremely difficult to interpret the complex emotional, behavioral, and environmental factors that impact the overall disease state.

Postherpetic neuralgia (PHN), along with painful diabetic neuropathy (PDN), is one of the best models for the clinical investigation of human neuropathic pain because numbers of patients are adequate and the condition provides a stable chronic pain state and a contralateral control. Trigeminal neuralgia is also a model frequently cited when assessing drug response in humans.

Information on the number needed to treat (NNT) has provided insight into the overall effect of drugs in groups of patients in different neuropathic pain states, and has become a common assessment parameter. NNT is an estimate of the number of patients that would need to be given a treatment for one of them to achieve a desired outcome; e.g. for postoperative pain the NNT describes the number of patients who have to be treated with an analgesic intervention for one of them to have at least 50% pain relief over 4–6 hr, and who would not have had pain relief of that magnitude with placebo. Which is to say, NNT represents the number of patients that must be treated, after correction for placebo responders, to obtain one patient with at least 50% pain relief (**46**).

NNT = 1 / (proportion of patients with at least 50% pain relief from analgesic–percentage of patients with at least 50% pain relief with placebo). Generally, NNTs between two and five are indicative of effective analgesic treatments.

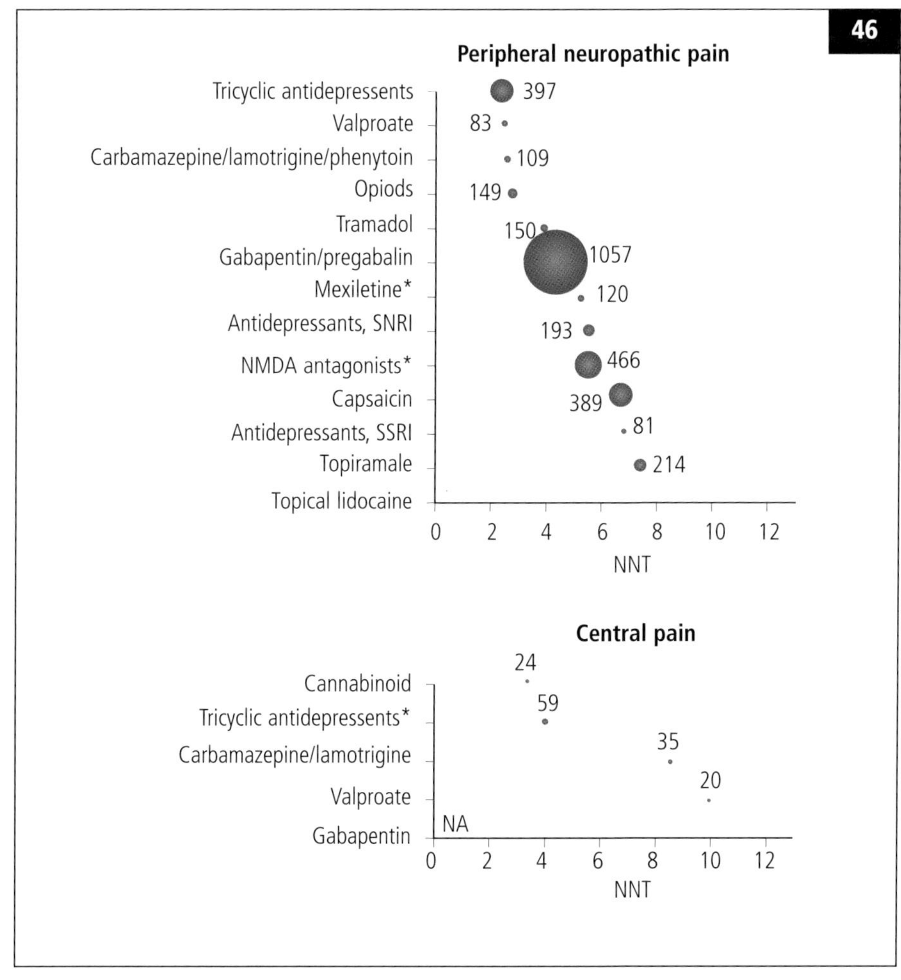

46 Numbers needed to treat in peripheral and central neuropathic pain. Circle size and related numbers indicate number of patients who received active treatment.[129]

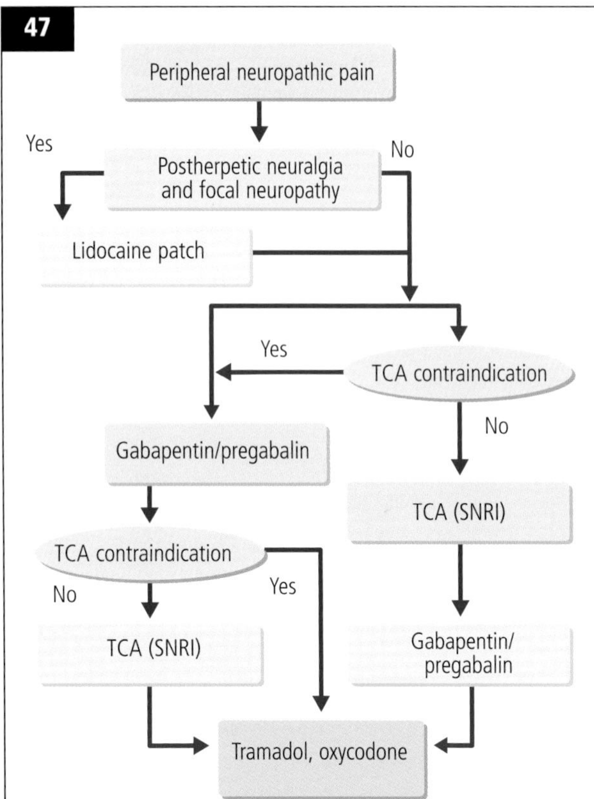

47 Treatment algorithm for peripheral neuropathic pain in humans. Topical lidocaine has been shown to be analgesic in patients with allodynia.[129]

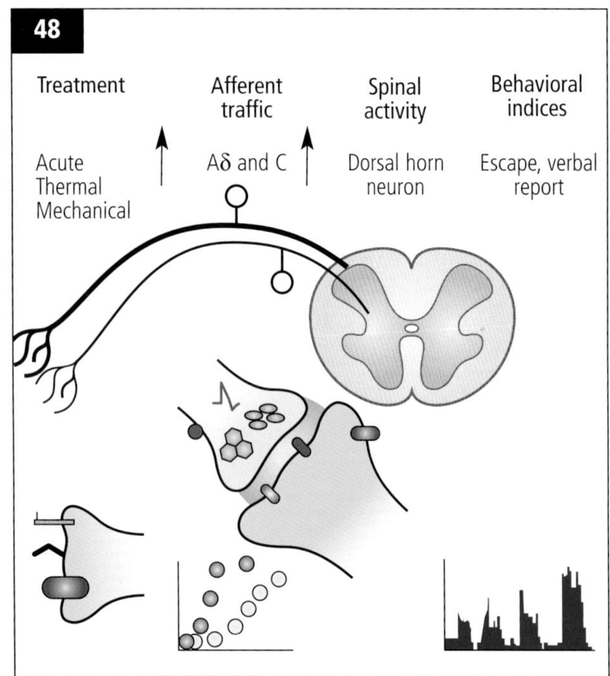

48 Activities associated with transient high-intensity stimuli.

Guidelines for the pharmacological treatment of neuropathic pain in humans have been published (**47**).[128,129]

TRACKING ELEMENTS INVOLVED IN POST TISSUE INJURY PAIN STATES

Damage to a peripheral nerve initiates a cascade of peripheral nerve molecular events, and tissue inflammation sensitizes the peripheral nerve to a more dramatic stimulation response. However, it is also recognized that inflammation or peripheral nerve injury will produce dramatic changes in the spinal cord. These include the release of neurotransmitters such as glutamate, sP, neurokinin A, and CGRP. This is followed by activation of certain receptors, such as the NMDA channel, which, in turn, initiate a further cascade of events within neurons. Such a cascade includes the activation of second messengers (calcium, PGs, and NO) and expression of particular genes, such as *c-fos*. The amount of protein product of the *c-fos* gene in the spinal cord correlates with the initial stimulus magnitude,[40] but it also mediates some of the adaptive responses of the spinal cord.

Neuropeptide levels in the spinal cord also change. The levels of GABA fall and the levels of cholecystokinin, a neuropeptide with antiopioid actions, increase dramatically with peripheral nerve damage. An increased production of novel sodium channels mediated by nerve injury and NGF adds further to excessive spinal cord excitability. This can result in a state of spinal cord disinhibition and increased receptivity to incoming stimuli.

Following nerve injury and inflammation, profound changes occur in neuronal phenotype. Large-diameter primary afferent neurons (which transmit non-noxious stimuli) begin to express sP. Since sP is associated with only small-diameter neurons (which give rise to C fibers and transmit pain and temperature) and transduction of noxious information, this may lead to misinterpretation of light touch and proprioception by the spinal cord and brain. Sprouting of the Aβ nerves within the spinal cord may also occur, with new contacts formed between the Aβ (laminae III–IV) and C fibers (superficial laminae). This may be a basis for the development of chronic pain and allodynia.

Activity in sensory afferents is largely absent under normal physiological conditions. Yet, peripheral thermal and mechanical stimuli will evoke intensity-dependent increases in firing rates of lightly myelinated (Aδ) or unmyelinated (C) afferent fibers (**48**). As a result, the nervous system maintains a specific intensity-, spatial- and modality-linked encoding of the somatic stimulus. In humans, the response parallels a psychophysical report of pain sensation and in animals it parallels the vigor of the escape response.

In the event that tissue is not actually injured, removal of the stimulus is accompanied by a rapid abatement of the afferent input and pain sensation. Herein the question arises, 'why do we hurt after injury even though the initiating stimulus is removed?'

There is no spontaneous activity of primary afferents. Following tissue injury there is an ongoing sensory experience associated with primary hyperalgesia (extremely noxious sensation with moderate stimulus applied to the injury site), and secondary tactile allodynia (very unpleasant sensation with mechanical stimulus applied adjacent to the injury site), i.e. tissue-injury-evoked afferent activity. When tissue injury involves trauma (crush) or an incision, such stimuli result in elaboration of active products that directly activate afferent local terminals innervating the injury region and facilitating their discharge to an ongoing afferent barrage (**49**). In addition, after local injury, afferent terminals increase their response to any given stimulus.

Tissue injury leads to localized extravasation of plasma and increased capillary wall permeability. Such a physiological response is manifest as the 'triple response' of redness (local arterial dilatation), edema (from capillary permeability), and hyperalgesia (left shift of the stimulus–response curve). Hormones, such as bradykinin, PGs, and cytokines (small secreted polypeptides/glycoproteins which mediate and regulate immunity, inflammation, and hematopoiesis) bind to specific membrane receptors, which then signal the cell via second messengers, often tyrosine kinases, to alter its function: activate local release of effector molecules/gene expression, or potassium or hydrogen ions released from inflammatory cells and plasma extravasation products. These result in stimulation and sensitization of free nerve endings that depolarize terminals, with the local release of sP and CGRP into the injured tissues. Thus, mild damage to cutaneous receptive fields results in significant increases in the excitability of polymodal nociceptors (C fibers) and high-threshold mechanoreceptors. Some C fibers have thresholds so high as to be activated only by intense physical stimuli: these are silent nociceptors.

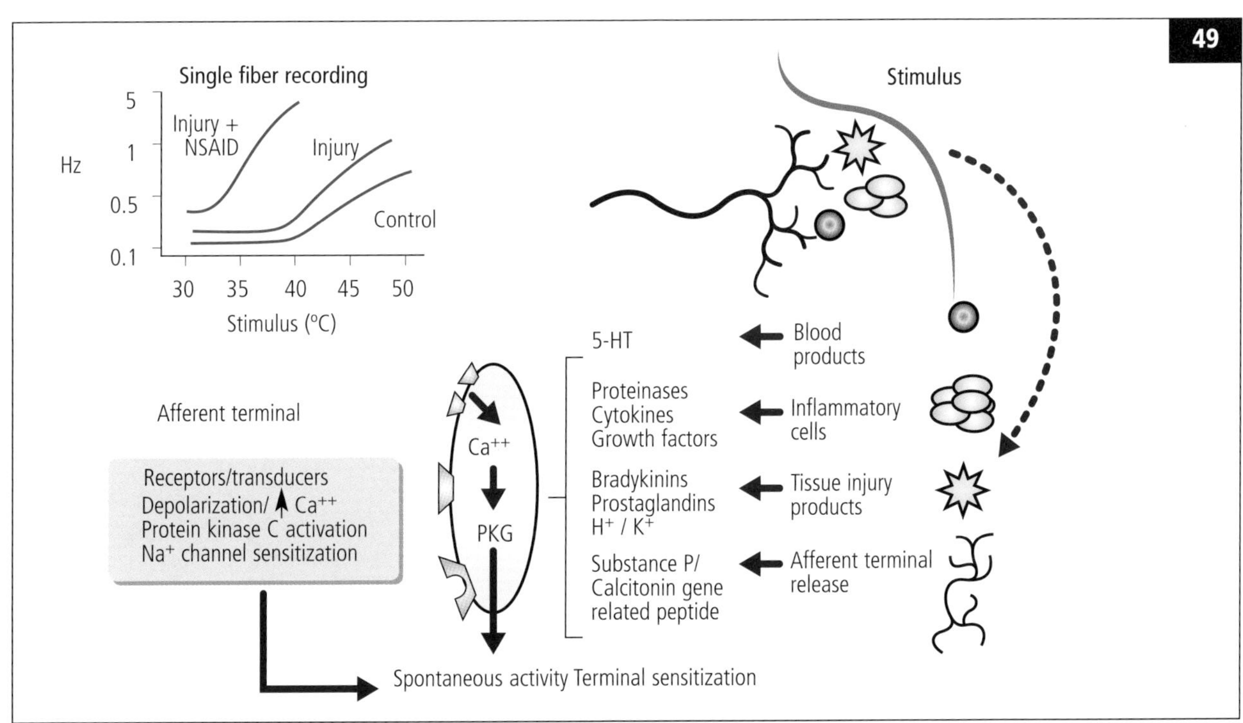

49 'Active' factors generated from peripheral injury and effect of NSAIDs on stimulus frequency (upper graph).

Under the influence of the inflammatory milieu these silent nociceptors are sensitized such that they become spontaneously active, with activity that can be enhanced by relatively mild physical stimuli.

Transduction of a physical stimulus occurs by terminal sensors (such as TRP for temperature, ATP and P2X for mechanical and hydorgen ions and acid-sensing ion channels (ASICs) for chemical), which convert the energy to local terminal neuronal depolarization (transduction) (**50**).

The increasing stimulus intensity increases channel opening for the passage of sodium or calcium ions that then depolarizes the membrane and leads to an action potential: nerve conduction. The greater the stimulus, the greater the depolarization and the greater the frequency of discharge.

Due to the plasticity of the spinal cord, this linear (monotonic) relationship between peripheral activity and activity of neurons that project out of the spinal cord to the brain, occurs as a nonlinear increase in spinal output.

A repetitive stimulation at a moderately fast rate given to WDR, afferent C fibers (but not A fibers), results in a progressively facilitated discharge. The exaggerated discharge of (lamina V) WDR neurons is recognized as windup, signaled by intracellular recording of a progressive and long sustained partial depolarization of the cell, allowing its membrane to be increasingly susceptible to afferent input.

Hereafter, a natural stimulus applied over a large area near the noxious insult displays the ability to activate the same WDR neuron. The WDR discharge, projecting through the same spinal tracts can augment response to a given stimulus. This facilitation by repetitive C-fiber input, accordingly, increases the subsequent neuronal response to low-threshold afferent input, and facilitates the response generated by a given noxious afferent input (**51**).

An increased receptive field size reflects contribution of sensory input converging upon dorsal horn neurons from adjacent noninjured dermatomes.

This is believed to be due to the presence of subliminal excitatory input between adjacent segments. Afferents arriving at the spinal cord have collateral projections to up to four to six segments, with a distal diminution of projection density (**52**). This neuroanatomy was termed 'long-ranging afferents' by Patrick Wall. After injury in a given receptive field, the primary associated neuron becomes sensitized. A collateral input from any long-ranging afferent might be able to initiate sufficient excitatory activity to activate that neuron through synergism. Now the receptive field of the original afferent is effectively the sum of both afferents. Clearly, there is an enhanced excitability of dorsal horn neurons initiated by small afferent input (**53**).

After tissue injury, inflammation and cellular/vascular injury lead to the local peripheral release of active factors producing a prolonged activation of C fibers that evokes a facilitated state of processing in WDR neurons and ongoing facilitation of nociceptive perception. These observations support

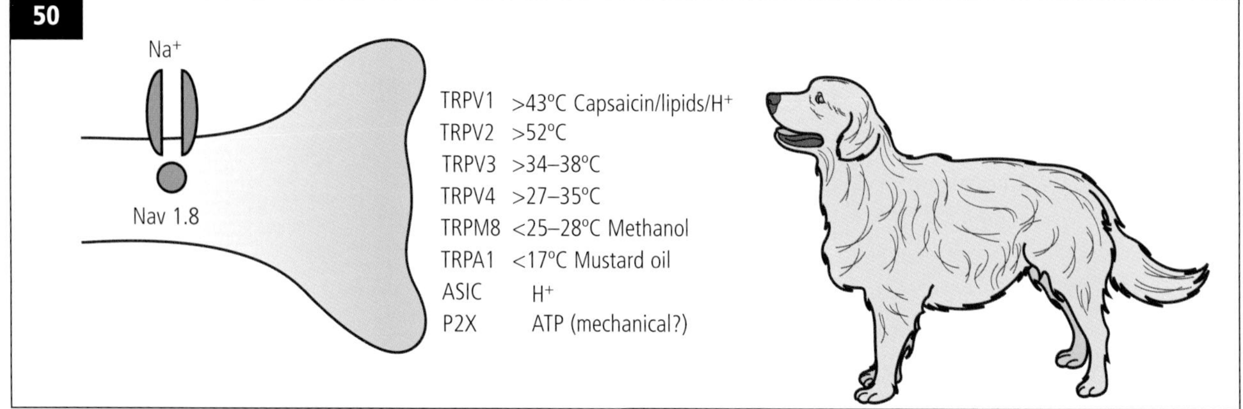

50 Terminal sensors are activated by various physical stimuli, giving rise to terminal depolarization. (TRP = transient receptor potential; ASIC = acid-sensing ion channel; P2X = subtype of ATP receptor; Nav 1.8 = TTX-resistant voltage-gated sodium channel)

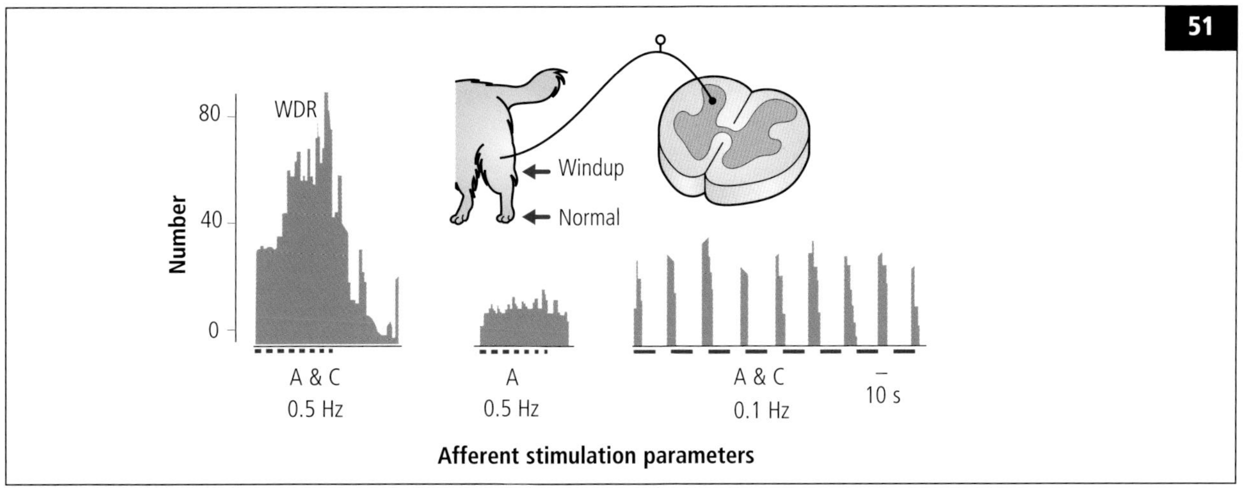

51 With WDR neurons in a state of windup, nonpainful stimuli applied near the noxious insult can activate the same WDR neuron, facilitating the nociceptive response.

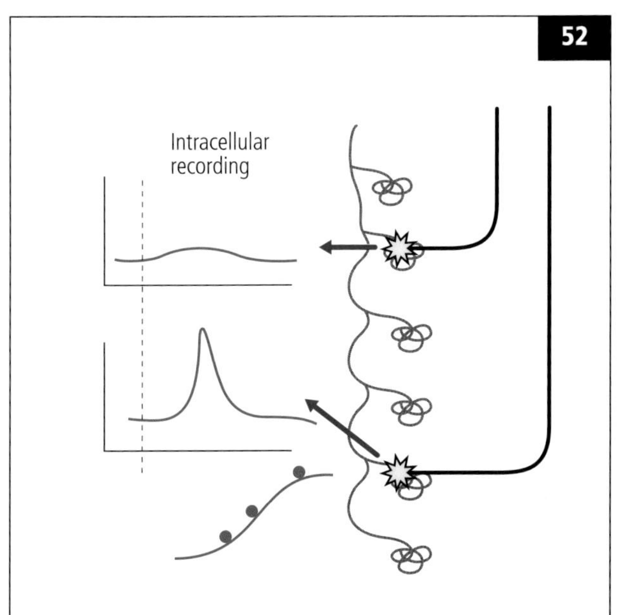

52 Afferents arriving at the spinal cord have collateral projections to up to four to six segments, yielding a receptive field representing the 'sum' of afferents (see text for explanation).

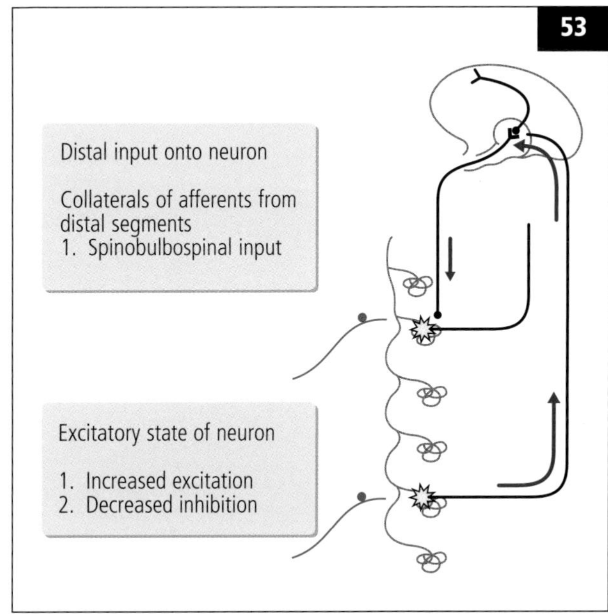

53 'Long-ranging afferents' influence the summation effect of excitatory activity.

speculation that afferent C fiber burst may initiate long-lasting events, changing the spinal processing that alters a response to subsequent input. However, the windup state reflects more than the repetitive activation of a simple excitatory system.

The unique pharmacology of NMDA antagonists first revealed the phenomenon of spinal windup (**54**). Such drugs showed no effect upon acute pain behavior, but reduced the facilitated states induced after tissue injury. Under normal resting membrane potentials, the NMDA receptor is in a state of 'magnesium block', where occupancy by the excitatory amino acid glutamate will not activate the ionophore. With a modest depolarization of the membrane (as during repetitive stimulation secondary to the activation of AMPA and sP receptors) the magnesium block is removed, glutamate now activates the NMDA receptor and the NMDA channel permits the passage of calcium ions (**55**). Increased intracellular calcium serves to initiate downstream components of the excitatory and facilitator cascade.

Primary afferent C fibers release peptides and excitatory amino acids that evoke excitation in second-order neurons. Afferent barrage induces additional excitation via product release of glutamate and prostanoids that markedly increase intracellular calcium and activation of various phosphorylating enzymes, including protein kinases A and C, as well as mitogen-activated kinases including p38MAP kinase and extracellular signal-regulated kinase (ERK) (**56**). Increased intracellular calcium leads to phosphorylation of several proteins, including the NMDA receptor and p38MAP kinase.

p38MAP kinase phosphorylates phopholipase A_2 that initiates the downstream release of arachidonic acid (AA) and provides the substrate for COX to synthesize PGs. It also activates a variety of transcription factors (e.g. NF-κB), which activates synthesis of a variety of proteins, including COX-2. COX derivatives and NOS products are formed and released that diffuse extracellularly and facilitate transmitter release (retrograde transmission) from primary and nonprimary afferent terminals.

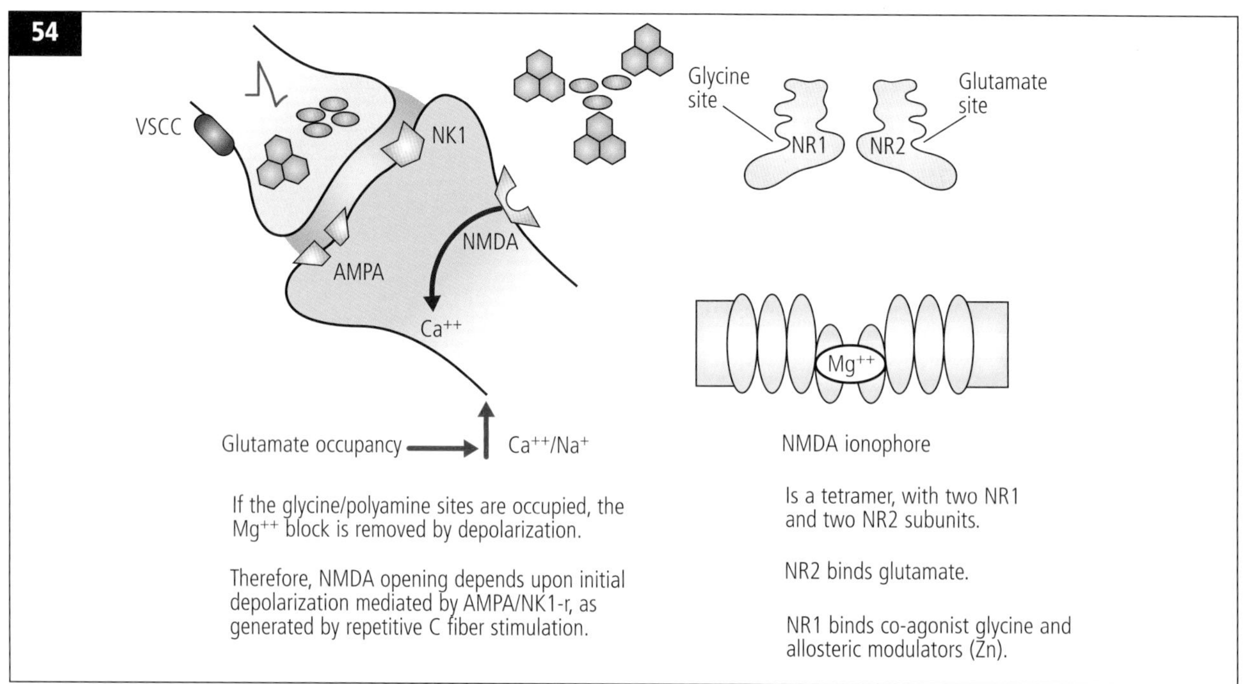

54 Pharmacology involved in spinal facilitation. (VSCC = voltage-sensitive calcium channel; NK1 = neurokinin 1)

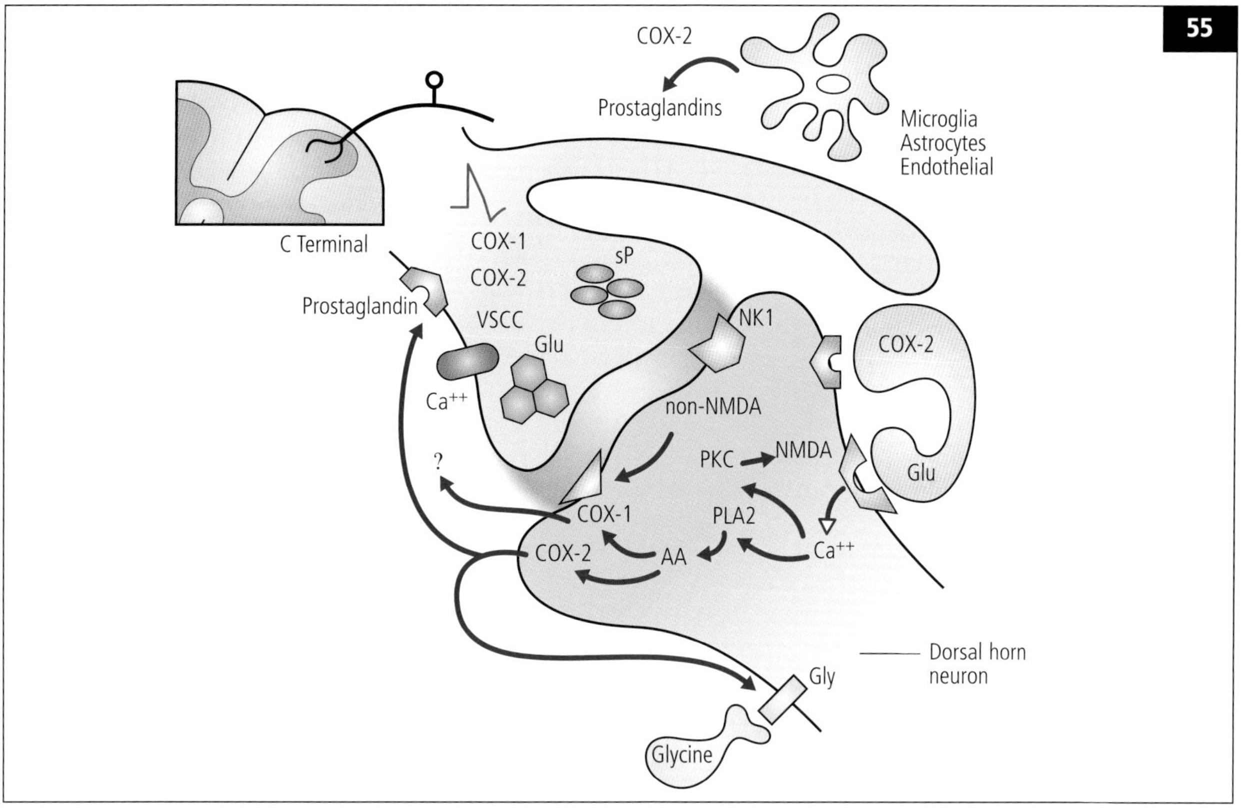

55

COX-2
Prostaglandins
Microglia
Astrocytes
Endothelial
C Terminal
COX-1
COX-2
sP
Prostaglandin
VSCC
Glu
Ca^{++}
NK1
COX-2
non-NMDA
PKC
NMDA
?
Glu
COX-1
PLA2
COX-2
AA
Ca^{++}
Dorsal horn
neuron
Gly
Glycine

55 Transmitter interaction at the dorsal horn neuron. (PLA2 = phospholipase A2; VSCC = voltage-sensitive calcium channel; NK1 = neurokinin 1)

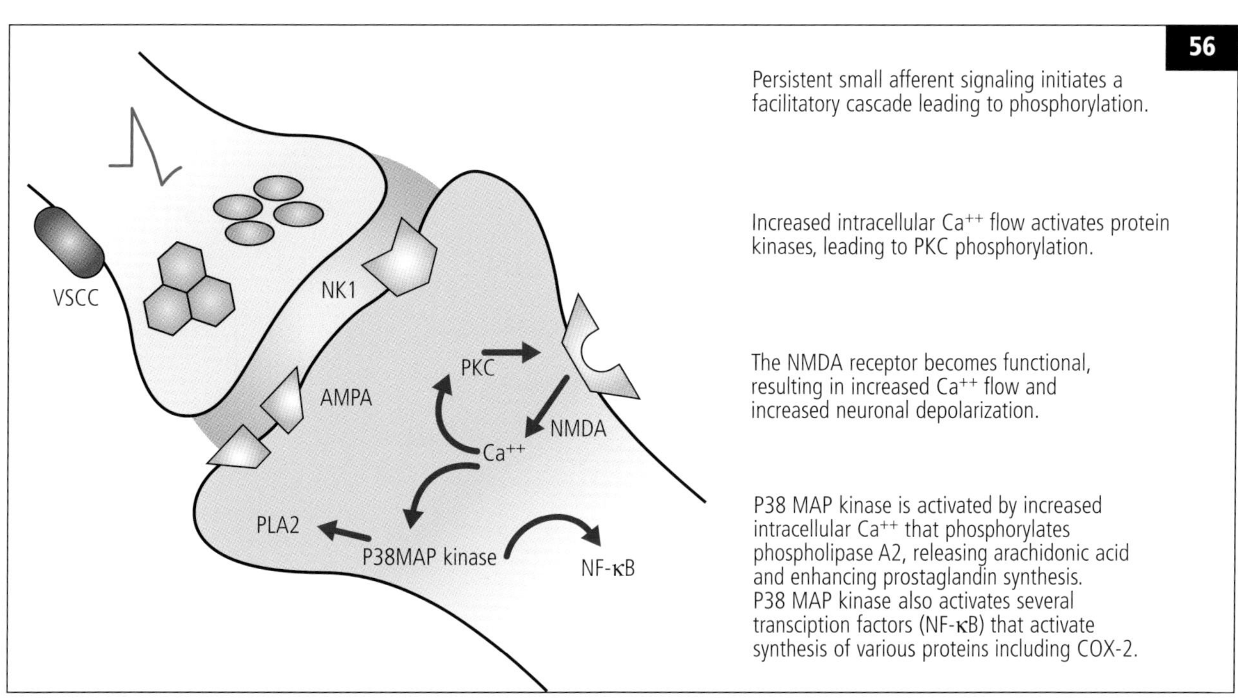

56 Persistent small afferent input contributes to spinal facilitation. (PLA2 = phospholipase A2; VSCC = voltage-sensitive calcium channel; PKC = protein kinase C)

Released PGs act presynaptically to enhance the opening of voltage-sensitive calcium channels that augment transmitter release. Additionally, PGs can act postsynaptically to block glycinergic inhibition (**57**).

The reduction in activation of inhibitory glycine or GABA leads to interneuron regulation resulting in a potent facilitation of dorsal horn excitability. It appears that the excitatory effect of large afferents is under a presynaptic $GABA_A$/glycine modulatory control, with removal resulting in a behaviorally defined allodynia.

Intrinsic interneurons containing peptides, such as enkephalin, inhibitory amino acids or bulbospinal pathways containing monoamines (norepinephrine, serotonin), and peptides (enkephalin, neuropeptides Y (NPY)) may be activated by afferent input and exert (reflex) a modulatory influence upon the release of C fiber peptides and postsynaptically hyperpolarize projection neurons.

Spinal facilitation is also believed to be under the influence of the bulbospinal serotonergic pathway (**58**). Bulbospinal NE (arising from the locus coreulus/lateral medulla) acts as an inhibitory link upon the α_2 receptors, which are pre- and postsynaptic to the primary afferent. Serotonin (5-HT, from the caudal raphe) may be inhibitory or excitatory on inhibitory interneurons (GABA).

The CNS contains a variety of non-neuronal cells including astrocytes and microglia. Microglia are resident macrophages that are present from development. Primary afferent and intrinsic neuron transmitters (glutamate, ATP, sP) can overflow from synaptic clefts to adjacent non-neuronal cells, leading to their activation (**59**).

57

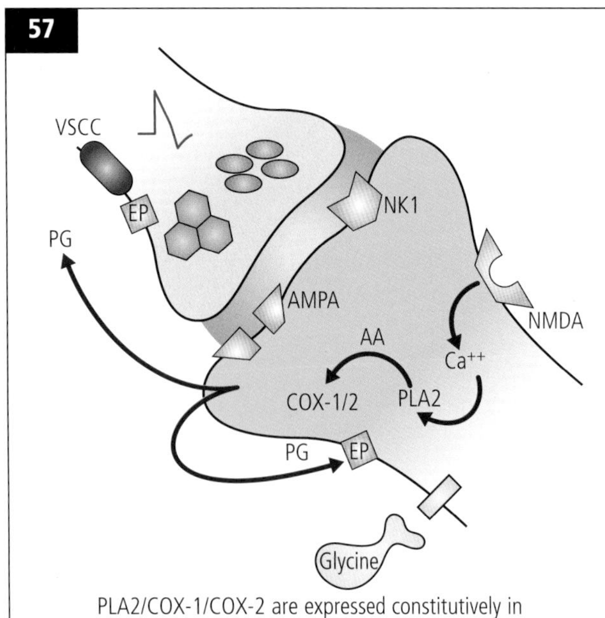

Glutamate/sP increase the activity of the NMDA/NK 1 receptor, with the result of increased intracellular flow of calcium.

This stimulates phospholipase A2 and the production of prostaglandians via the arachidonic acid cascade and cyclooxygenase 2.

Intracellular flow of calcium is further enhanced by the EP receptor, with the consequence of increased transmitter release and increased evoked neuronal depolarization.

Transmitters		Receptors
Glutamate	→	AMPA
	→	NMDA
sP	→	NK1
ATP	→	P2

57 PGs act both pre- and postsynaptically to facilitate the cascade of afferent transmission. (PLA2 = phospholipase A2; VSCC = voltage-sensitive calcium channel; NK1 = neurokinin1; EP = prostaglandin receptor)

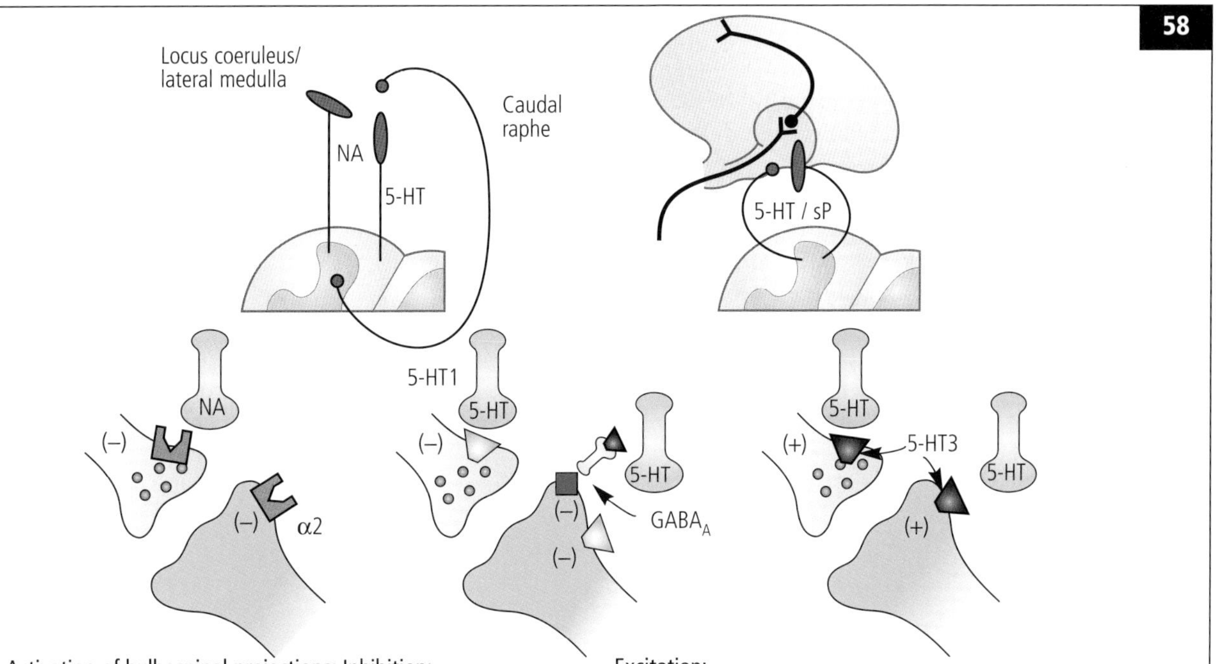

58

Activation of bulbospinal projections: Inhibition:

NA $\alpha 2$: inhibition on primary terminal/secondary cell body
5-HT1: inhibition of cell body and terminals
5-HT3: activates inhibitory (GABA) neurons

Excitation:

Small afferent input excites laminar 1 cell into medullary raphe.

Activates bulbospinal 5-HT projection on to 5-HT3 receptor on laminar V projection neuron.

Lamina V: windup is blocked by destruction of bulbospinal 5-HT projections and by IT 5-HT3 inhibitor (Ondansetron).

58 Dorsal horn influence from bulbospinal pathways.

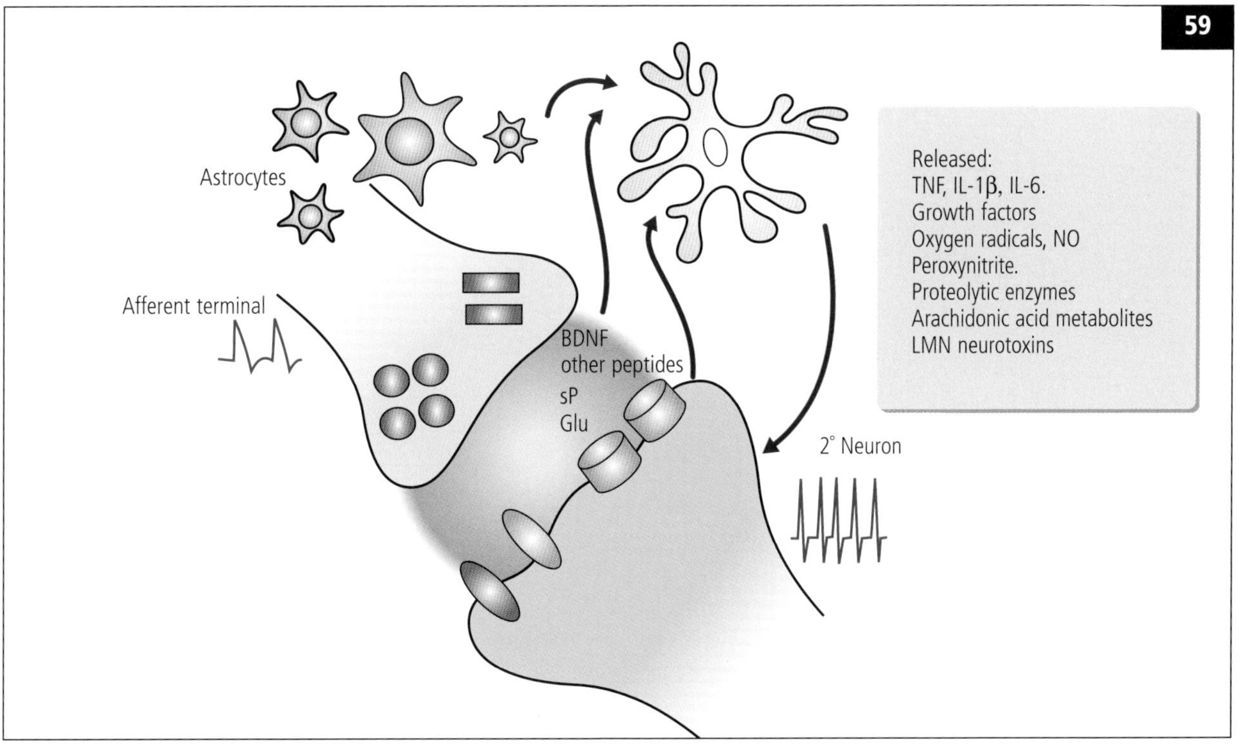

59

Released:
TNF, IL-1β, IL-6.
Growth factors
Oxygen radicals, NO
Peroxynitrite.
Proteolytic enzymes
Arachidonic acid metabolites
LMN neurotoxins

59 Activation of microglia is associated with the release of various neurotransmitters.

In the process of 'neuroinflammation', neurons may activate microglia by the specific release of membrane chemokine (fractalkine), which is expressed extracellularly on neurons and freed by neuronal excitation (constitutively) which, subsequently, binds to spinal microglia. Astrocytes may communicate over a distance by the spread of excitation through local nonsynaptic contacts of 'gap junctions', and may communicate with microglia by the release of a number of products including glutamate/cytokines. Non-neuronal cells can influence synaptic transmission by release of various active products such as ATP and cytokines. They regulate extracellular parenchymal glutamate by their glutamate transporters which can serve to increase extracellular neuronal glutamate receptors. Additionally, following injury and inflammation, circulating cytokines (i.e. IL-1β/TNF-α) can activate perivascular astrocytes/microglia. Although these cells are constitutively active, they can be upregulated after peripheral injury and inflammation (**60**).

The post tissue injury pain state reflects sensitization of the peripheral terminal responding to release of various factors that initiate spontaneous activity, as well as sensitize the peripheral terminal. Potent central (spinal) sensitization leads to facilitated

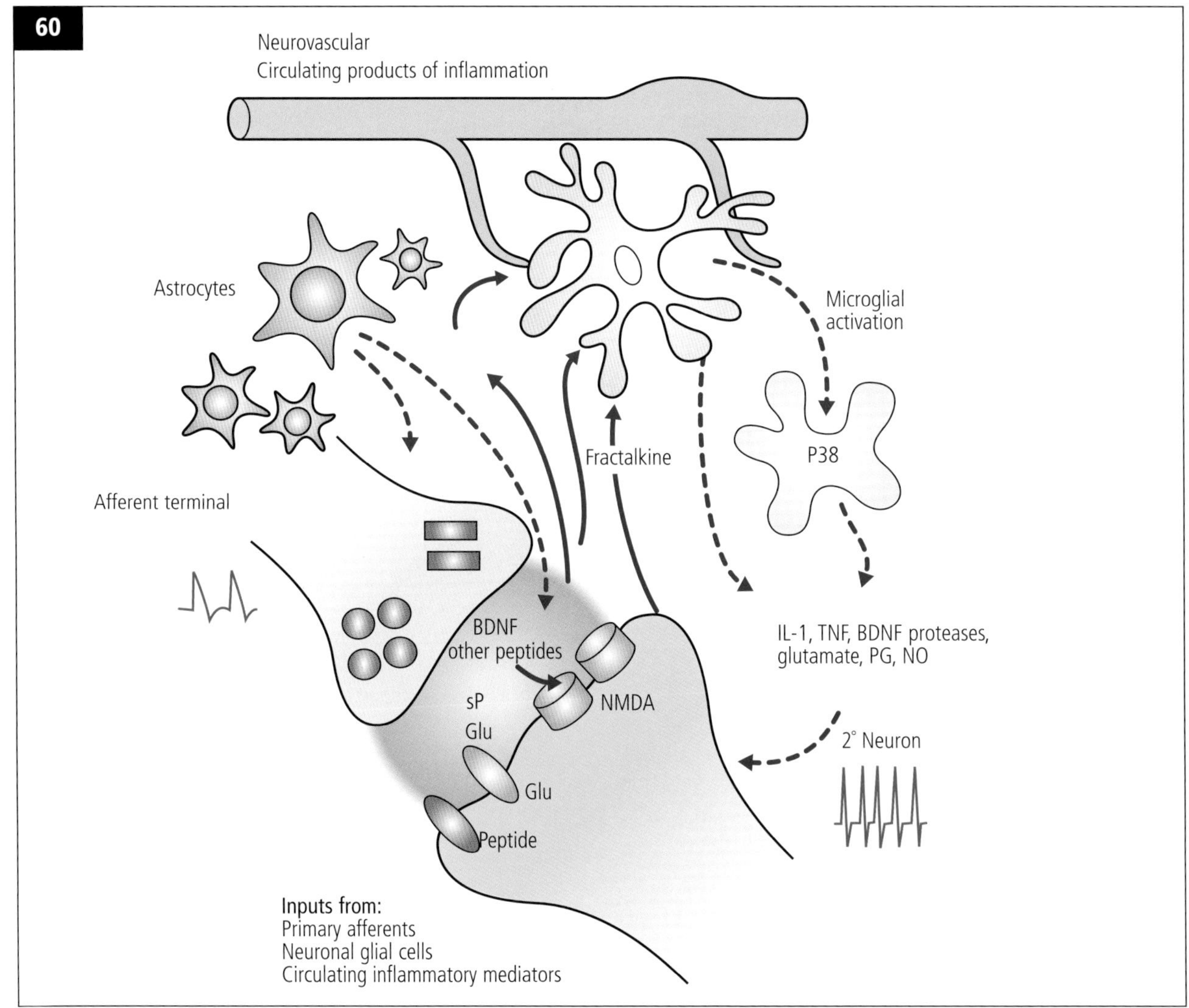

60 Following injury and inflammation, perivascular nonneuronal cells, including astrocytes and microglia, contribute to nociceptive processing.

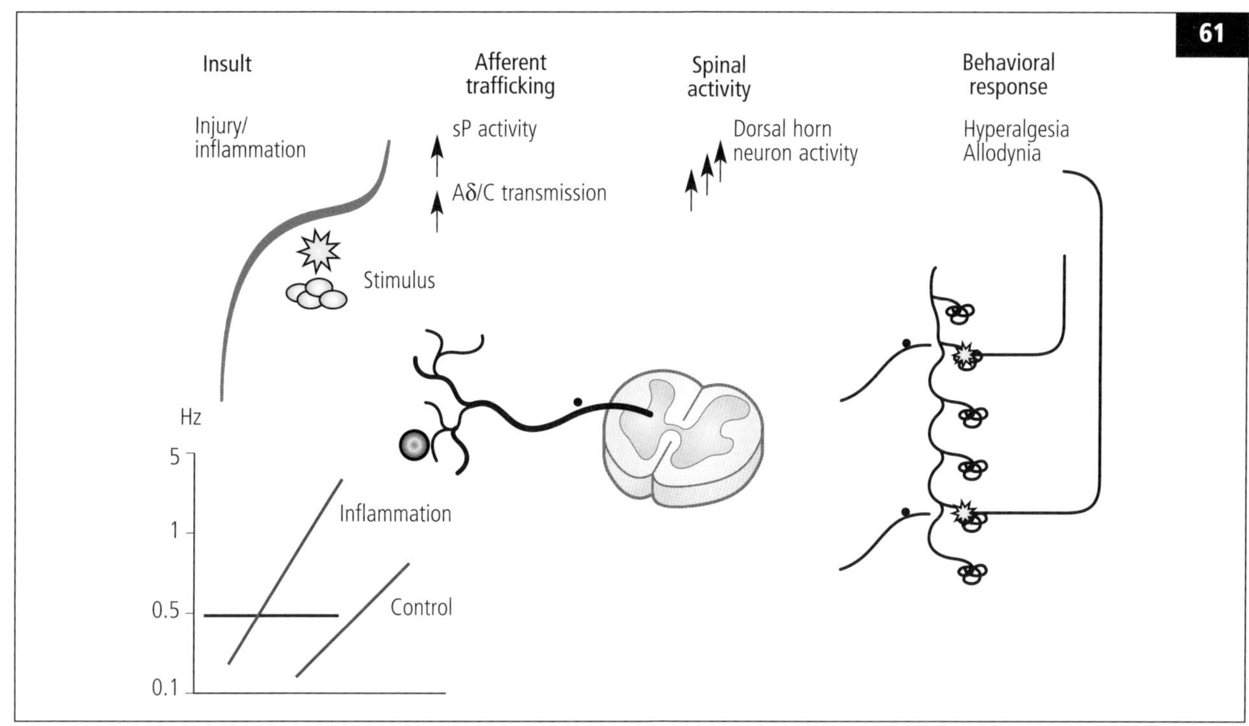

61 Overview of nociceptive processing from injury to responsive behavior. Graph represents relative responses to the pain state following sensitization of inflammation.

responsiveness from the dorsal horn neurons that receive ongoing small afferent traffic (**61**). Sequential cascades lead to an enhanced response to injured receptive field input, but also enlarge the peripheral fields that are now capable of activating those neurons with originally ineffective subliminal input. Augmentation reflects not only local synaptic circuitry (glutamate/sP), but also spinobulbospinal linkages (5-HT) and byproducts released from local non-neuronal cells.

The common symptom of pain following tissue injury and inflammation disappears consequential to the healing process. In contrast, after a variety of injuries to the peripheral nerve over time, a shower of painful events ensues, including tactile allodynia–abnormal painful sensations in response to light tactile stimulation of the peripheral body surface. Tactile allodynia provides evidence that the peripheral nerve injury has led to a reorganization of central processing.

The mechanisms underlying such spontaneous pain and the miscoding of low-threshold afferent input are poorly understood; however, increased spontaneous activity in axons of the injured afferent nerve and/or the dorsal horn neuron and exaggerated response of dorsal horn neurons to normally innocuous afferent input are recognized. Dysesthesia (spontaneous pain) and allodynia (pain evoked by light touch) can result from various peripheral nerve injuries due to: sectioning or stretching, as with trauma; compression, as with tumor or mechanical insult; chemical, as with anticancer agents and pesticides; radiation, as with plexopathies; metabolic, as with diabetes; viral, as with PHN or human immunodeficiency virus (HIV); and immune, as with paraneoplastic activity.

Following mechanical injury to a peripheral nerve, there is an initial dying back of the axon (retrograde chromatolysis) for some distance, at which point the axon begins to sprout growth cones that then proceed forward. Growth cones often fail to make contact with the original target, and as if in frustration, proliferate significantly with formation of neuromas. This phenomenon gives rise to ectopic activity and alteration in transported factors from the terminal sprouts to the DRG. Yang *et al.*[130] have shown that within 14 days following nerve injury, there is considerably increased expression of many proteins in the spinal cord and DRG (*Table 10*) (overleaf).

Neuromas, formed by failed efforts of injured peripheral nerve sprouts, become ectopic generators of neural activity. Additionally, the DRG cells of such axons begin to demonstrate ongoing discharge. These discharges are believed to arise from the over-expression of sodium channels and a variety of receptors which sense the inflammatory products in the injured environment.

There are multiple populations of sodium channels, differing in their current activation properties and structures. VGSCs mediate the conducted potential in both myelinated and unmyelinated axons. Following nerve injury, there is an increased presence of various VGSCs, particularly in a neuroma and the DRG of unmyelinated axons, which likely support the ectopic activity observed in regenerating fibers. Lidocaine, at doses which do not block conduction, will block ectopic activity in neuromas and the DRG, reducing neuropathic thresholds and behaviors.[131,132] Injured nerves have also shown a decreased expression of potassium channels in axons and the DRG. Potassium channels contribute to membrane hyperpolarization, and a decreased expression would contribute to increased afferent excitability.

Following nerve injury, various amines, lipid mediators (PGs) and pro-inflammatory cytokines (IL-1β, TNF-α) influence an accentuated effect on neuromas and the DRG. Local inflammatory cells such as macrophages as well as Schwann cells release cytokines such as IL-1β and TNF-α (**62**).

TNF-α binding protein attenuates nerve injury-induced allodynia. A clinical example would be avulsed disk, where inflammatory products, such as TNF-α, have been shown to be released that activate adjacent DRGs and nerves (**63**).

Table 10 Receptors and channels showing increased activity within 14 days following nerve injury. (SK1 = small conductance channel–a gene-specific delayed-rectifier-type potassium channel)

Receptors	
5-HT receptor 5B	$GABA_A$ receptor alpha-5 subunit
Cholinergic receptor, nicotinic, alpha polypeptide 5	Glutamate receptor, ionotropic, AMPA3
Cholinergic receptor, nicotinic, beta polypeptide 2	Glutamate receptor, ionotropic, 4
CSF-1 receptor	Glycine receptor alpha 2 subunit
Channels	
Calcium channel, voltage-dependent, L-type, alpha 1E subunit	Pyrimidinergic receptor P2Y
Calcium channel, voltage-dependent, alpha2/delta subunit 1	G protein-coupled, scavenger receptor class B
Chloride channel, nucleotide-sensitive, 1A	Neurotrophic tyrosine kinase, receptor, type 2
Sodium channel, nonvoltage-gated 1, beta (epithelial)	Homolog to peroxisomal PTS2 receptor
Potassium channel KIR6.2 Potassium voltage-gated channel, SK1-related subfamily, member 1	Prostaglandin D2 receptor
Protein kinase C-regulated chloride channel	Purinergic receptor P2Y, G protein-coupled 1
ATPase, Na^+K^+ transporting, alpha 2	Vasopressin V2 receptor
Calcium channel, voltage-dependent, alpha 1C subunit	Cholinergic receptor, nicotinic, delta polypeptide
Chloride channel protein 3 long form	C-kit receptor tyrosine kinase isoform
Potassium channel KIR6.2 Potassium voltage-gated channel, Isk-related subfamily, member 1	Interleukin 13 receptor, alpha 1
Sodium channel, voltage-gated, type 1, alpha polypeptide	Neurotensin receptor
Sodium channel, voltage-gated, type 6, alpha polypeptide	Opioid receptor, kappa1
Potassium channel KIR6.2 Potassium related, subfamily relationship not yet defined	Opioid receptor-like

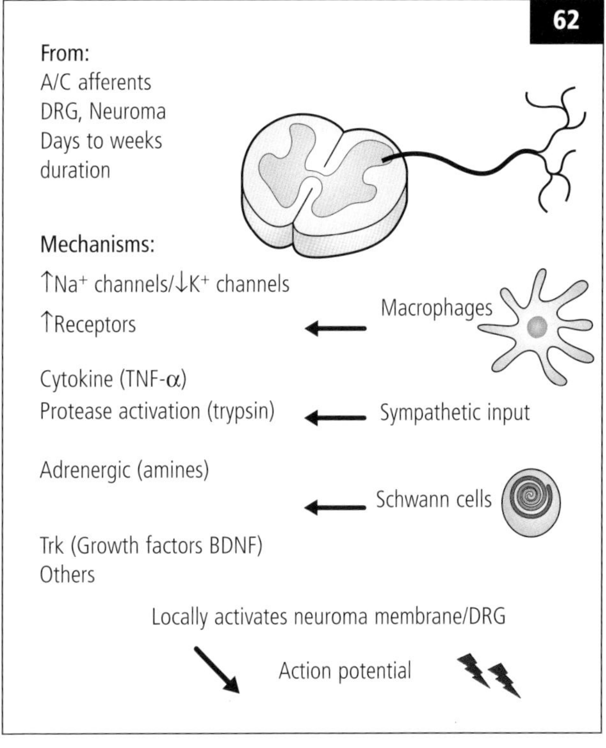

62 Overview of afferent activity resultant from nerve injury.

62
From:
A/C afferents
DRG, Neuroma
Days to weeks
duration
Mechanisms:
↑Na+ channels/↓K+ channels
↑Receptors
Cytokine (TNF-α)
Protease activation (trypsin)
Adrenergic (amines)
Trk (Growth factors BDNF)
Others
Macrophages
Sympathetic input
Schwann cells
Locally activates neuroma membrane/DRG
Action potential

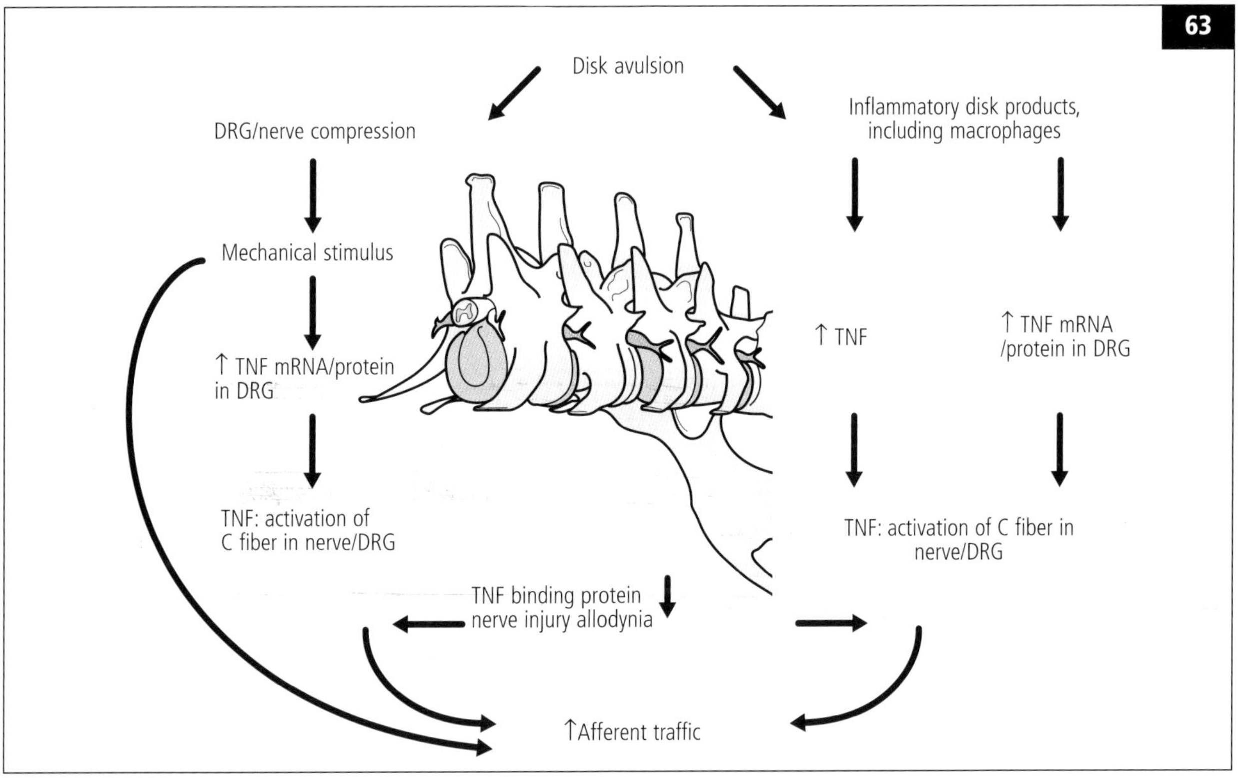

63
Disk avulsion
DRG/nerve compression
Inflammatory disk products, including macrophages
Mechanical stimulus
↑ TNF mRNA/protein in DRG
↑ TNF
↑ TNF mRNA /protein in DRG
TNF: activation of C fiber in nerve/DRG
TNF: activation of C fiber in nerve/DRG
TNF binding protein nerve injury allodynia
↑Afferent traffic

63 TNF-α in back pain.

After peripheral injury, the DRG is markedly changed. There is activation of immediate early genes, an increase in the expression of various injury-related transcription factors, activation of local satellite (glial) cells, and a massive alteration in DRG neuron protein expression of receptor channels and enzymes. Further, the DRG neuron is mechanically sensitive to local compression that will lead to ectopic activity, as in the clinical condition of an avulsed disk fragment.

In summary, the concept of low-threshold tactile stimulation yielding a pain state is quite intriguing. Mechanisms proposed to account for this linkage include: (1) direct interactions between large and small (nociceptive) afferents; (2) altered connectivity of the dorsal horn, such that Aβ afferents drive nociceptive systems; and (3) altered excitability of dorsal horn systems activated by large afferents. Afferents in the DRG and in the neuroma develop a 'cross-talk' following nerve injury. Depolarizing currents in one axon generate a depolarizing voltage in an adjacent quiescent axon. Herein, a large low-threshold afferent would drive activity in an adjacent high-threshold afferent. In the presence of ongoing spontaneous activity in large afferents, there is significant local depolarization of afferent terminals in the dorsal horn initiating local release of GABA. GABA/glycinergic terminals are frequently presynaptic to the large central afferent terminal complexes and these amino acids normally exert an important tonic or evoked inhibitory control over the activity of Aβ primary afferent terminals and second-order neurons in the spinal dorsal horn. Following nerve injury, spinal neurons regress to a neonatal phenotype in which $GABA_A$ activation becomes excitatory. This results from a reduction in the expression of the chloride transporter protein in dorsal horn neurons following afferent nerve injury.

Normally, transmembrane chloride is at equilibrium or just negative to resting membrane potentials. Increasing membrane chloride permeability by activation of $GABA_A$ or glycine receptors normally yields hyperpolarization and inhibition. Following peripheral nerve injury, there is a loss of chloride transporter, which normally exports chloride. This leads to an intracellular accumulation of chloride. Under such conditions, increasing chloride permeability, as by opening the $GABA_A$ or glycine receptor ionophore, there is no inhibitory effect, but instead, an excitatory effect on the second-order neuron may occur (**64**).

After nerve injury there is a significant enhancement in resting spinal glutamate secretion, glutamate having a major impact on the NMDA receptor, which in turn, is a major player in windup. Following peripheral nerve injury, there is an increased expression of the peptide dynorphin. Dynorphin can initiate the concurrent release of spinal glutamate and a potent tactile allodynia. Also, a significant increase in activation of spinal microglia and astrocytes occurs in the ipsilateral spinal segments receiving input from injured nerves. These cells play a powerful constitutive role in the increase of synaptic excitability through release of a variety of active factors. Particularly in bone cancer, these cells are active. It is also noted that there is an ingrowth of postganglionic sympathetic terminals into the dorsal

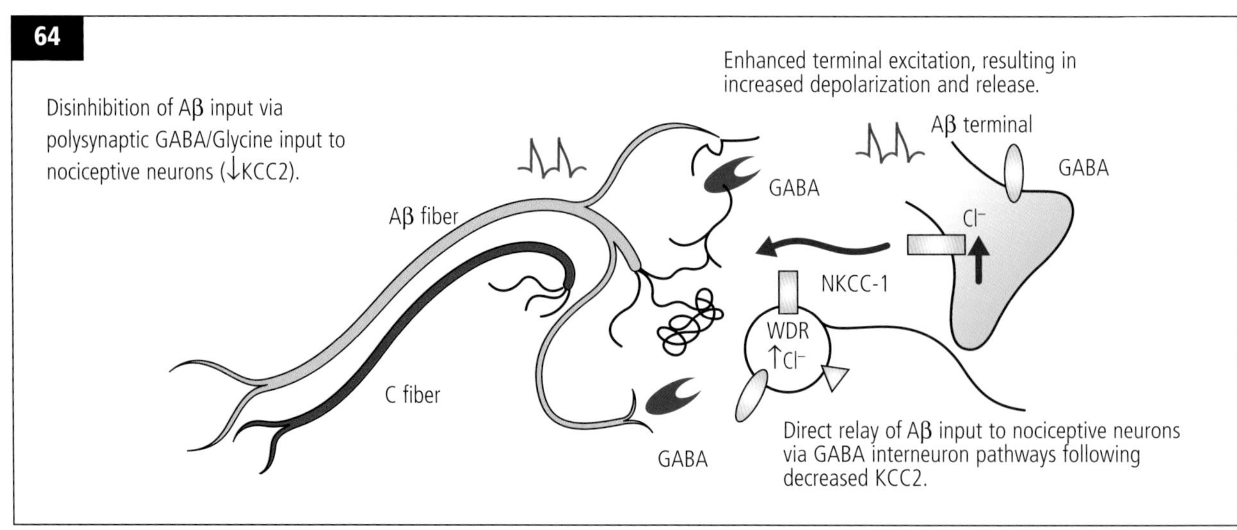

64 Influence of spinal chloride transporters on allodynia.

root ganglia of injured axons, forming baskets of terminals around the ganglion cells.

To paraphrase Albert Einstein, 'The significant problems that we face today cannot be solved at the level of thinking that we were at when we identified them.'

COMMON QUESTIONS RELATED TO CHRONIC PAIN

What is the difference between pain and suffering?

Pain is a sensation plus a reaction to that sensation. Suffering is more global. Suffering is an overall negative feeling that impairs the sufferer's quality of life. Both physical and psychological issues are involved in suffering, and pain may be only one component. Arguably, clinical suffering depends less upon the magnitude of the hurting and more upon the uncertainty over how long the hurting will last.

What is nociceptive pain?

Nociceptive pain results from the activation of nociceptors (Aδ and C fibers) by noxious stimuli that may be mechanical, thermal, or chemical. Nociceptors may be sensitized by endogenous chemical stimuli (algogens) such as serotonin, sP, bradykinin, PGs, and histamine.

Under normal circumstances, where are algogenic substances found?

Serotonin, histamine, potassium ions, hydrogen ions, PGs, and other members of the arachidonic acid cascade are in tissues: kinins are in plasma; and sP is in nerve terminals of primary afferents. Histamine is found in the granules of mast cells, in basophils, and in platelets. Serotonin is present in mast cells and platelets.

What are the most widely used classifications for pain?

The most recognized categories are based on inferred neurophysiological mechanisms, temporal aspects, etiology, or region affected.

What is meant by an etiological classification?

This classification pays more attention to the primary disease process in which pain occurs, rather than to the pathophysiology or temporal pattern. Examples include cancer pain and arthritis.

What is the basis of the regional classification of pain?

The regional classification is strictly topographic and does not infer pathophysiology or etiology. It is defined by the part of the body affected, then subdivided into acute and chronic.

What is the temporal classification of pain, and what are its shortcomings?

Temporal classification is based on the time course of symptoms and is usually divided into acute, chronic, and (perhaps) recurrent. The major shortcoming is that the division between acute and chronic is often arbitrary.

What is acute pain?

Acute pain is temporally related to injury and resolves during the appropriate healing period. It often responds to treatment with analgesic medications and treatment of the precipitating cause (e.g. treatment of bacterial infection with antibiotics).

What is chronic pain?

Chronic pain is often defined as pain that persists for more than 3 months or that outlasts the usual healing process. Some authors choose 6 months as a cut-off. Chronic pain serves no useful biological purpose. Many of us were schooled to believe that chronic pain is simply acute pain of extended duration. Our present understanding of pain physiology has demonstrated that this is not the case. *Acute pain is as different from chronic pain as Mars is from Venus.*

What is the advantage of classifying pain?

It provides the clinician with information about the possible origin of the pain. More important, it steers the clinician toward a proper pharmacological treatment plan. For example: neuropathic pain generally responds to adjuvant medications, whereas nociceptive pain states are often controlled by NSAIDs alone or in combination with opioids.

NOCICEPTOR SIGNALING: THERAPEUTIC TARGETS

Nociceptors express mechanically gated channels that upon excessive stretch, initiate a signaling cascade. These cells also express several purinergic receptors capable of sensing ATP, released from cells during excessive mechanical stimulation. In sensing noxious chemical stimuli, nociceptors express a wide range of receptors that detect inflammation-associated factors released from damaged tissues, including protons, endothelins, PGs, bradykinin, and NGF.

CYCLO-OXYGENASE

Tumor cells and tumor-associated cells secrete a variety of factors that sensitize or directly excite primary afferent neurons: PGs, endothelins, IL-1 and IL-6, epidermal growth factor, transforming growth factor (TGF), and platelet-derived growth factor. Identification of these factors provides potential blocking strategies for treatment. One such strategy is focused at COX-2. COX-2 inhibitors (coxib-class NSAIDs) are currently used to inhibit inflammation and pain. Further, experiments suggest coxibs may have the added advantage of reducing the growth and metastasis of cancer.[133]

ENDOTHELIN

Endothelin-1 is a second pharmacological target for cancer pain. Clinical studies in humans have shown a correlation between prostatic cancer pain and plasma levels of endothelins.[134] Similar to PGs, endothelins that are released from tumor cells are also thought to be involved in regulating angiogenesis and tumor growth.[135,136]

ACID-SENSING ION CHANNELS

A hallmark of tissue injury is local acidosis, and tumor cells become ischemic and apoptotic as the tumor burden exceeds its vascular supply. Two major ASICs expressed by nociceptors, the TRPV1 and ASIC-3, are sensitized by the acidic tumor environment. This is likely accentuated by osteolytic tumors where there is a persistent extracellular microenvironment of acidic pH at the osteoclast and mineralized bone interface. Further, studies showing that osteoprotegerin[137] and a bisphosphonate,[138] both of which induce osteoclast apoptosis, are effective in decreasing osteoclast-induced bone cancer pain.

SENSORY NEURON DYNAMICS

To appreciate the complexity of cancer pain is to understand that the biochemical and physiological status of sensory neurons is a reflection of factors derived from the innervated tissue, and therefore changes in the periphery associated with inflammation, nerve injury or tissue injury influence changes in the phenotypes of sensory neurons. NGF and glial-derived neurotrophic factor (GDNF) influence such changes. The medley of growth factors to which the sensory neuron is exposed will change as the growing tumor invades the peripheral tissue innervating the neuron. With the potential for changing phenotype and response characteristics, it is understandable that the same tumor in the same individual may be painful at one site of metastasis but not at another. It follows that different patients with the same cancer may have vastly different symptoms.

PAIN ASSESSMENT

Pain management is a cardinal example of integrating the science of veterinary medicine with the art of veterinary practice. New graduate veterinarians are well schooled in the science, whereas the art comes only with experience. This is particularly true in managing pain because pain is a subjective phenomenon. *In man, pain is what the patient says it is, whereas in animals, pain is what the assessor says it is!* Because pain is subjective, an abstract, multi-attribute construct similar to intelligence or anxiety, pain management does not lend itself to a 'cookbook' approach. For example: following surgery, if the dog is lying quietly in its cage, is it doing so because it is very content, or because it is too painful to move? Further, trained as scientists, veterinarians are schooled to assess responses based on the mean ± standard deviation, yet effective pain management suggests we target the least-respondent patient within the population, so as to ensure no patient is denied the relief it needs and deserves. There are many clues the attentive assessor may note to suggest an animal is in pain (*Table 11*).

As a rule of thumb, any change in behavior can signal pain, however *the most reliable indicator of pain is response to an analgesic*. Physiological parameters, including heart rate, respiratory rate, blood pressure, and temperature, are not consistent or reliable indicators of pain. Various acute pain assessment measures have been used by researchers to quantify pain. These include verbal rating scales (VRS), simple descriptive scales (SDS), numeric rating scales (NRS), and visual analog scales (VAS); all of which have their limitations. Historical limitations of scales used to assess pain have been assessment of pain on intensity alone. Such limitations have led to development of multidimensional scales, taking into account the sensory and affective qualities of pain in addition to its intensity. The 'Glasgow Pain Scale'[140] is such a multidimensional scheme, and although it is detailed, its ongoing refinement may result in greater utilization. Currently, there are no 'scales' to assess chronic pain. Several investigators have suggested exploring this area of interest through creation of novel questionnaires as an instrument for measuring chronic pain in dogs through its impact on health-related quality of life (HRQL).[141–143]

Table 11 Characteristics associated with pain in cats and dogs (modified from reference 139).

Characteristic	Example
Abnormal posture	Hunched up guarding or splinting of abdomen 'Praying' position (forequarters on ground, hindquarters in air) Sitting or lying in an abnormal position Not resting in a normal position
Abnormal gait	Stiff No to partial weightbearing on injured limb Slight to obvious limp
Abnormal movement	Thrashing Restless Inactivity when awake Escape behavior
Vocalization	Screaming Whining Crying None
Characteristic	**Example**
Miscellaneous	Looking, licking, or chewing at painful area Hyperesthesia or hyperalgesia Allodynia Failure to stretch or 'wet dog shake' Failure to yawn Failure to use litter box (cat)
*May also be associated with poor general health	Restless or agitated Trembling or shaking Tachypnea or panting Weak tail wag Low carriage of tail Depressed or poor response to caregiver Head hangs down Not grooming Decreased or picky appetite Dull Lying quietly and not moving for long durations Stupor Urinates or defecates without attempt to move Recumbent and unaware of surroundings Unwilling or unable to walk Bites or attempts to bite caregivers

– Continued on next page

Table 11 Characteristics associated with pain in cats and dogs (modified from reference 139) – *continued.*

*May also be associated with apprehension or anxiety	Restless or agitated Trembling or shaking Tachypnea or panting Weak tail wag Low tail carriage Slow to rise Depressed Not grooming Bites or attempts to bite caregiver Ears pulled back Restless Barking or growling Growling or hissing Sitting in back of cage or hiding (cat)
May be normal behavior	Eye movement, but reluctance to move head Stretching when abdomen touched Penile prolapse Licking a wound or incision
Physiological signs that may be associated with pain	Tachypnea or panting Tachycardia Dilated pupils Hypertension Increased serum cortisol and epinephrine

Expanding on the value of owner assessment, a client-specific outcome measures scheme has been developed.[144] In this scheme, five very specific problems related to osteoarthritis (OA) were identified, which are recorded, and the intensity of the problem is monitored as treatment progresses. Because the questions are very specific to the individual animal in its environment, this measurement system appears to be very sensitive.

Table 12 shows an example of a very specific questionnaire used at North Carolina State University Comparative Pain Research Laboratory to assess pain associated with clinical OA in cats. Activity or behavior that is suspected to have become altered as a result of the pain and specific to the animal and its home environment are defined. Activities are graded at the start of treatment and after analgesic treatment is started. A left shift corresponds to pain relief.

Current methods of classifying pain are considered unsatisfactory by some[145] for several reasons. Foremost is that pain syndromes are identified by parts of the body, duration, and causative agents, rather than the mechanism involved. The argument holds that anatomical differences should be disregarded in favor of mechanisms that apply to either particular tissues or all parts of the body, rather than a particular part of the body. For example: the term cancer pain relates only to the disease from which the patient suffers, not the mechanism of any pain the patient may experience. A *mechanism-based approach* is likely to lead to specific pharmacological intervention measures for each identified mechanism within a syndrome. Advances in pain management are, then, contingent on first determining the symptoms that constitute a syndrome and, then, finding mechanisms for each of these. The clinical approach for a mechanism-based classification of pain is illustrated in **65**.

Table 12 Client-specific outcome measures – activity.

Problems in mobility related to osteoarthritis in your cat	No problem	problematic	A little problematic	Quite problematic	Severely Impossible
1. Jumping on to sofa		∇	√		
2. Jumping on to kitchen counter			∇		√
3. Walking up steps on back deck	∇		√		
4. Jumping on bed	∇				√
5. Using litter tray	∇	√			

√ = start of treatment: ∇ = after treatment

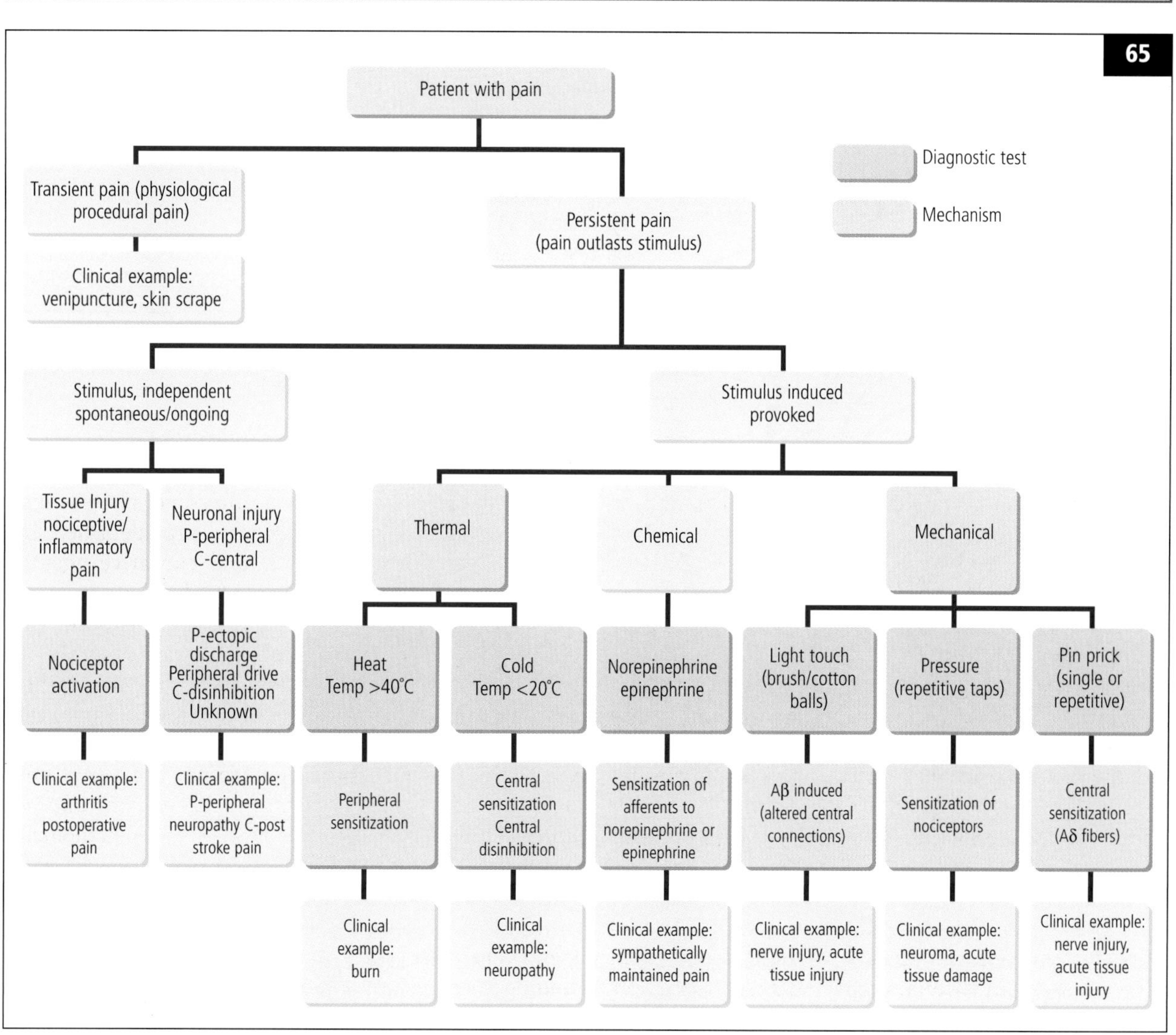

65 Proposed scheme for a clinical approach to a mechanism-based classification of pain.[145]

65 illustrates how a patient with pain could be analysed from a pain-mechanism perspective. It is the mechanism that needs to be the target for novel drugs, rather than particular disease states. Herein lies the greatest potential for advancement in pain management (*Table 13*).

Clearly, the mechanisms associated with pain are complex. However, only through the understanding of these mechanisms can we best manage our patient's pain with an evidence-based confidence (66).

The real mandate of medical care is not the saving of lives, but the dispensing of comfort. We cannot expect to extend life forever. Yet, we can hope to extend lives free of suffering. *When treating pain, knowledge is still the best weapon.*

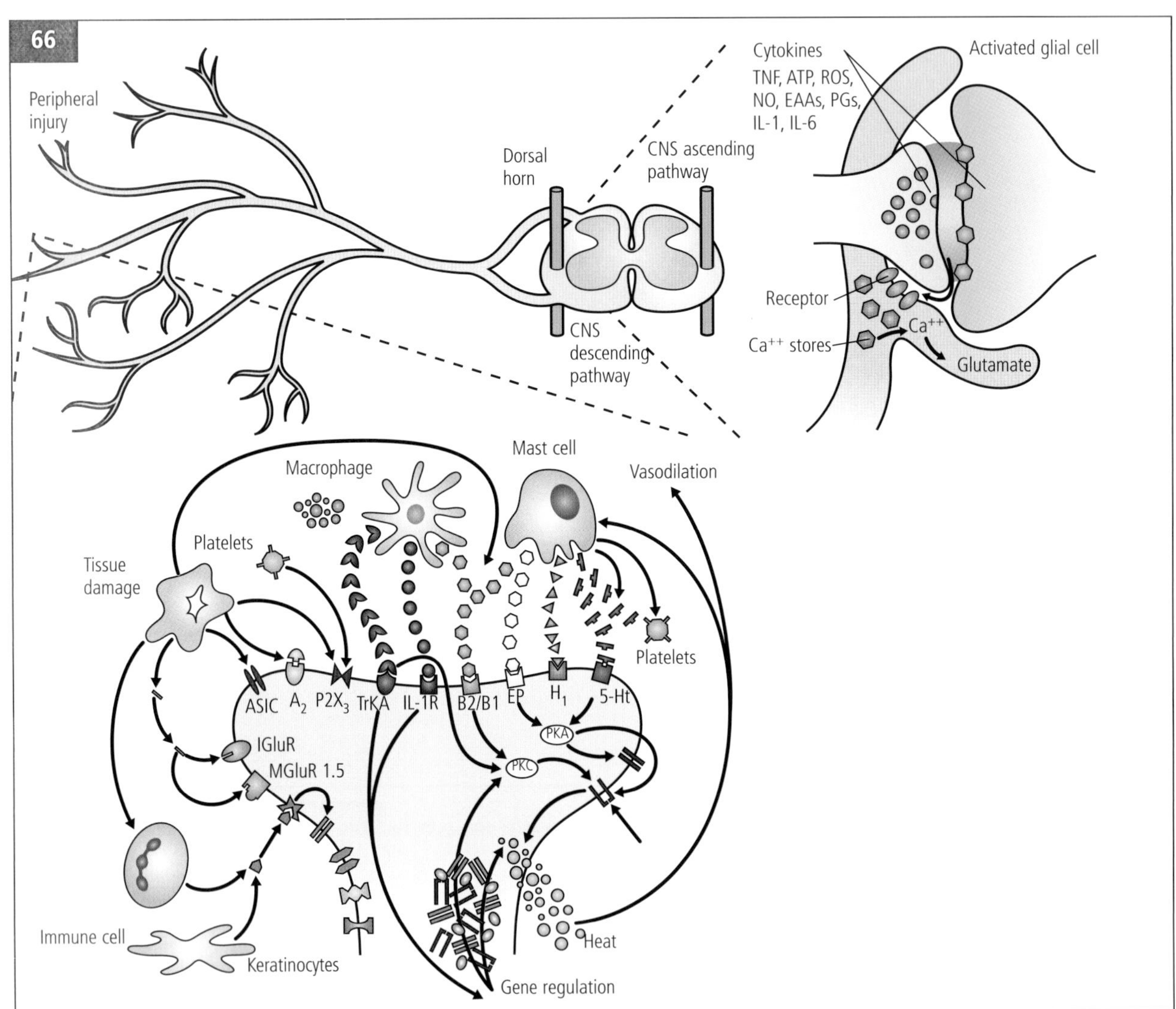

66 The moving target of pain management. Well characterized receptors in the periphery are activated by noxious stimuli, acute inflammation, and tissue injury, sending afferent information to the dorsal horn of the spinal cord where synaptic transmission to ascending pathways is subject to modulation by descending pathways, local neuronal circuits, and a variety of neurochemicals. (A_2 = adenosine A_2 receptor; ATP = adenosine triphosphate; B1/2 = bradykinin receptors 1 and 2; EAAs = excitatory amino acids; EP = prostaglandin E receptor; H_1 = histamine H_1 receptor; IGluR = glutamate ionotropic receptor; IL-1R = interleukin 1 receptor; MGluR = glutamate metabotropic receptor; $P2X_3$ = purinergic receptor X_3; PKA = protein kinase A; PKC = protein kinase C; ROS = reactive oxygen species; TrkA = tyrosine receptor kinase A)

Table 13 Summary of various pain states.

Pain categories	Pain conditions	Pain mechanisms	Potential drug /targets	Animal models	Proof-of-concept
1. Transient stimulus-induced pains (nociceptive pain)	Procedural pain (injections/ minor injuries)	Nociceptor activation	VRs; Na^+-TTXs; MOR, nAChR	Thermosensitivity, mechanosensitivity, chemosensitivity	Minor surgical procedures
2. Tissue damage (inflammatory pain); spontaneous and provoked pain	Trauma/ postoperative pain; arthritis/ infection	Nociceptor activation; peripheral sensitization; central sensitization; phenotype switch	COX-2, EPR, 5-HTR, P_{2x}, BKR; IL-β TNR-α, TrkA, TrkB; Na^+-TTXr, ASIC, α_2, MOR, DOR, A1, N-Ca^{++}, NK1, nAChR, NMDA-R, GluR5, mGluR, PkCγ	Chemical irritants: capsaicin, mustard oil, formalin Experimental inflammation: carrageen, UVB, Freund's adjuvant, cytokines/growth factors	Dental postoperative pain; abdominal postoperative pain; thoracotomy; joint replacements; osteoarthritis
3. Injury: primary afferent (neuropathic pain); spontaneous and provoked pain	Peripheral nerve diabetic injury; neuropathy (human); toxic neuropathy; postherpetic neuralgia (human)	Ectopic activity; phenotype switch; central sensitization; structural reorganization; disinhibition	Na^+-TTXr/ TTXs; α_2, NMDA-R, N-Ca^{++}, PKCγ; NGF/GDNF; GABA, AEAs, gabapentin; TCA, SNRIs	Peripheral nerve section; partial nerve section; loose ligatures; experimental diabetes, toxic neuropathies	Diabetic neuropathy (human); postherpetic neuropathy (human); radicular pain
4. Injury: central neuron (neuropathic pain); spontaneous and provoked pain	Spinal cord injury; stroke (humans)	Secondary ectopic activity; disinhibition; structural reorganization	GABA-R; Na^+-TTXs; AEAs; TCA, SNRIs	Spinal cord injury; ischemia; central disinhibition (e.g. strychnine/ bicuculline)	Spinal cord injury
5. Unknown mechanism	Irritable bowel syndrome; fibromyalgia (humans)	? Altered gain	COX-2, NMDA-R, Na^+ channels		Irritable bowel syndrome/ fibromyalgia

Na^+-TTXs, tetrodotoxin-sensitive sodium ion channels; MOR, μ-opiate receptors; nAChr, nicotine acetylcholine receptor; EPR, prostaglandin receptors; 5-HTR, serotonin receptors; P_{2x}, ligand-gated purino receptors/ion channels; BKR, bradykinin receptors; TrkA, TrkB, high-affinity neurotrophin tyrosine kinase receptors; Na^+-TTXr, tetrodotoxin-resistant sodium ion channels; α_2, adrenergic receptors; DOR, delta opiate receptors; A_1, adenosine receptors; N-Ca^{++}, voltage-gated calcium ion channels; NK1, neurokinin receptors; NMDA-R, N-methyl-D-aspartic acid receptors; GluR5, kainate receptors; mGluR, metabotropic glutamate receptors; PKCγ, protein kinase C gamma; AEAs, antiepileptic agents, GABA-ergic compounds; TCA, tricyclic antidepressants; SNRIs, serotonin and norepinephrine reuptake inhibitors.

2 PATHOPHYSIOLOGY OF OSTEOARTHRITIC PAIN

OVERVIEW

In late 2003, a special report entitled 'Usefulness, completeness, and accuracy of Web sites providing information on osteoarthritis in dogs' appeared in the Journal of the American Veterinary Medical Association.[1] Five popular search engines (AltaVista, Google, Lycon, Netscape, and Microsoft Network) were searched with the key words: dog, degenerative joint disease, canine, and osteoarthritis. From this exercise, the authors concluded that although most of the sites conveyed some conventional information with reasonable accuracy, the information was incomplete, of minimal use, and often considered counterproductive. Further, those (veterinarians and clients) seeking information about OA may have access to faulty or misleading information.

Cranial cruciate ligament deficiency (CrCLD) in dogs is only one of many etiologies for OA, however Wilke *et al.* estimate that dog owners spent approximately \$1.32 billion for the treatment of CrCLD alone in the US in 2003.[2] These insights reveal the prominence OA has in veterinary medicine. OA affects more than 80% of Americans over age 55[3] and approximately one in five adult dogs in America.[4] It is the number one cause of chronic pain in dogs, and approximately 10–12 million dogs in the US show signs of OA.

In 1999 the 'average' veterinary practice saw approximately 45 arthritic dogs per month, 21% of which were considered 'severe', 38% were considered 'moderate', and 41% were considered 'mild' as assessed by their clinical presentation (**67**).[5]

The demographics of dogs with OA is broad-reaching. Although the condition tends to be over-represented in older, heavy dogs, it can be a clinical problem in any dog. The 'poster child' for OA in dogs is the middle-aged to older (>4 years), large breed (>25 kg) dog that is overweight to obese. OA is often secondary to either abnormal forces on normal joints (e.g. trauma, instability) or normal forces on abnormal joints (e.g. dysplasias, development disorders). In the case of obesity, which is often seen in older dogs, abnormal stress on the joints is accentuated.

Cats, being light and agile, can compensate for fairly severe orthopedic disease, including musculoskeletal conditions such as OA. They are noted for hiding signs of lameness in the veterinarian's office. Clinical signs of chronic pain at home, as reported by owners, include change of attitude (e.g. grumpiness, slowing down) and disability (decreased grooming, missing the litter box on occasion, and inability to jump on to counters), rather than overt signs of lameness. Prevalence of radiographic signs of feline degenerative joint disease (DJD) ranges from 22–90% of investigated populations.[6–8] Freire *et al.* reported that 74% of 100 cats selected randomly from a data base of 1,640 cats

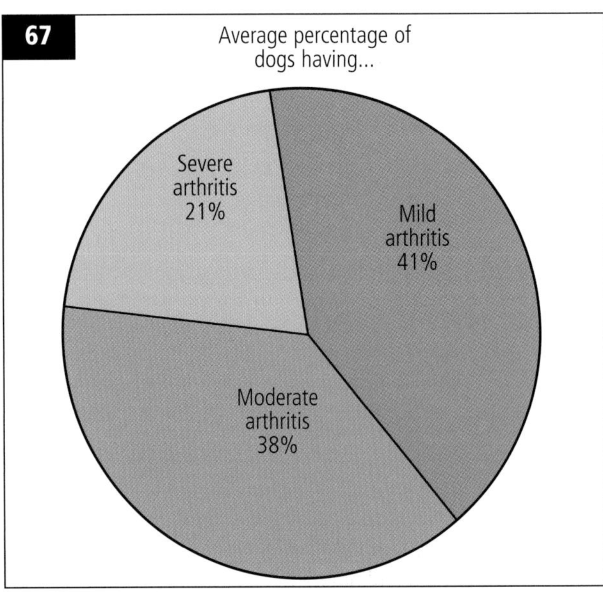

67 Prevalence of canine osteoarthritis in the US (1999).

in a single practice had DJD somewhere in the skeleton.[9] Freire *et al.* also reported that radiographic appearance does not accurately predict whether or not feline joints show lesions associated with DJD.[10] In the latter report, 31 of 64 joints (elbow, hip, stifle, and hock) assessed from eight postmortem, euthanized animal shelter cats had radiographic signs of DJD. The absence of osteophytes did not predict appearance of cartilage pathology, with 35 joints showing no radiographic signs of osteophytosis, but showing macroscopic cartilage lesions. There was no agreement between cartilage damage and the presence of sclerosis in the radiographs. In stifle, hock, and hip joints, no sclerosis was identified, even in those joints with moderate and severe cartilage damage. The best correlations and agreements between radiographic osteophyte score and macroscopic osteophyte score were in the elbow and hip. In the elbow, moderate cartilage damage was present before any sclerosis was identified in the radiographs and only mild sclerosis was identified in joints with severe cartilage damage. Although OA is a commonly recognized disease in dogs, it is frequently under-diagnosed in cats. However, it is now being recognized as a disease of senior aged cats.[11]

DEFINITION

OA can be defined as a disorder of movable joints characterized by: deterioration of articular cartilage; osteophyte formation and bone remodeling; pathology of periarticular tissues including synovium, subchondral bone, muscle, tendon, and ligament; and a low-grade, nonpurulent inflammation of variable degree. OA is differentiated from rheumatoid arthritis, which is the classic example of a primary immune-mediated systemic condition characterized by bone destruction and articular cartilage erosion. Rheumatoid arthritis is considered to be a more destructive, progressive, and debilitating condition than OA.

OA is not a single disease, and is often misperceived as a disease of cartilage. Herein, the joint can be considered as an 'organ', where all components of the 'organ' are affected by the disease process (**68**).

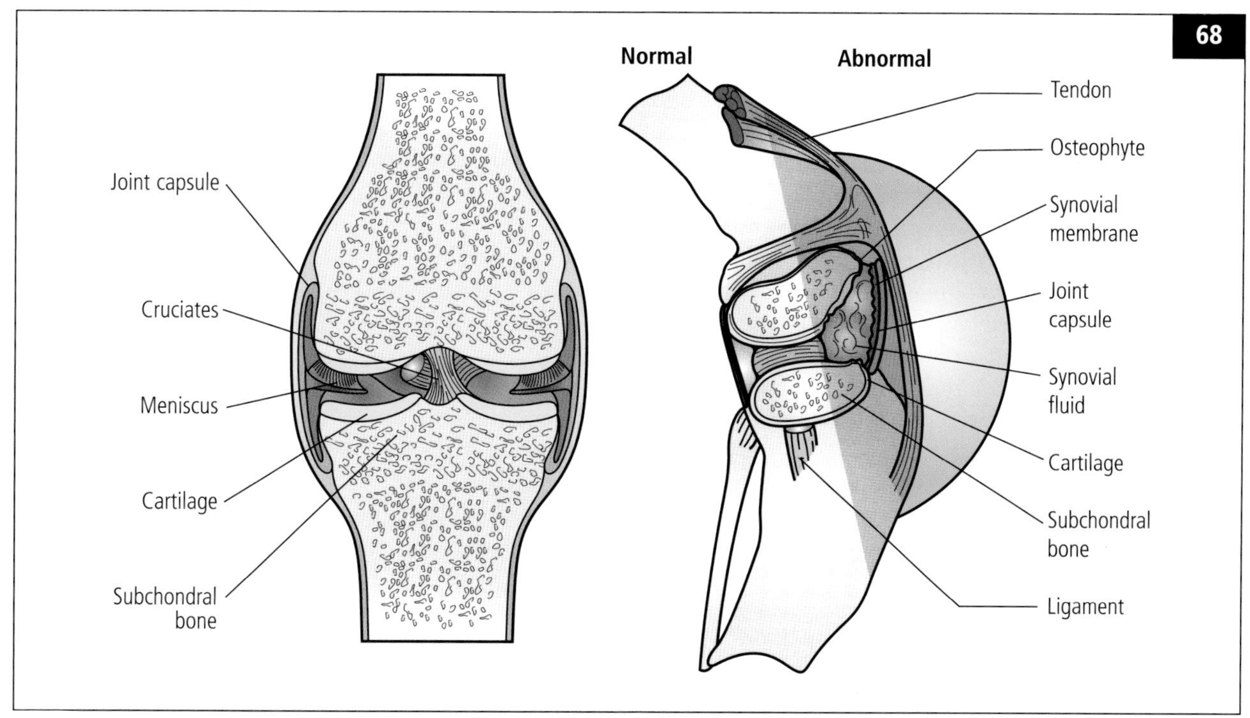

68 Anatomy of the femoral-tibial joint. The arthritic joint is analogous to a totally diseased 'organ', with loss of cartilage, sclerosis of subchondral bone, inflammation of the synovial membrane, osteophyte formation, and pain.

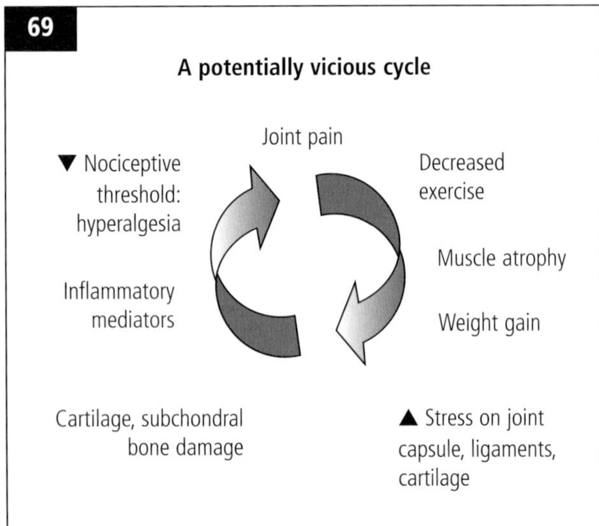

69 OA is a degradative cycle.

OA is a syndrome characterized by pathological changes of the synovial or diarthrodial joint expressed by disability and clinical signs of pain. It is a complex condition involving multiple biochemical and biomechanical interactions. Often termed DJD, OA can be classified by the joint involved and whether it is primary or secondary. It appears to be mechanically driven but chemically mediated, with endogenous attempts at aberrant repair.

OA and DJD are synonyms, however, these two terms and arthritis, arthrosis, rheumatism, and others are often used interchangeably and incorrectly. Historically recognized as 'noninflammatory', OA is now recognized as an inflammatory condition, but the inflammation is not that classically mediated by neutrophils as in other types of arthritis.[12] OA is associated with destruction and loss of cartilage, remodeling of bone, and intermittent inflammation. Changes in subchondral bone, synovium, and ligaments are detectable at an early stage, and cartilage matrix synthesis occurs concurrently with increased degradation. Synovial and cartilage-derived proteases are major players in cartilage matrix degradation, with metalloproteases and aggrecanases, seemingly, key catabolic agents. The vicious catabolic/anabolic cycle of OA (**69**) is not yet comprehensively understood.

ETIOLOGY

Degradation and synthesis of cartilage matrix components are related to the release of mediators by chondrocytes and synoviocytes, including the cytokines, IL-1 and TNF, NO, and growth factors.[13] Release of these mediators is related to joint loading, nutrition, and matrix integrity (**70**). A minor injury could start the disease process in a less resistant environment, whereas in other individuals the joint may be able to compensate for a greater insult. Although cartilage assuredly has the potential for endogenous repair, damage may become irreversible when compensation is exhausted.

INFLAMMATION

Inflammation in joints causes peripheral sensitization, with an upregulation of primary afferent neuron sensitivity, and also central sensitization, with hyperexcitability of nociceptive neurons in the CNS (see Chapter 1).[14] Peripheral sensitization is produced by the action of inflammatory mediators such as bradykinin, PGs, neuropeptides, and cytokines. Quantitative sensory testing in human OA patients shows that there is diffuse and persistent alteration of nociceptive pathways, irrespective of the level of severity associated with the underlying disease.[15] Inflammatory mediators play a role either by directly activating high-threshold receptors or more commonly by sensitizing nociceptive neurons to subsequent daily stimuli. Damaged joints and sensory nervous system interactions may not only produce pain, but may actually influence the course of the disease.

The inflammatory component is more prevalent at different phases of the disease. The synovial fluid of most OA patients shows increased numbers of mononuclear cells and increased levels of immunoglobulins and complement. The synovial membrane shows signs of chronic inflammation including hyperplasia of the lining with infiltration of inflammatory cells. Inflammation likely plays an important role in the painful symptoms of OA.[16]

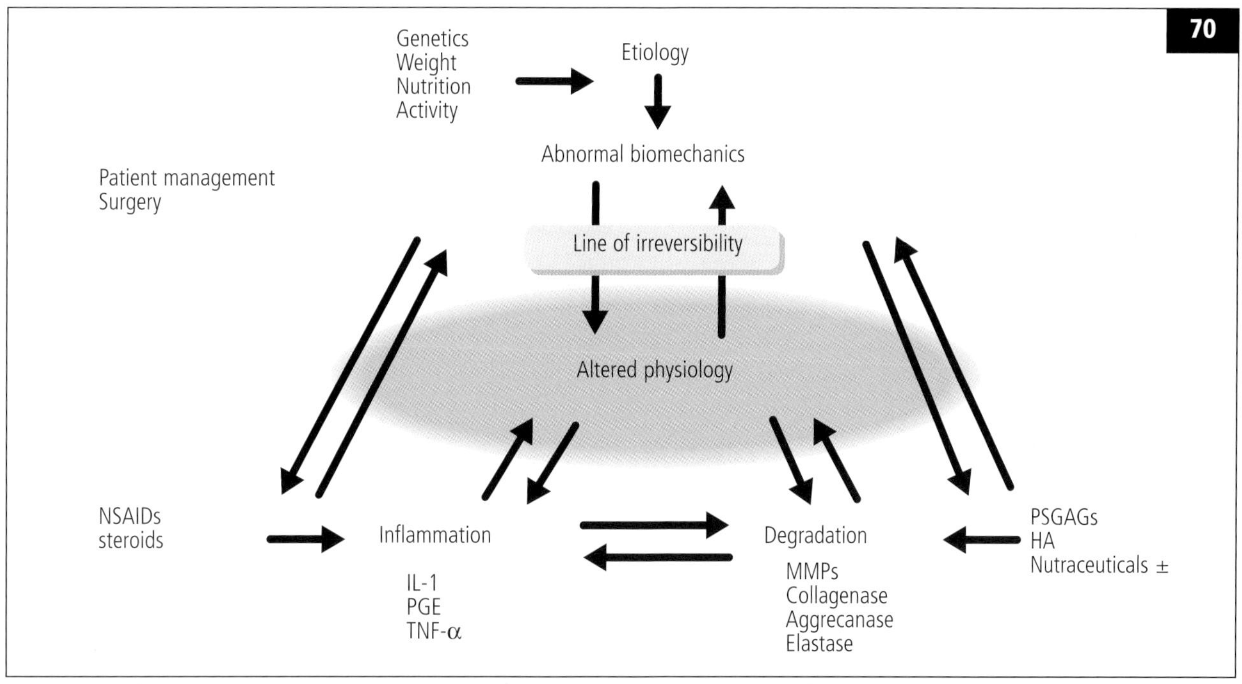

70 Etiology of osteoarthritis. Damage may become irreversible when compensation fails.

The discovery of COX-2 was linked to the finding that it was upregulated as a result of inflammatory stimuli. As a consequence, COX-2 inhibitors are marketed on the premise that they may be more effective for the treatment of OA pain. This is supported by the assumption that COX-2 activity is upregulated in the joint tissues of dogs suffering from OA, and is the primary COX enzyme responsible for pain in OA. Although this is corroborated within the human literature,[17–19] there is sparse evidence for this assumption in naturally occurring canine OA, and nothing is known about the expression of lipoxygenase (LOX) in naturally occurring OA. Lascelles et al.[20] have investigated this area by comparing the levels of COX-1, COX-2, and LOX protein in joint tissues (joint capsule/synovium, osteophytes, and subchondral bone), as well as levels of PGE_2 and leukotriene $(LT)B_4$ in joint tissues (joint capsule/synovium and subchondral bone) between a limited number (three each) of normal vs. arthritic dogs. Results showed that significantly more COX-2 protein was present in hip joint capsule from joints with OA than normal joints. Further, there was a significantly greater concentration of LTB_4 from coxofemoral joints with OA compared to normal dogs. Significantly more COX-1, COX-2, and LOX protein was present in subchondral bone from the femoral head of joints in OA than in normal joints. There was no difference in PGE_2 or LTB_4 concentration in normal femoral head tissue compared to femoral head from coxofemoral joints with OA. Overall, there was significantly more PGE_2 and LTB_4 in hip joint capsule than in femoral head samples.

JOINT STRUCTURE INTERACTIONS

Cartilage is void of vessels, lymphatics, and nervous tissue. It derives its nutrition from the diffusion of synovial fluid. The diffusion of synovial fluid into the hyaline cartilage (and evacuation of cartilage waste products) is enhanced by the loading and unloading of cartilage by daily activities. This is analogous to the movement of water in and out of a sponge while being squeezed within a bucket of water.

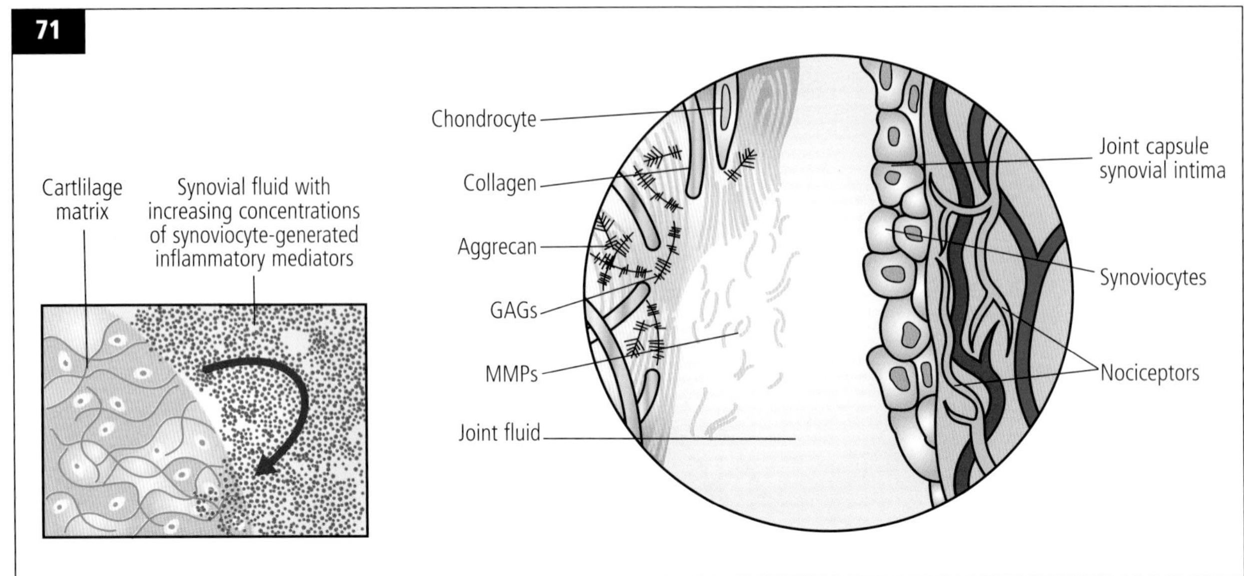

71 As matrix metalloproteinases (MMPs) are released from diseased cartilage, they stimulate the generation of additional inflammatory mediators and cytokines from synoviocytes located in the synovial intima. (GAGs = glycosaminoglycans)

The synovial intima (lining layer) of the joint capsule is normally only one to two cell layers thick, and contains type A and B synoviocytes. Type A synoviocytes are macrophage-like cells that have a role in removing debris from joints and processing antigens. Type B synoviocytes are fibroblast-like cells that are responsible for production of hyaluronan, but also are capable of producing degradative enzymes. Both types of synoviocytes produce cytokines and other mediators.[21] Therefore, as inflammatory mediators and cytokines are released into the joint fluid, they stimulate synoviocytes in the synovial intima to produce additional degradative enzymes that find their way back into the cartilage by diffusion, and the catabolic cycle becomes self-perpetuating (**71**). The subsynovial layer, lying immediately below the intima, contains free nerve endings. With such close proximity of these nociceptors within the subsynovium to inflammatory mediators in the synovial fluid, the process of noxious stimulation is practically intuitive.

OA pain is the result of a complex interplay between structural change, biochemical alterations, peripheral and central pain-processing mechanisms, and individual cognitive processing of nociception. Bony changes at the joint margins and beneath areas of damaged cartilage can be major sources of OA pain. Chondrophyte and osteophyte growth result in elevation and stretching of richly innervated periosteum, which is also a common origin of expansile bone tumor pain. Human OA patients report pain, even at rest, associated with raised intraosseous pressure.[22]

So, what is the source of pain in OA? The source of pain in the joint 'organ' is multifocal: direct stimulation of the joint capsule and bone receptors by cytokines/ligands of inflammatory and degradative processes, physical stimulation of the joint capsule from distention (effusion) and stretch (laxity, subluxation, abnormal articulation), physical stimulation of subchondral bone from abnormal loading, and (likely) physical stimulation of muscle, tendon, and ligaments.

JOINT COMPONENTS AND PHYSIOLOGY

Cartilage is a physiologically complex, yet structurally simple tissue. It is composed mostly of water. Type II collagen contributes to structural integrity, the functional cell is the chondrocyte, and the aggrecan aggregate of proteoglycans forms the functional unit. The term aggrecan has been given to the proteoglycan monomer that aggregates with hyaluronan and is found in articular cartilage (**72**).

It is the major proteoglycan by mass of hyaline cartilage. The aggrecan has a 'bottle brush' appearance with a hyaluronan backbone and 'bristles' of hydrophylic glycosaminoglycans (GAGs) that retain the water. An aggrecan aggregate may contain over 100 aggrecan monomers (**73**).

Cartilage exists in three forms: hyaline, fibrocartilage, and elastocartilage. Hyaline cartilage is an avascular, aneural, and alymphatic tissue found at the end of long bones. It is a perfect example of the structure–function relationship, where compromise of one directly affects the other.

The *chondrocyte* is the cellular element of articular cartilage. Chondrocytes are metabolically active cells responsible for the production, organization, and maintenance of the extracellular matrix.[23] This cell type exists within a lacuna, which together with its perilacunar rim comprises the structural and functional entity called the chondron. The chondrocyte not only synthesizes extracellular matrix components, but also generates the proteinases that degrade these extracellular matrix components, dependent upon changing properties of the surrounding matrix.[23] Chondrocytes make up 5% of the tissue volume by composition.

Collagen exists in 19 different forms.[24] Collagen type II is the predominant form of collagen in articular cartilage. Type IX collagen is thought to link collagen type II fibrils together and limit their separation by proteoglycan swelling, to limit fibril diameter, and also possibly to bind proteoglycan molecules to collagen type II.[25] The deepest collagen fibers of hyaline cartilage, which are embedded in the zone of calcified cartilage immediately above the subchondral bone, appear to help in securing the cartilage to the bone. These fibers are arranged perpendicular to the subchondral bone and constitute

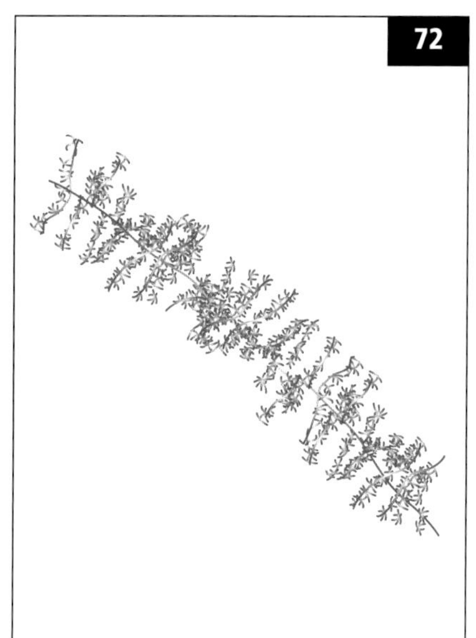

72 Aggrecan refers to the proteoglycan monomer that aggregates with hyaluronan, appearing as a 'bottle brush'.

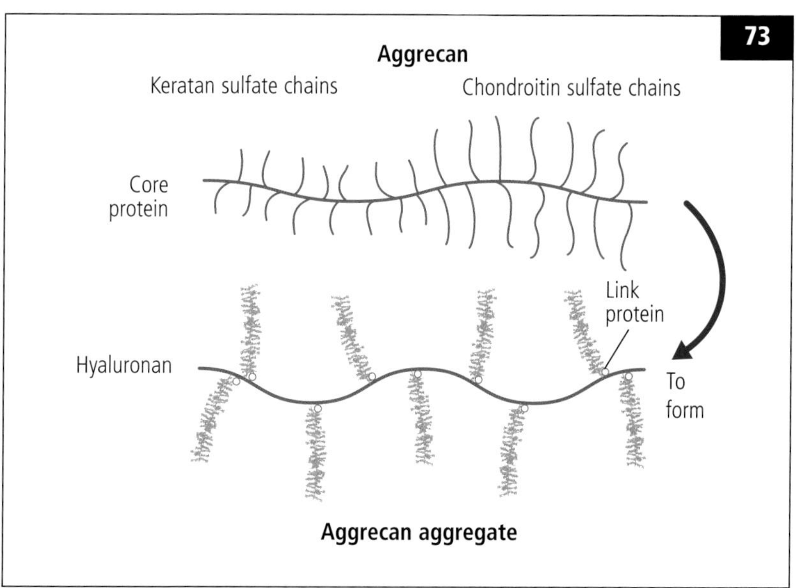

73 The aggrecan aggregate is the 'functional unit' of cartilage, containing over 100 aggrecan monomers.

the radial zone. The most superficial fibers form a thin layer parallel to the articular surface and comprise the tangential zone. Between these is an intermediate zone in which the fibers appear to have a random oblique orientation (74).

These zones of collagen orientation produce an arcade-like arrangement and correspond to the distribution of chondrocytes seen in histological sections of normal articular cartilage. The arrangement of collagen fibers within the matrix accounts for the physical properties of the cartilage (elasticity and compressibility). The triple helices of collagen types II, IX, and X are susceptible to collagenase cleaving by matrix metalloproteinases (MMPs): MMP-1 and MMP-3 (stromelysin).[26]

Hyaluronan is a GAG, although it is not sulfated and does not bind to a core protein like chondroitin and keratan sulfate. It is an important component of both the articular cartilage matrix and synovial fluid.

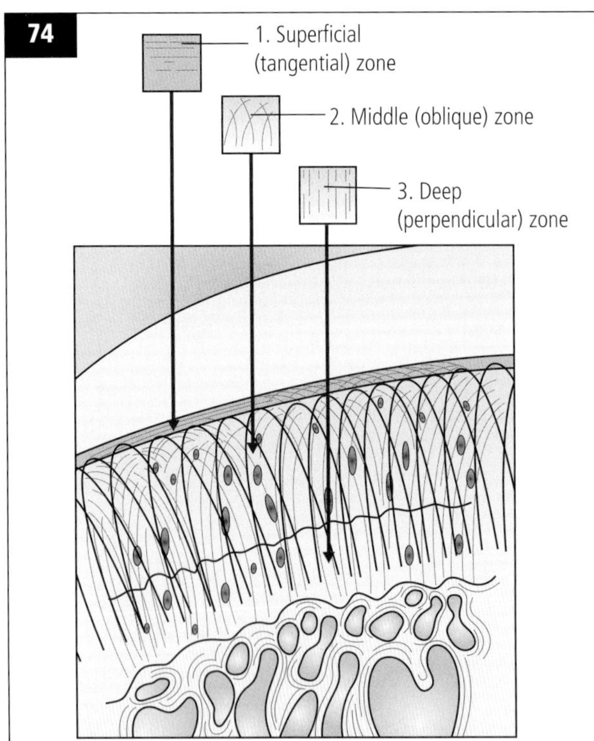

74 The three zones of collagen orientation account for the elasticity and compressibility of cartilage, allowing cartilage to more evenly distribute forces to the underlying, shock-absorbing subchondral bone.

Hyaluronan found in the extracellular matrix is produced by chondrocytes, whereas hyaluronan found in synovial fluid is produced by type B synoviocytes. Synovial fluid hyaluronan functions as both a lubricant and molecular barrier. Due to its steric configuration, hyaluronan acts as a molecular sieve, excluding macromolecules from its space.

Proteoglycans comprise most of the extracellular matrix that is not collagen and make up 22–38% of the dry weight of adult articular cartilage.[27] The common GAGs of articular cartilage are chondroitin sulfate, keratan sulfate, and dermatan sulfate. They are chains of variable length made up of repeating disaccharide subunits covalently attached to a protein core (75).

The GAGs are negatively charged due to the carboxyl and sulfate groups of these subunits. This negative charge causes the GAGs to remain separated, thereby occupying a large volume. The anionic charge also contributes to the hydrophilic properties of cartilage. Adult cartilage is 75–80% water by weight. Retention of water by proteoglycan within the extracellular matrix creates a swelling pressure and turgidity that are integral to normal articular cartilage function. Proteoglycans can occupy a volume up to 50 times their dry weight volume when hydrated.[28] Their expansile potential is limited to 20% of their potential by the collagen framework. This constraint keeps the cartilage turgid, helping to resist deformation when a compressive load is applied.

There are no covalent links between collagen and the proteoglycans.[29] The size of the hydrated proteoglycans ensures their retention within the articular cartilage, with the hydrophobic collagen network constraining their escape. The interrelationship between the proteoglycans and collagen is also critical to the ability of the articular cartilage matrix to respond to a compressive load (76). Upon loading, the compressive force placed upon the articular cartilage forces the fluid phase to flow through the permeable solid phase. The hydraulic pressure increases as the compressive force increases. This is due to decreased pore size as the solid matrix is compressed causing increased resistance to fluid flow until an equilibrium is reached with the compressive force, resulting in a ceasing of cartilage deformation. Further contributing to this equilibrium is the increasing negative charge density within the matrix as water is extruded from the matrix in response to increasing compression. Upon removal of the compression, water and nutrients re-enter the cartilage matrix allowing the proteoglycans to swell and the cartilage to recover to its nondeformed configuration.

Normal cartilage turnover and OA will result in proteoglycan fragment release. Further, susceptibility of the various proteoglycan monomers to cleavage at different sites leads to diversity of fragments, some of which may serve as potential markers for distinguishing the nature, cause, and severity of proteoglycan cleavage.

Subchondral bone is a thin layer of bone that joins hyaline cartilage with cancellous bone supporting the bony plate. The undulating nature of the osteochondral junction allows shear stresses to be converted into potentially less damaging compressive forces on the subchondral bone. The subchondral/cancellous region has been found to be approximately 10 times more deformable than cortical bone, and plays a major role in the distribution of forces across a joint.[30] Compliance of subchondral bone to applied joint forces allows congruity of joint surfaces for increasing the contact area of load distribution, thereby reducing peak loading and potential damage to cartilage.[31] Cartilage itself makes a poor shock absorber, however subchondral bone serves such a role well. Thickening of the subchondral bone plate and cancellous trabeculae occurs during OA, thereby limiting the distribution of loads across the joint.

Subchondral bone contains unmyelinated nerve fibers, increasing in number with OA.[32] Increased pressure on subchondral bone associated with OA articular cartilage degradation results in these nociceptors being stimulated. This is thought to contribute to the vague but consistent pain frequently associated with OA. In humans OA is believed to be responsible for increased interosseous pressure, which may contribute to chronic pain, particularly nocturnal pain.[12]

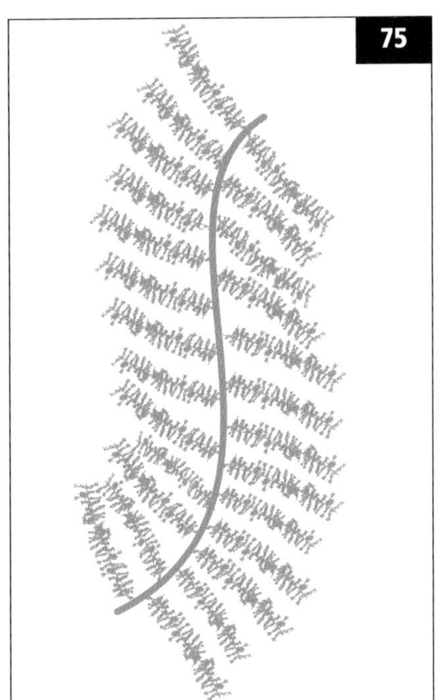

75 Proteoglycans (chondroitin sulfate, keratan sulfate, and dermatan sulfate) are chains of variable length covalently attached to a protein core.

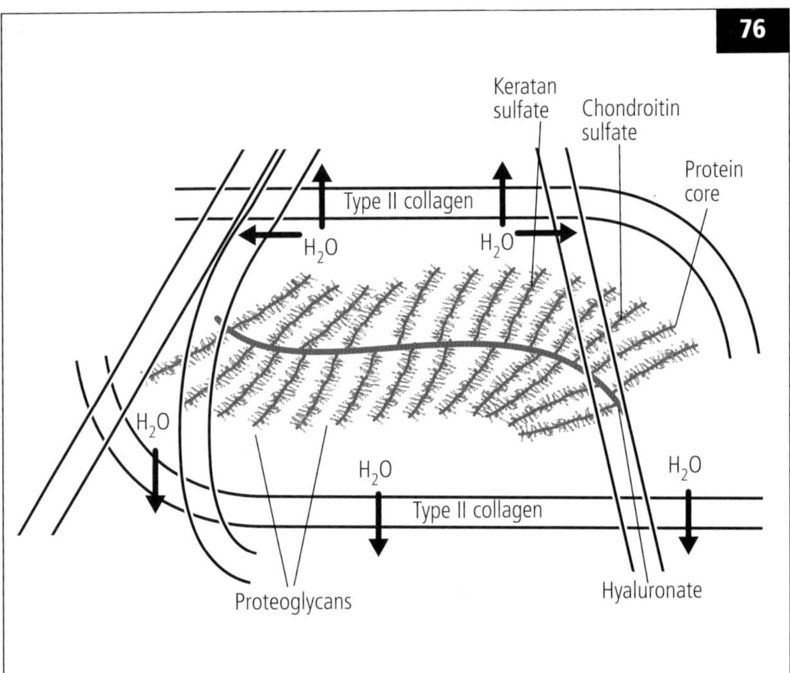

76 The aggrecan aggregates, collagen, and water interact, allowing the articular cartilage matrix to respond to compressive loads.

OA frequently results in osteophyte formation (77). *Osteophytes* are a central core of bone that blends in with the subchondral bone. They are covered by hyaline and fibrocartilage and are formed by a process similar to enchondral ossification.[33] Although they may occur centrally in the joint, they are most frequently found at the junction of the synovium, perichondrium, and periosteum.[34]

Mechanical instability is believed to be the predisposing cause of osteophyte formation; however, synovial membrane inflammation may play a role as well. Other etiologies include venous congestion and blood vessel invasion. Experimental models have demonstrated osteophyte formation as early as 3 days to 1 week after creation of instability.[35]

The *periosteum of bone* is richly innervated with nociceptors, and stimulation of these nociceptors with elevation of the periosteum by osteophytes is likely (78). Additional stimulation of these nociceptors is likely as OA progresses and friction between soft tissues and periosteum increases due to decreased boundary lubrication.

OA is a disease condition of the entire diarthrodial joint, including the articular (hyaline) cartilage, synovial membrane, synovial fluid, subchondral bone, and surrounding supporting structures (muscles and ligaments) (79). The term *enthesiophytes* refers to bony proliferations found at the insertion of ligaments, tendons, and capsule to bone. Ligaments and muscles surrounding the OA joint are contributors to the pain of OA. Although ligamentous neuroreceptors serve mainly to determine spatial orientation of the joint, tissue strain incites the pain state. Muscle weakness accompanying OA is also associated with pain and disability. Stimulation of neuroreceptors within the damaged OA joint can stimulate a reflex arc resulting in constant stimulation of muscle tissue. Muscle spasm and muscle fatigue may greatly contribute to the pain of OA. Mild muscle trauma thereafter likely releases

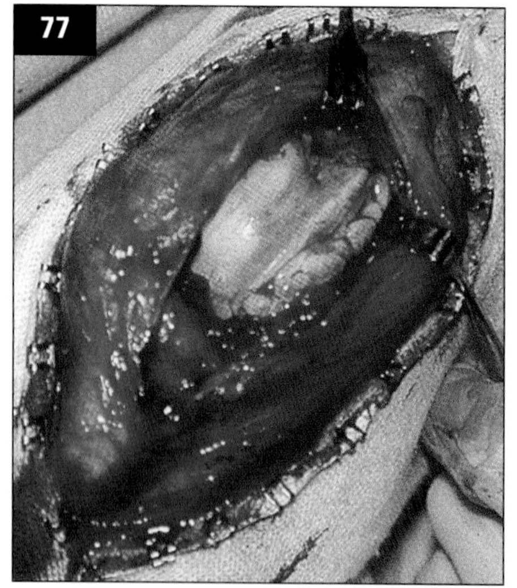

77 Osteophytes are common sequelae of OA.

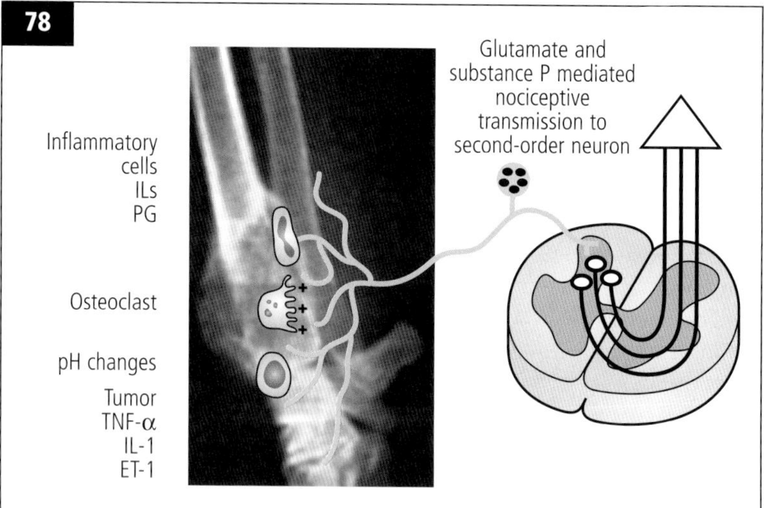

78 Bone periosteum is rich with nociceptors that are stimulated with stretching by osteophytes or tumors. In the case of tumors, additional nociceptive mediators are also involved. (ET-1 = endothelin-1)

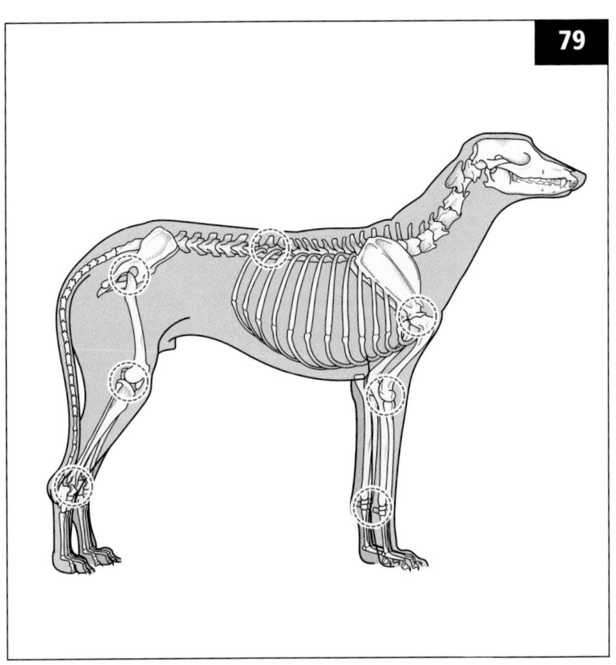

79 OA is a 'total joint disease', and can be found in a number of diarthrodial joints.

inflammatory mediators sensitizing muscle nociceptors to further mechanical stimulation. Local tenderness often results from the release of inflammatory mediators such as bradykinin and PGE_2. Nociceptors are found in muscle, fascia, and tendons, and since afferent nerve fibers from muscle distribute over a relatively large region of the dorsal spinal horn, poor localization of muscle pain is common.

The *synovium* is composed of the synovial lining, which containes both type A and B synoviocytes. The subsynovial layer contains fibroblasts, is vascular, contains free nerve endings, and functions to enhance motion between the fibrous joint capsule and the synovial membrane.[36] Menisci in the stifle are contiguous with the joint capsule and are composed of fibrocartilage.[37] Pain from meniscal tearing and disruption comes from stimulation of joint capsule pain receptors and perhaps from stimulation of C fibers in the outer one-third of the meniscus.[38]

Synovial fluid is frequently referred to as a dialysate of plasma, in that it contains electrolytes and small molecules in similar proportions as in plasma. The release of inflammatory mediators results in synovial vasculature increased permeability.[39] This upregulates the synovial vasculature protein content with resultant disturbance of the normal oncotic balance and change of synovial fluid volume. As the synovial membrane is distended and increased synovial blood flow accompanies the synovitis of OA, there becomes an increased exchange of small molecule proteins across the synovial membrane. Proteins are then cleared by joint lymphatic drainage.[40] The increased rate of removal of these molecules, along with variable rates of release from cartilage, reflects the difficulty in using these markers as indicators of disease severity.[41]

AGING CARTILAGE

Normal age-related changes occur in articular cartilage throughout life. Data from porcine articular cartilage have shown a decrease in hydration, a decrease in collagen on a dry matter basis, a decrease in GAG concentration especially chondroitin sulfate, and a decrease in proteoglycan size with age.[42] Although the total GAG concentration may not vary much with increasing age, the ratio of keratan sulfate to chondroitin sulfate increases.[43] Chondroitin sulfate, the four-sulfated compound, decreases, while the six-sulfated compound increases. The link proteins are also subject to proteolytic cleavage as aging progresses.[44] The end result of these normal age-related changes is a matrix with reduced capability to withstand the forces associated with normal joint functioning.

MORPHOLOGICAL CHANGES

The tangentially oriented collagen fibrils of the superficial cartilage zone (**74**), along with relatively low proteoglycan content, have the greatest ability to withstand high tensile stresses, thereby resisting deformation and distributing load more evenly over the joint surface. Loss of this superficial layer, as occurs in the early stages of cartilage *fibrillation* of OA, alters the biomechanical properties of the articular cartilage. One of the first changes of OA, recognized microscopically, is fibrillation of the superficial cartilage layer.[45] Fibrillation occurs as a flaking of the superficial cartilage layers, following the course of collagen fibrils parallel to the joint surface.

Once integrity of the stiff cartilage outer layer is lost by the progression of fibrillation, abnormal stresses give rise to fissures into the deeper layers (**80**). These fissures develop in a vertical plane, again following the orientation of mid-zone collagen fibrils. Such fissures can extend to the subchondral bone. Concurrently, chondrocytes become larger and begin to cluster.

INFLAMMATORY MEDIATORS

OA-induced pathological changes in joints include ulceration, fibrillation, softening, and loss of articular cartilage. Excessive production of MMPs by chondrocytes is one of the major causes of altered cartilage homeostasis and cartilage degradation.[46] In OA cartilage, proinflammatory cytokines, such as TNF-α, IL-1, and IL-6, mediate the transcription of MMPs.[36] Synovial lining cells are likely the primary source of these proinflammatory cytokines, as these cytokines have been demonstrated in the synovial membrane and synovial fluid of OA joints.[47,48] Studies suggest that (under experimental conditions) TGF-β, the synovial membrane, and synovial macrophages contribute to osteophyte formation.[49,50] Inflammatory changes within OA joints are proposed to be secondary to cartilage-soluble, cartilage-specific macromolecule degradation products.[51] Phagocytosis of these products by synovial macrophages induces chronic inflammation of the synovial membrane and joint capsule with subsequent synthesis of proteases and proinflammatory cytokines such as TNF-α, IL-1, and IL-6.[52] In addition to the role of synovial macrophages in osteophyte formation, synovial macrophages play an important role in the development and maintenance of synovial inflammation as supported by the observation that vascular endothelial growth factor derived from synovial macrophages promotes vascular endothelial growth factor immunoreactivity and endothelial cell proliferation.[53] In a study[54] of 17 dogs (with naturally occurring rupture of the cranial cruciate ligament) macrophages and the cytokines TNF-α and IL-6 were detected in the synovial membranes and joint capsule at concentrations reflecting the chronicity of the OA. Such observations have led to the development of therapeutic agents for human rheumatoid patients, the mechanism of action of which includes neutralization of cytokines, cytokine receptor blockade, and folate-mediated drug delivery to macrophages.[55]

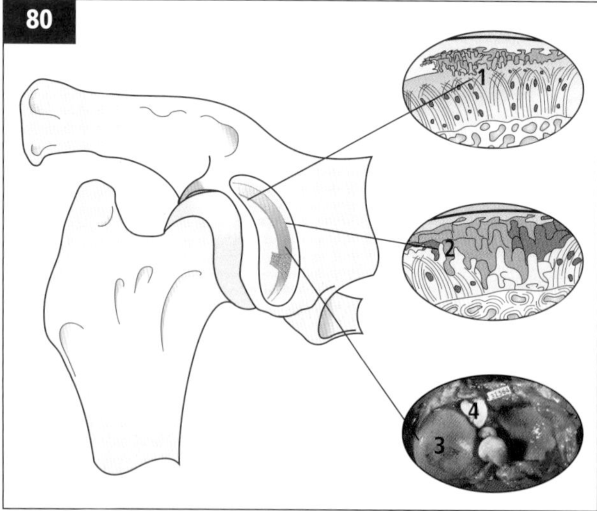

80 Morphologically, arthritic hyaline cartilage undergoes fibrillation (1) that progresses to deep cartilage fissures (2), and is ultimately replaced with structurally inferior fibrocartilage (3). Joint mice (4) might be present if osteochrondrosis dissecans fragments have maintained viability from the synovial fluid.

The release of free cartilage fragments initiates a synovitis (**81**) as they are phagocytized by type A synoviocytes.[56] This is followed by the release of additional inflammatory mediators such as cytokines and PGs which enhance the inflammatory process to varying severity.[57] Despite the increase of proteoglycan synthesis, catabolism exceeds the anabolic rate. As collagen breakdown progresses, proteoglycans are no longer constrained of their expansile potential and the water content of the cartilage increases.[58] One of the earliest changes seen in OA is an increase in hydration (2–3%).[59] This hydration appears to be the result of the cleavage of type II collagen by collagenase. The functional collagen network is disrupted thereby permitting the proteoglycans, the hydration capacity of which is no longer restricted by the collagen network, to bind increased amounts of water resulting in the cartilage swelling.[60] At this point proteoglycans are lost into the synovial fluid. Cartilage at this stage is grossly softer than normal and more susceptible to mechanical injury.

Chondromalacia is an early sign of degeneration and is attributed to a decrease in sulfated mucopolysaccharide content in the ground substance of the cartilage matrix. As previously indicated, fibrillation is the term applied to the exposure of the collagen framework through the loss of ground substance (matrix) and is one of the earlier

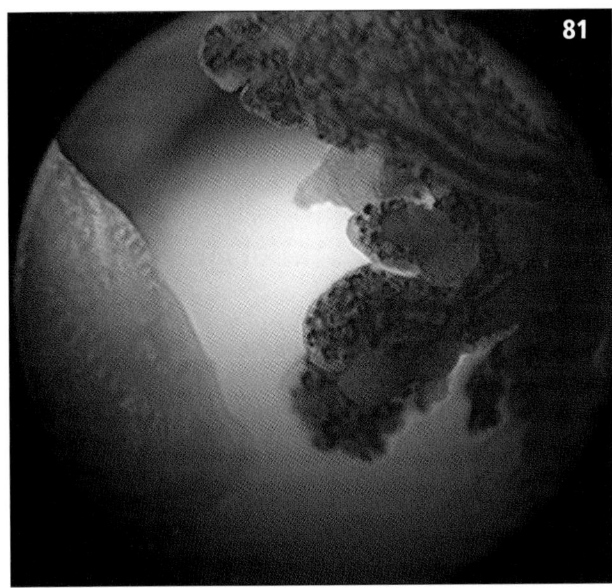

81 Synovitis is a common arthroscopic finding in OA patients. The cauliflower-like red mass contained in the upper-right quadrant is the characteristic intimal proliferation associated with synovitis.

pathological features of OA. As fibrillation progresses, the cartilage may fragment and erode. Erosion may continue until all the cartilage is worn away and the subchondral bone is exposed. The subchondral bone becomes sclerotic from mechanical pressure and/or the effect of the synovial fluid, and takes on the appearance of polished ivory, a process called *eburnation*.

With the progression of OA, chondrocytes undergo apoptosis and necrosis. Extracellular matrix synthesis decreases while degradation increases. Chondrocyte activity is stimulated in part by release of growth factors (e.g. insulin-like growth factor), however the newly synthesized proteoglycans have an abnormal composition, and newly synthesized proteoglycan subunits do not normally aggregate with hyaluronic acid (HA).[61] The collagen network becomes increasingly disorganized and disintegrated, with the content of collagen and proteoglycans reduced. The removal of functional proteoglycans from the extracellular matrix results in decreased water content of the cartilage and subsequent loss of biomechanical properties. Mechanical stress and trauma to chondrocytes perpetuates the OA process.

MMP AND TIMP IMBALANCE

In the osteoarthritic cartilage an imbalance develops between active MMP levels and tissue inhibitors of metalloproteinase (TIMPs), resulting in cartilage catabolism. Although synoviocytes and some inflammatory cells produce proteases, most are derived from chondrocytes.[62] MMPs exist as a number of different molecules and play a major role in cartilage destruction. Collagenases act on collagen fibers to break down the cartilage framework, while stromelysin cleaves the aggrecan leading to the loss of matrix proteoglycan. In the process of OA cytokines, acting as chemical messengers to maintain the chronic phase of inflammation and tissue destruction, are upregulated. Whereas these degradative enzymes and cytokines are normally found within chondrocytes, they are normally inactive or only produced in response to injury.[63] IL-1, IL-6 and TNF-α are believed to be of great importance in this process. Among other functions, cytokines further stimulate chondrocytes and synoviocytes to produce and release more degradative enzymes.

Proteoglycan and collagen breakdown is mediated by an increase in MMPs, serine proteases, lysosomal enzymes, and other proteases at the articular surface early in the degenerative process. Extensive matrix degeneration is the consequence of these proteases. The production of metalloproteinases greatly exceeds the ability of heightened TIMPs released to maintain homeostasis. Cytokines such as IL-1 and TNF-α further stimulate metalloproteinase and serine protease chondrocyte synthesis that further degrades the extracellular matrix.[64] IL-1 also stimulates chondrocyte and synovial cell release of PGE_2, LTB_4 and thromboxane: AA metabolites that enhance inflammation. IL-1 stimulates fibroblasts to produce collagen types I and III, which contribute to fibrosis of the joint capsule in the OA joint.[65]

SYNOVITIS

It is proposed that the chondrocyte is the most active source of degradative protease production; however this is stimulated primarily by cytokines and LTs produced by the synovium.[66] Yet it appears that synovitis alone is insufficient as the sole etiology of OA, and that physical trauma is also necessary.[67] Nevertheless, the impact strict hemostasis makes on the development of degenerative articular change in the cruciate-deficient model (i.e. producing less inflammatory stimulus) illustrates the importance of the synovium in the development of OA changes.[68] *It is therefore logical to assume that intervention in the inflammatory process of OA will slow the disease process.* This substantiates the legitimacy of NSAID therapy in OA disease.

JOINT CAPSULE DYNAMICS

Progressive alterations of the synovium include thickening of the synovial intima from one to two cell layers thick to three to four cell layers thick, development of synovial villi, and increased vascularity and infiltration of the subsynovial stroma by lymphocytes.[69] Apparently, changes in the synovium precede changes in the articular cartilage. In the cruciate-deficient canine model initial change, including increased cellularity of the synovial lining layer and infiltration of the subsynovial layer by mononuclear cells, is noted as early as 1 week.[70] Increased vascularity of the subsynovial layer and synovial villi development was seen at the same time. At 3–4 weeks following ligament transection, fibrosis of the joint capsule is observed, most pronounced on the medial aspect of the joint. Phagocytosis of proteoglycan and collagen fragements in synovial fluid by synovial intima macrophages may undermine the synovium changes,[55] which may, in turn, stimulate synoviocytes to produce cytokines and metalloproteinases, perpetuating the cycle of further degeneration.[71]

INTRA-ARTICULAR STRUCTURE DEGRADATION

ARACHIDONIC ACID CASCADE

The inflammation associated with DJD upregulates cytokines, such as IL-1 and TNF-α, which in turn activate the AA cascade. The AA cascade stimulates the synovium to produce various inflammatory mediators such as PGs, thromboxanes, LTs, and kinins (82).[72]

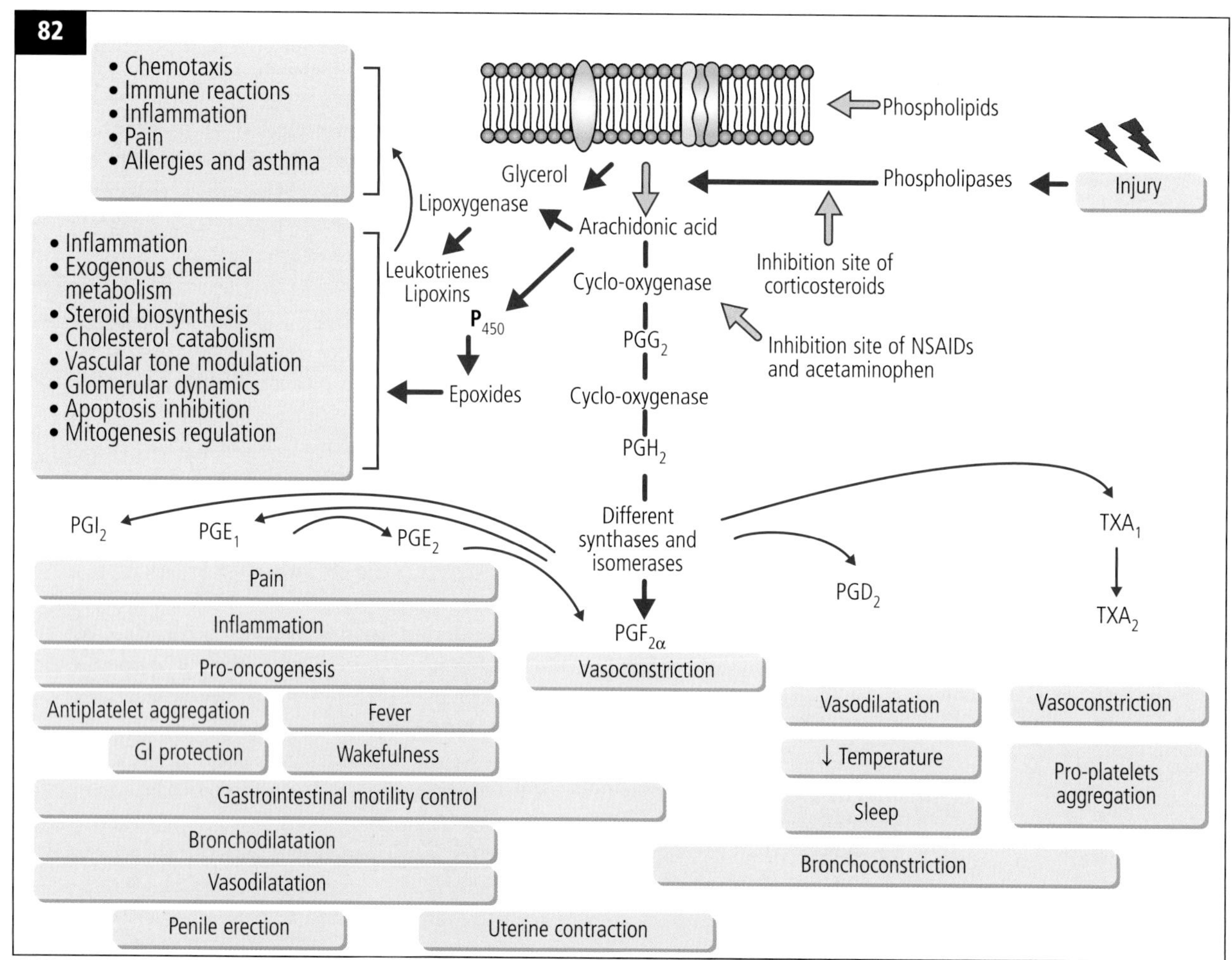

82 The arachidonic acid pathway produces a number of eicosanoids that impact on the physiology of joint inflammation.

A major inflammatory mediator is PGE_2, which influences vasodilatation and permeability of small blood vessels leading to erythema, sensitizes peripheral nociceptors,[73] stimulates the formation of new blood vessels,[74] and stimulates expression of MMPs via promotion of plasminogen activators.[75] A primary group of MMPs active in the cleavage of type II collagen are the collagenases (MMP-1, -8, and -13).

PGE_2 in synovial fluid is believed to originate from articular tissue, rather than blood, since no relationship has been established between PGE_2 concentrations and total leukocyte count in blood samples.[76] PGE_2 depresses proteoglycan synthesis by chondrocytes, thereby accelerating GAG loss from articular cartilage.[77]

POTENTIAL BIOMARKERS

As OA progresses, numerous factors play consistent roles in the catabolic process, offering potentially quantifiable markers (**83**). Most investigators suggest that components that may serve as molecular markers of OA can be categorized based on their origin and function during the process.[78] The first group includes enzymes released from periarticular macrophages or synoviocytes as well as degradative enzymes from chondrocytes: stromelysin (MMP-3), collagenase (MMP-1), TIMPs, and the cytokines IL-1 and IL-6. A second group includes the degradation products of OA, which may mimic the normal homeostatic degradation products of cartilage. Herein, a differentiation might be made in the quantity of degradative products and/or a qualitative

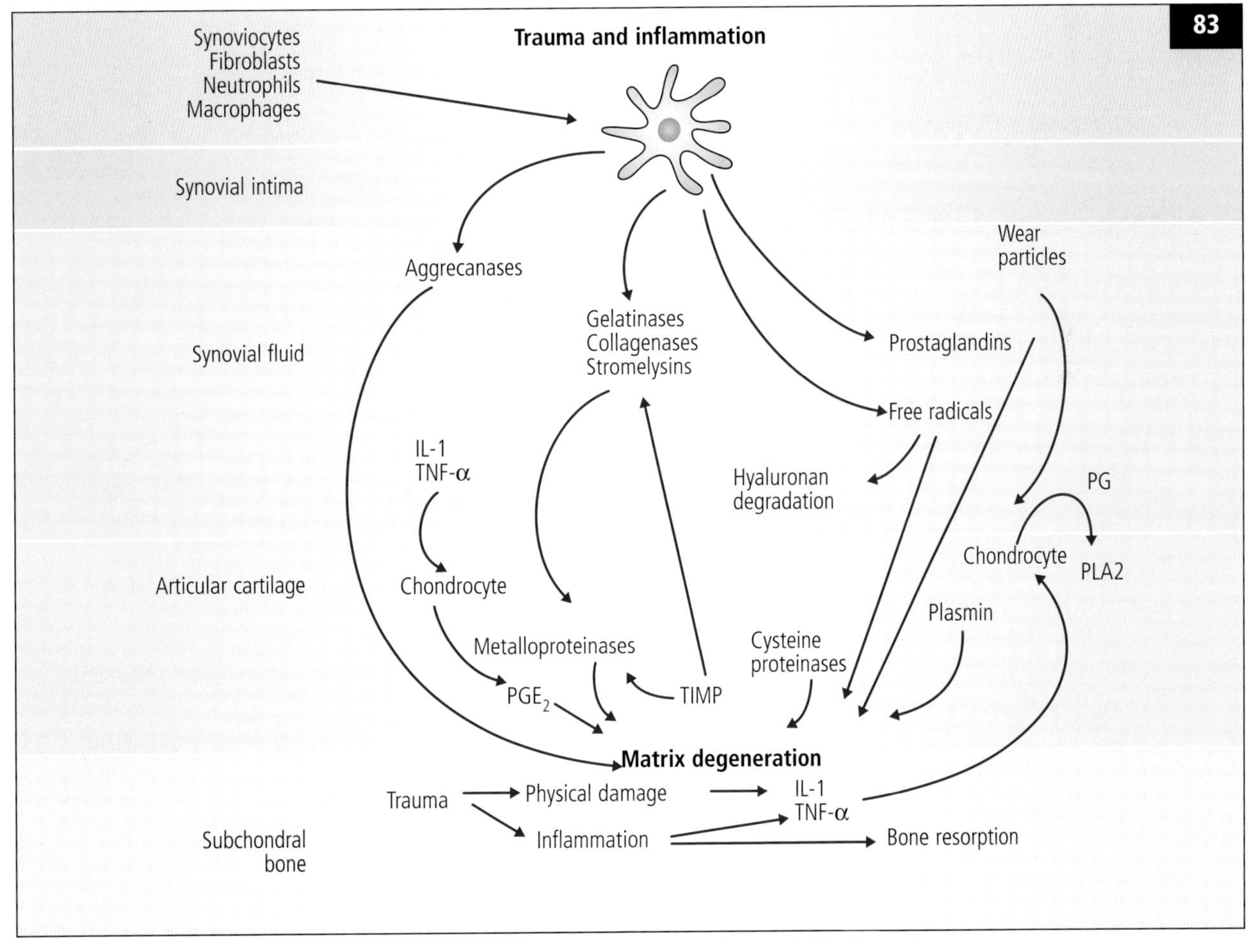

83 The catabolic process of OA is quite complex, offering several potential quantifiable biomarkers.

difference in proteoglycan fragments associated with variations in proteoglycan cleavage sites. OA-related molecules include keratan sulfate, chondroitin sulfate, aggrecan fragment components, cartilage matrix glycoprotein, and cartilage oligometric matrix protein. A third group of potential OA markers includes anabolic components: specific types of chondroitin sulfate, link protein, and collagen X. Currently, the synovial fluid is favored for measuring concentrations of potential OA markers, rather than serum or urine.[68]

The Osteoarthritis Biomarkers Network Consortium is developing and characterizing new biomarkers and redefining existing OA biomarkers.[79] The scheme is represented by the acronym BIPED: Burden of disease, Investigative, Prognostic, Efficacy of intervention, and Diagnostic (**84**).

- Burden of disease markers assess the severity or extent of disease, typically at a singe point in time, among individuals with OA.
- An investigative marker is one for which there is insufficient information to allow inclusion into one of the existing categories.
- The key feature of a prognostic marker is the ability to predict the future onset of OA among those without OA at baseline or the progression of OA among those with existing disease.
- An efficacy of intervention biomarker chiefly provides information about the efficacy of treatment among those with OA or those at high risk of developing OA.
- Diagnostic markers are defined by the ability to classify individuals as either diseased or nondiseased.

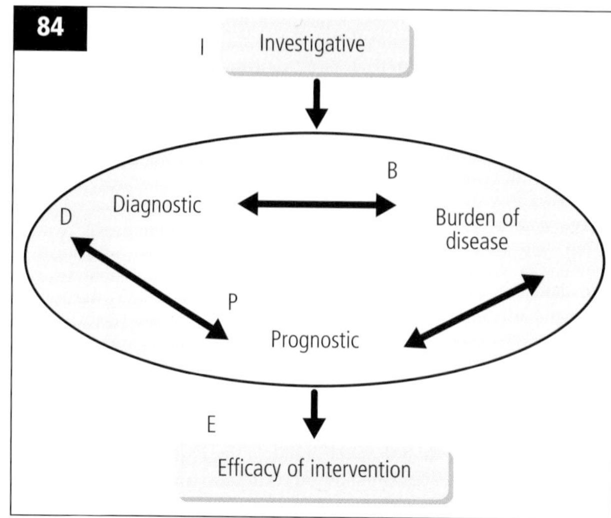

84 The BIPED scheme, proposed by the Osteoarthritis Biomarkers Network Consortium, is designed to characterize OA biomarkers.

THE PAIN OF OSTEOARTHRITIS

Pain is the clinical symptom most frequently associated with OA.[80] The clinical manifestation of this pain is lameness. When an animal presents with clinical lameness, a determination must be made whether the animal is unable to use the limb, or is unwilling to use the limb. Inability to use the limb may be attributable to musculoskeletal changes, such as joint contracture or muscle atrophy. These anomalies are best addressed with physical rehabilitation. On the other hand, unwillingness to use a limb is most often attributable to pain. Herein, lameness is an avoidance behavior.

Ironically, articular cartilage is frequently the focus of studies in OA. However, clinical treatment of the OA patient is most often focused on the alleviation of pain. Appreciating that articular cartilage is aneural, the focus of OA pain management resides in the pathophysiology of periarticular structures. No pain is elicited by stimulation of cartilage, and stimulation of normal synovial tissue rarely evokes pain.[81]

NOCICEPTORS

The major sources of clinical pain in deep tissues such as joint structures are inflammatory disease, trauma, overload, and degenerative diseases. Joint structures and muscles are innervated by nociceptors that are mostly activated under normal conditions by nonphysiological painful stimuli such as overload, twisting, strong pressure, and ischemic contraction, which may cause deep structure damage. Most joint nociceptors are chemosensitive for inflammatory mediators such as bradykinin and PGs, and in the presence of inflammation, joint and muscle nociceptors show pronounced sensitization to mechanical stimuli. There are two types of second-order dorsal horn neurons, nociceptive-specific and WDR neurons (see Chapter 1).[82] WDR neurons respond to various stimuli, whereas nociceptive-specific neurons respond only to noxious stimuli. Spinal cord neurons processing nociceptive input from joint and muscle are often convergent with inputs from skin and other deep tissue (85). During inflammation in muscle and joint, these convergent spinal cord neurons develop pronounced hyperexcitability, with enhanced mechanical stimulation from different foci and an expansion of the receptive field. Accordingly, these neurons are under strong descending inhibition as well.

Although there is considerable sensory information transmitted from muscle and joint, most involves the sense of movement and position, evading consciousness. Pain in the normal joint is commonly elicited by twisting or traumatizing the joint. Clearly, the processing of nociceptive inputs from deep tissues of muscle and joint differs from the processing of inputs from cutaneous structures.[83]

JOINT AFFERENTS

Typical joint nerves contain thick myelinated Aβ, thinly myelinated Aδ, and a high proportion (~80%) of unmyelinated C fibers. Articular Aβ fibers terminate as corpuscular endings in fibrous capsule, articular ligaments, menisci, and adjacent periosteum. Articular Aδ and C fibers terminate as noncorpuscular or free nerve endings in the fibrous capsule, adipose tissue, ligaments, menisci, and the periosteum.[84] Within muscle, most of these endings are located in the wall of arterioles in the muscle belly and surrounding connective tissue.[85] The major neuropeptides in joint and muscle nerves are sP, CGRP, and somatostatin, although these neuropeptides are not specific for deep afferents.

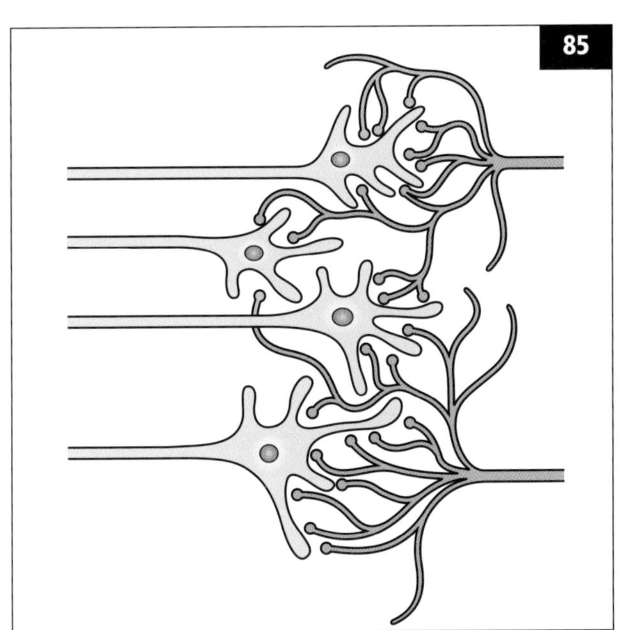

85 The CNS is made up of hundreds to thousands of neuronal pools. Each input fiber (right) divides thousands of times, spreading over a large area in the pool to synapse with dendrites or cell bodies of neurons (left) in the pool. Each input fiber arborizes such that large numbers of its synaptic knobs lie on the centermost neurons in its 'field', while fewer lie on adjacent neurons. Therefore, an input stimulus can be either an excitatory stimulus (threshold stimulus) or a subthreshold stimulus to a neuron, depending upon the required knobs needed for stimulation. A neuron made more excitable, but not to the point of discharge, is said to be *facilitated*, and can reach threshold when complemented by input from other input fibers. Subthreshold stimuli can *converge* from several sources and *summate* at a neuron to cause an excitatory stimulus.

86 Sensory receptors are end organs of afferent nerves and belong to one of two main physiological groups: 1) exteroceptors, which detect stimuli that arise external to the body; and 2) interoceptors, which detect stimuli that are within the body. Proprioceptors are a special class of interoceptors that signal conditions deep within the body to the CNS. Proprioceptors are located in skeletal muscles, tendons, ligaments, and joint capsules. Free nerve endings act as thermoreceptors and nociceptors (pain). Merkel endings are pressure-sensitive touch receptors. Pacinian corpusles respond to pressure and are widely distributed throughout the dermis and subcutaneous tissue, joint capsules, and other pressure sites. Meissner corpuscles are highly sensitive to touch. Ruffini corpuscles in subcutaneous connective tissue respond to tension. Krause end bulbs are cold sensitive. See also ***Table 14***.

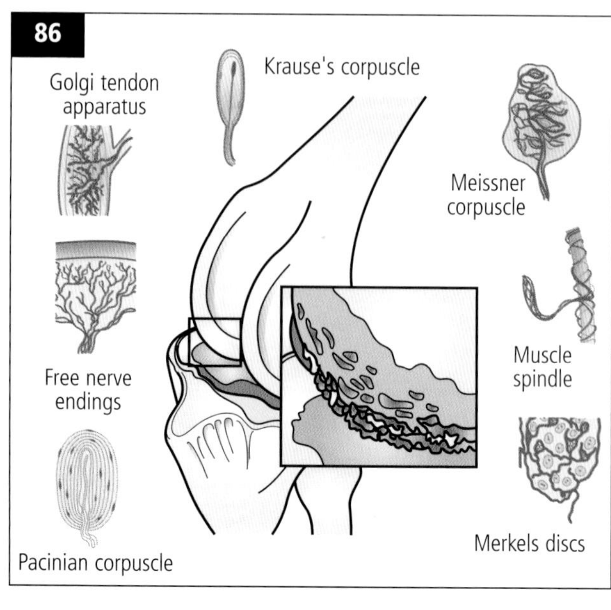

Table 14 Classification of articular receptor systems. See also 86.

Type	Morphology	Location	Parent nerve fibers	Behavioral characteristics
I	Thinly encapsulated globular corpuscles (100 μm × 40 μm), in clusters of three to six corpuscles	Fibrous capsule of joint (mainly superficial layers)	Small myelinated (6–9 μm)	Static and dynamic mechanoreceptors; low threshold, slowly adapting
II	Thickly encapsulated conical corpuscles (280 μm × 120 μm), in clusters of two to four corpuscles	Fibrous capsule of joint (mainly deeper layers). Articular fat pads	Medium myelinated (9–12 μm)	Dynamic mechanoreceptors; low threshold, rapidly adapting
III	Thinly encapsulated fusiform corpuscles (600 μm × 100 μm)	Joint ligaments (intrinsic and extrinsic)	Large myelinated (13–17 μm)	Dynamic mechanoreceptors; high threshold, very slowly adapting
IV	Plexuses and free nerve endings	Fibrous capsule. Articular fat pads. Ligaments. Walls of blood vessels	Very small myelinated (2–5 μm) Unmyelinated (<2 μm)	Pain receptors; high threshold,nonadapting

Wyke[86] has described four types of sensory receptors associated with joints (**86**, *Table 14*). Located in the joint capsule, type I and II receptors respond to mechanical stimuli such as pressure or tension, and are therefore known as mechanoreceptors. Type I and II receptors are located in the superficial layers and deep layers of the capsule, respectively, and rapidly transmit information via myelinated fibers. Type II (mostly Aβ) receptors are more rapidly adapting, thereby serving a more dynamic function than the slowly adapting type I receptors.[76] In combination with other receptors in the muscle and skin, type I and II receptors allow recognition of limb and joint orientation in space.[87] Type III receptors are not actually in the joint, but are found on the surface of ligaments.

They are associated with large myelinated afferent (Aα) fibers, allowing rapid transmission, and are inactive during normal joint activity. Type III receptors become active when a strong mechanical stimulus threatens damage.[76]

In contrast to type I and II mechanoreceptors, type IV receptors are high-threshold, slowly adaptive, polymodal free nerve endings. These receptors also respond to thermal and chemical stimuli associated with inflammation. They are typically stimulated by tension and pressure. Therefore, they play a major role in discomfort associated with increased intra-articular pressure of motion, increased synovial fluid volume seen in chronic OA and cruciate ligament rupture patients, and a relative increase due to decreased atmospheric pressure associated with weather changes. These receptors also respond to subluxation of the joint, causing tension in or pressure on the joint capsule. Type IV receptors are found in all joint tissues, including subchondral bone, but not cartilage, which is aneural. Afferent signaling from type IV receptors is via thinly myelinated Aδ or unmyelinated C fibers.[76] Some type IV receptors are considered to be silent nociceptors,[88] contributing to central sensitization.

Joint afferents have been best described in cat and rat stifle and tarsus joints, revealing proportions of different fibers in different sensitivity classes (**87**).

Many low-threshold Aβ and Aδ fibers in the fibrous capsule and in ligaments, including the anterior cruciate ligament, fire in the innocuous range, but they have their strongest response in the noxious range.[89] An additional group of sensory neurons is mechanoinsensitive under normal conditions, but becomes mechanosensitive during inflammation: silent nociceptors. The mechanosensitivity of these afferents, changes during

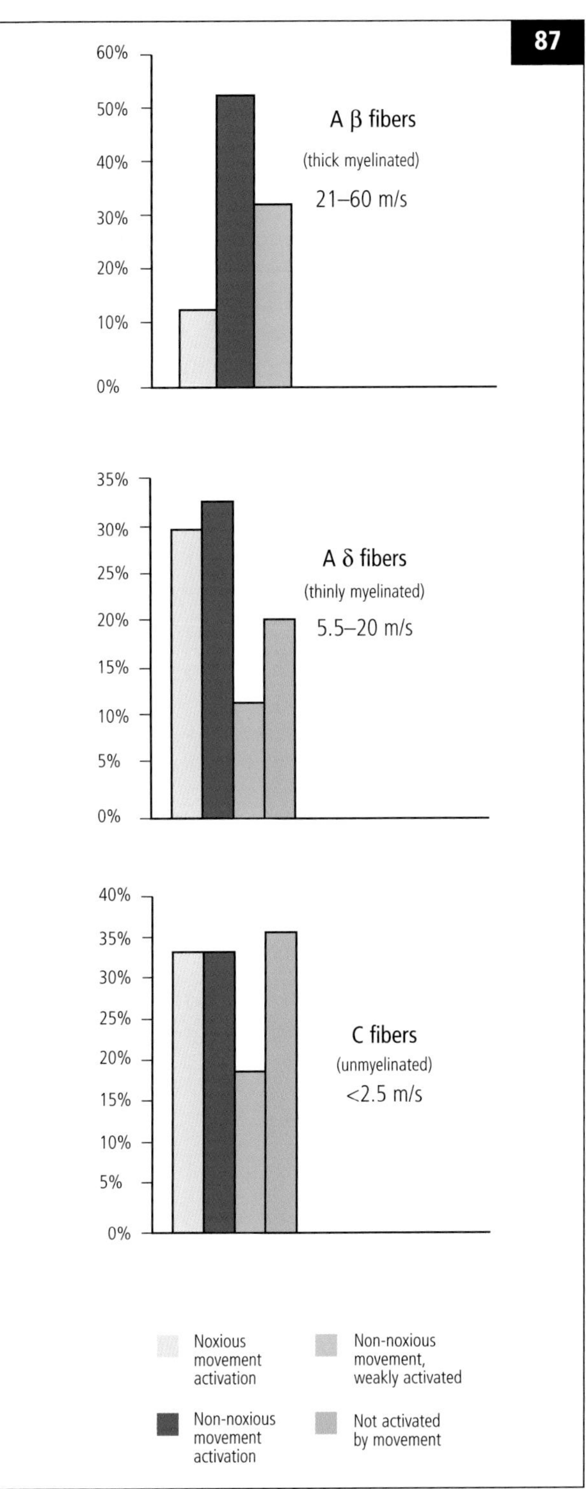

87 Mechanosensitivity of primary afferent neurons supplying normal cats' stifle joint. The bar graphs show the proportion of fiber types in the different sensitivity classes.[73]

inflammation of the joint. Many low-threshold Aδ and C fibers, as well as a large proportion of high-threshold afferents, respond to movements in the working range of the joint. Noteworthy is the recruitment of silent nociceptors for mechanosensitivity, encoding for noxious events during an inflammatory process.[90]

INFLAMMATORY MEDIATORS

A large proportion of Aδ and C fibers express receptors for endogenous compounds associated with pathophysiological conditions (*Table 15*). The classical inflammatory mediators, bradykinin, PGE_2 and PGI_2, and serotonin, excite joint afferents and sensitize them to mechanical stimuli. Such mediators affect Aδ and C fibers, but not Aβ fibers. Although each mediator has its own profile of effect, they can interact and yield synergistic responses.[92]

CONVERGENCE MAY AMPLIFY AFFERENT NOCICEPTION

Nociceptive information from joint and muscle, which is transmitted to neurons in the superficial and deep dorsal horn, is processed either from exclusively deep tissue input or neurons that exhibit convergent inputs from skin and deep structures. Some neurons may also input convergence from the viscera. Neurons exclusively driven from deep tissue often include receptive fields of the joint and adjacent muscle. Some convergent neurons are excited by mechanical stimuli applied to deep tissue (muscle, tendons, joint structures) and by mechanical stimulation of the skin.

NEUROGENIC INFLAMMATION

Once a stimulus is received by the second-order neuron in the dorsal spinal horn, an ascending signal

Table 15 Chemosensitivity of Aδ and C fibers from normal joints.

Mediator	Resting activity	Mechanosensitivity	Source
Bradykinin	⇑	⇑	91, 92, 93
Prostaglandin E_2	⇑	⇑	93, 94, 95, 96
Prostaglandin I_2	⇓	⇓	93, 95, 96, 97, 98
Serotonin	⇑	⇑	99, 100
Capsaicin/anandamide	⇓		101, 102
NO	⇓		103
ATP	⇑		104, 105
Adenosine	⇑		105
Substance P	(⇑) ⇓		106, 107
NK2 receptor agonist			108
Somatostatin		⇓	109
Galanin		⇑ ⇓	110
Neuropeptide Y	⇑	⇑ ⇓	111
Nociceptin		⇑ ⇓	112

is sent to the third-order neuron in the brain and a reflex arc back to the joint may also be initiated. The reflex arc may result in stimulation of muscles surrounding the joint and/or neurogenic inflammation (88).

Release of sP and NGF into the periphery causes the tissue reaction termed neurogenic inflammation. Neurogenic inflammation is driven by events in the CNS and does not depend on granulocytes or lymphocytes as with the classic inflammatory response to tissue trauma or immune-mediated cell damage. Cells in the dorsal horn release chemicals that cause action potentials to fire backwards down the nociceptors. The result of this dorsal root reflex is that nociceptive dendrites release sP and CGRP into peripheral tissues, causing degranulation of mast cells and changing vascular endothelial cell characteristics. The resultant outpouring of potent inflammatory and vasodilatating agents causes edema and potentiates transmission of nociceptive signals from the periphery.

CENTRAL SENSITIZATION AT THE DORSAL HORN

Central sensitization refers to chronic activation of primary afferent C fibers resulting in increased excitability of neurons in the spinal cord. A consequence of central sensitization is an increase in the magnitude of the response of postsynaptic ascending spinal neurons to noxious stimuli and increased response to low-threshold stimuli such as those arising from Aβ fibers, normally conveying information such as position and stress. Consistent with this phenomenon is expansion of the receptive field, explaining why tissues surrounding the joint are sensitive to stimuli. For example, an affected joint may show increased sensitivity to flexion and extension, but will also show sensitivity to light touch, and with an exaggerated response. This painful response to what would normally be an innocuous stimulus is termed allodynia. Allodynia is, in fact, an extreme left shift in the pain–response curve (89). (See Chapter 1 for further discussion and explanation.)

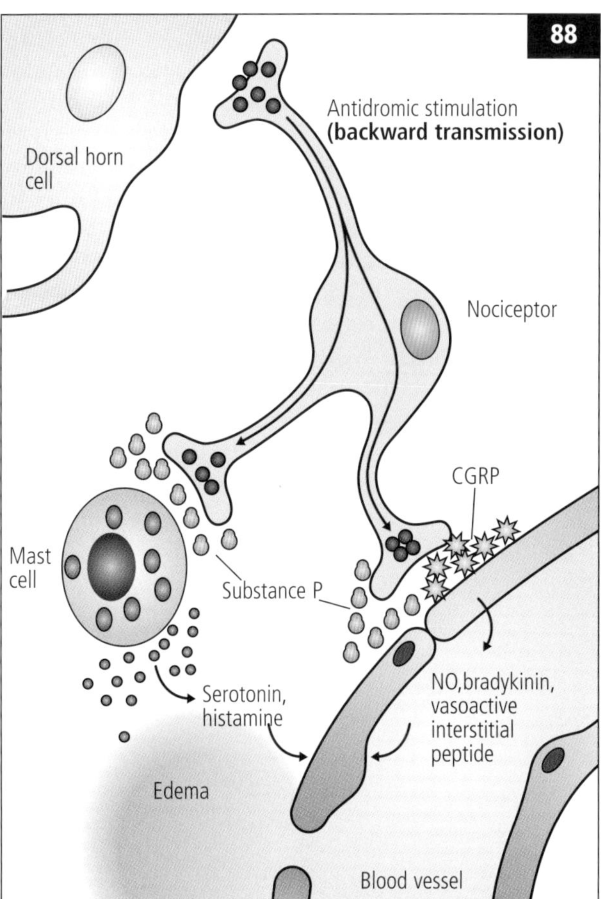

88 Neurogenic inflammation.

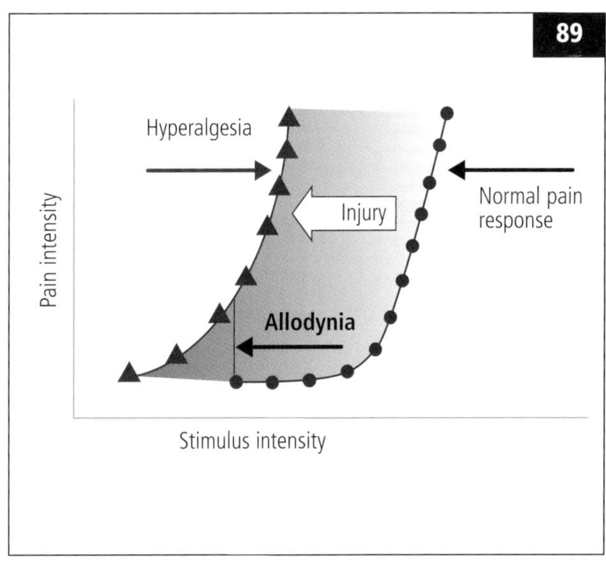

89 Allodynia is an extreme left shift in the pain–response curve.

During joint or muscle inflammation, spinal cord neurons receiving deep tissue input develop a state of hyperexcitability, contributing to central sensitization (**90, 91**). Mense[113] has illustrated the process of central sensitization from input of the stifle. Initially, the monitored spinal cord neuron responded only to noxious pressure applied to the stifle and adjacent muscles. Response to noxious compression of the stifle increased markedly after induction of inflammation by injection of kaolin and carrageenan into the stifle joint. Within 1 hour, the receptive field expanded from the knee, such that the neuron responded to pressure applied to the tarsus and paw, and the previously high-threshold neuron was now activated by gentle innocuous pressure.

Muscle fatigue and muscle spasm are often seen as a contributing cause or resultant feature of OA,[114] and are frequently associated with pain and disability.[115] Spasm can be part of the reflex arc neuroreceptor stimulation. Muscle soreness may also be a consequence of abnormal biomechanics across an arthritic joint.

ROLE OF MUSCLE FATIGUE AND SPASM

Spinal cord neuron central sensitization from muscle input appears to be similar to that of deep joint tissue. The population of neurons responding to stimulation of muscle expands during inflammation. Studies have shown the neurons in segments L3–6 of the cat are increased from normal in the inflamed muscle. It can be concluded that many synapses are too weak to activate the neuron under normal conditions, however these synapses are effective once the neuron becomes hyperexcitable. It has been proposed that

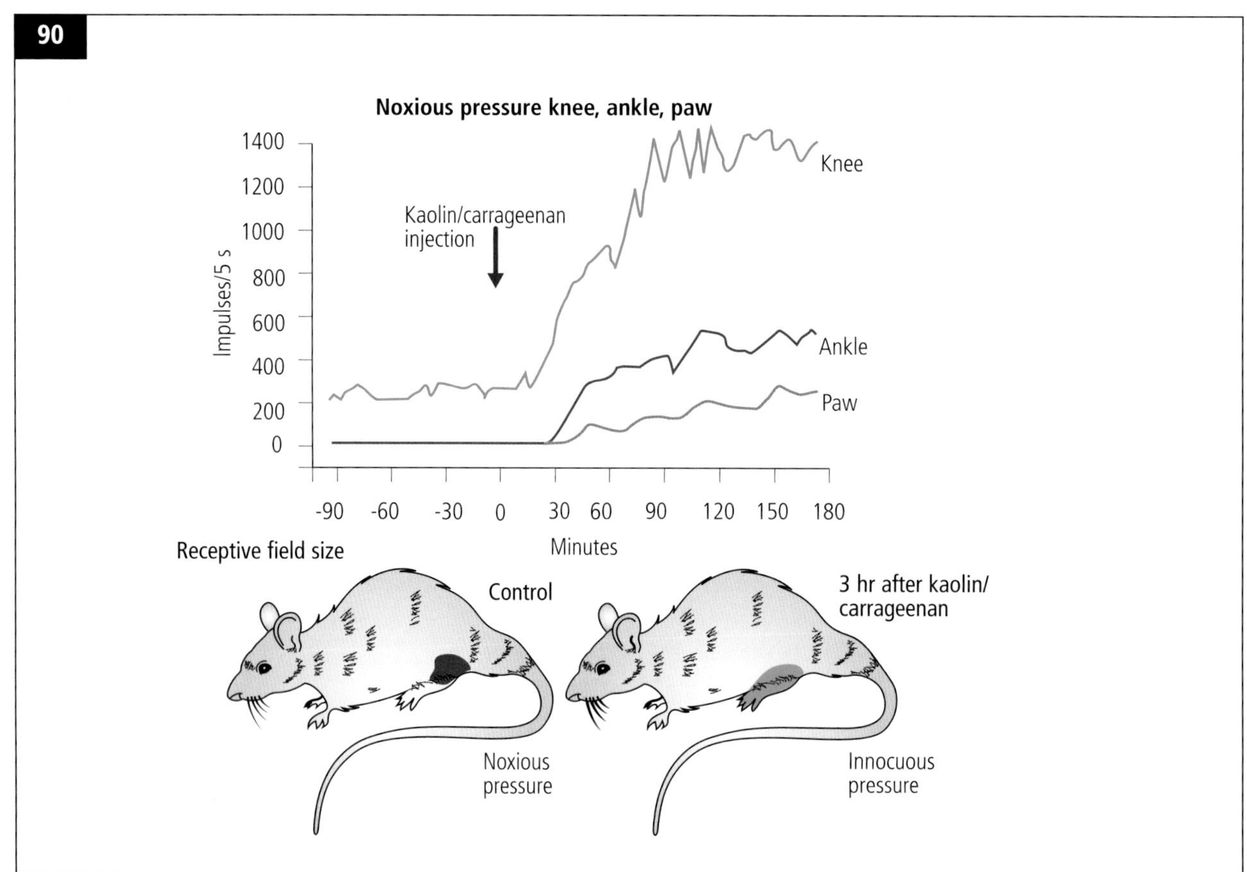

90 Development of a spinal cord neuron hyperexcitability. Histogram shows spinal cord neuron response to noxious pressure applied to the knee, ankle, and paw before and after the injection of kaolin and carrageenan into the knee joint. Shaded areas on the animal show the receptive field of the neuron before and during knee joint inflammation.[113]

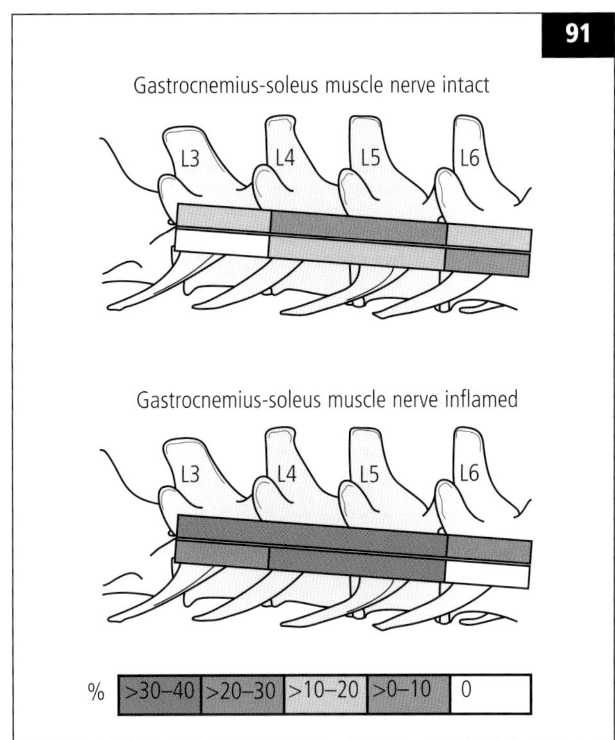

91 Proportion of spinal cord neurons that respond to gastrocnemius-soleus muscle electrical nerve stimulation in the normal and inflamed state.[113]

such spinal cord changes account for pronounced forms of referred pain from noxious stimulation of deep tissue in humans.[116] Central sensitization can persist during chronic inflammation and deep input is particularly able to induce long-term changes in the nociceptive system. Spinal sensitization is also enhanced by upregulation of transmitters and mediators of synaptic activity. The intraspinal release of glutamate is enhanced in joint inflammation, and antagonists of both the AMPA/kinase and NMDA receptors prevent the development of hyperexcitability and can reduce responses of the neurons to mechanical stimulation of the joint after inflammation is established.[117] Inflammation of the joint also impacts on the release of neuropeptides. Under inflammatory conditions a cocktail of transmitters and modulators such as sP, neurokinin A, and CGRP is released in large quantities that contribute to synaptic processing,[118] likely opening synaptic pathways such that more neurons respond to stimulation.[82] PGE_2 is also released within the dorsal and ventral horns during joint inflammation, likely a result from upregulation of spinal COX-2, seen within 3 hours after induction of knee joint inflammation.[119]

OSTEOARTHRITIS AND JOINT INSTABILITY

DJD can, simplistically, be identified as consequential sequelae to cartilage degeneration and the persistent trigger from instability of a joint. Surgically induced instability models of OA have been described in various animal species. Humans with a traumatic injury generally decrease use of the affected limb until restabilization has occurred. In animals, where restabilization has not occurred, the disease progression is usually much more rapid, making it much less amenable to therapeutic intervention.[120,121] Surgically induced models of OA, especially in rodents and rabbits, usually have rapid and severe cartilage degeneration after the instability is created, and generally, the greater the instability, the greater the lesion.[122] Surgical instability models of OA have been performed in rats, guinea pigs, rabbits, sheep, goats, and dogs.[123–126]

The most frequently described canine model of OA-related joint degeneration is the cranial cruciate ligament transection (CCLT) model. In the CCLT model, joint instability is the driving force in the development of degenerative features. Joint degeneration, as a result of acutely altered biomechanics, is perpetuated by inflammatory responses. These responses are secondary to the inflammation from poor resistance to shear mechanical stress of hyaline cartilage and due to the ligament endings in the joint, triggering an inflammatory response.[127–129] In 53–74% of CCLT dogs, medial meniscal damage occurs,[130] which, itself, is a driving force of joint degeneration modeling.[131] Accordingly, the combination of CCLT and meniscal damage constitutes a robust destabilizing drive for development of OA.[132] In the CCLT model, permanent instability in the knee joint is followed by degenerative changes in cartilage and changes in synovial tissue (representing secondary synovitis) that, over the course of several years, leads to canine OA.[128] Separating the two etiologies (instability and cartilage damage), the canine 'groove' model of OA has been proposed to exclude the influence of instability.[133]

Though not objectively evaluated, it has long been assumed that capsular thickening in a cranial cruciate ligament (CCL)-deficient canine knee functions to stabilize the joint over time.[134–136] The goal of reconstructive surgical methods should be not only to alleviate the existing instability of the unstable stifle joint, but also to mimic normal kinematics as closely as possible. Extracapsular suture techniques provide stifle joint stability through static neutralization of cranial drawer without alteration of stifle joint anatomy.[137] The tibial plateau leveling osteotomy has been used to provide dynamic stability to the stifle joint by alteration of the tibial plateau angle.[138] Recently, the tibial tuberosity advancement technique has been proposed to stabilize the stifle joint during weightbearing by neutralizing cranial tibial thrust.[139,140]

Studies indicate that passive hip joint laxity is the primary risk factor for development of DJD in dogs with hip dysplasia.[141,142] It is hypothesized that, in some dogs, passive joint laxity is transformed into functional laxity during weightbearing, thereby exposing the cartilaginous surfaces of the joint to excessive stresses. Such stresses cause cartilage damage and microfracture, release of inflammatory mediators, and, ultimately, the changes associated with DJD. Functional laxity appears to be both necessary and sufficient for the development of DJD.[143] Surgical management for hip dysplasia may involve corrective osteotomies or arthroplasty techniques, all designed to improve joint congruency and stability. Total hip arthroplasty may be performed in adult dogs with chronically painful hips that cannot be treated satisfactorily by other methods.

As with the knee and hip, instability is considered a primary etiological factor in elbow dysplasia.[144] Elbow incongruity is the term to describe poor alignment of the elbow joint surfaces. Two illustrative features are: (1) an abnormal shape of the ulnar trochlear notch, and (2) a step between the radius and ulna, caused by either a short radius or a short ulna. The suggestion is that both an elliptical notch and a step can cause increased local pressure within the joint, resulting in fragmentation at different locations, clinically recognized as ununited anconeal process, fragmented coronoid process, and osteochondrosis dissecans of the humeral condyle. Collectively, these lesions are referred to as 'elbow dysplasia'. Several surgical techniques have been proposed, and are currently under development to restore joint congruity and improve function.[145] It is proposed that incongruity worsens the prognosis after surgery to remove loose fragments,[146] accounting for 30–40% of postoperative patients still showing lameness.

SURGICAL INTERVENTION

It must be recognized that surgical intervention is necessary for some patients. Surgery most often involves extraction of inciting causes (e.g. ununited anconeal process, fragmented coronoid, joint mouse osteophytes, osteochondrosis dissecans lesions) and/or attempts to stabilize an affected joint. Clear indications for surgery include, but are not limited to:

- Cruciate ligament deficient stifle and/or meniscal tears.
- Symptomatic medial or lateral patellar luxation.
- Fragmented medial coronoid process and ununited anconeal process.
- Hip dysplasia that is nonresponsive to 'conservative management'.
- End stage: tarsal or carpal disease, stifle disease, hip disease, and elbow disease.
- Chronic shoulder luxation.
- Osteochondrosis dissecans lesions.

SUMMARY

The pain associated with OA results from a complex dynamic interaction of the musculoskeletal and nervous systems. Pain relief involves strategies for restoration of mechanical integrity, suppression of peripheral inflammation, and exogenous modulation of neurotransmission. This mandates a multimodal approach.

3 PATHOPHYSIOLOGY OF CANCER PAIN

IN PERSPECTIVE

The word *cancer* means 'crab' and was given to the disease because of its tenacity, a singular ability to cling to its victim like a crab's claws clinging to its prey. The all-important reality of cancer pain is witnessed in John Steinbeck's book, *The Grapes of Wrath*, where the character Mrs. Wilson, who is dying of cancer, states, 'I'm jus' pain covered in skin.'

Frank Vertosick, MD, states, 'From the Darwinian point of view, cancer is an unimportant disease. Since it preferentially afflicts animals beyond their child-bearing years, cancer poses no threat to animals in the wild, since natural populations experience death in other ways long before they are old enough for cancer to be a concern. We feel the sting of advanced prostate cancer because we are fortunate enough to live into our seventh decade and beyond, a feat rarely achieved even a hundred years ago. During the evolution of the nervous system, we developed pain to help us heal reversible insults: cracked vertebrae, pinched nerves, temporarily blocked colons, broken legs. To our great sorrow, this same pain also works against us when irreversible diseases like cancer strike; consequently, death becomes a painful affair. We die with all of our pain alarms impotently sounding. It is said that we are all born in another's pain and destined to die in our own.'[1]

TAXONOMY

In 1994 the International Association for the Study of Pain (IASP) revised a classification for chronic pain.[2] This classification includes five axes:

- Location of the pain.
- Involved organ or tissue system.
- Temporal pattern of pain.
- Pain intensity and time since onset of pain.
- Etiology of pain.

A distinct group of syndromes, therapies, and other etiologies of pain occur in cancer patients[3] such that neither the IASP nor any other diagnostic scheme distinguishes cancer pain from nonmalignant causes of chronic pain. Because the classification of cancer pain may have important diagnostic and therapeutic implications, a promising concept is a mechanism-based treatment approach, determining the sequence of analgesic agents based on the underlying etiopathology of cancer pain.

SCHEMES FOR CLASSIFYING CANCER PAIN

See *Table 16 (overleaf)*.

Etiological classification

Four different etiologies of cancer pain are:

- That directly produced by the tumor.
- That due to the various treatment modalities.
- That related to chronic debility.
- That due to unrelated, concurrent disease processes.[4]

Identification of these etiologies is important, as they reflect distinct treatment options and prognoses.

A tumor may compress a nerve fiber (**92**). Pain relief from debulking tumors suggests that mechanical distortion is a component of tumor pain.

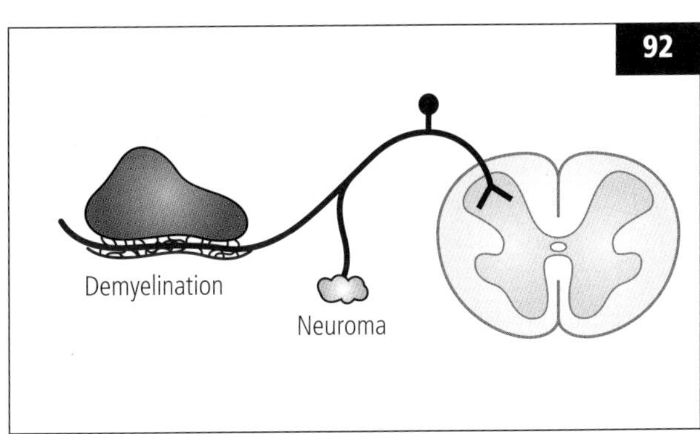

92 Tumors may compress a nerve fiber.

Table 16 Classifications for cancer pain.

Etiological classification	Primarily caused by cancer Treatment of malignancy Debility Concurrent pathology
Pathophysiological classification	Nociceptive (somatic, visceral) Neuropathic Mixed pathophysiology
Location of cancer pain syndromes	Head and neck Chest Vertebral and radicular pain Abdominal or pelvic Extremity
Temporal classification	Acute Breakthrough Chronic
Severity-based classification	Mild Moderate Severe

Compression of a peripheral nerve can cause local demyelination, Wallerian degeneration of the nerve, secondary axon sprouting, and neuroma formation. Physiological studies have demonstrated that DRG compression can initiate a continuous afferent barrage that becomes self-sustaining.

When tumors are identified as a foreign body, they can give rise to paraneoplastic neuropathy (93). It is postulated that expression of onconeuronal antigens by cancer cells results in an autoimmunity. When the tumor develops, the body produces antibodies to fight it, by binding to and helping the destruction of tumor cells. Such antibodies may cross-react with epitopes on normal nervous tissue, resulting in an attack on the nervous system.

Neoplasms of the spinal cord may be either intramedullary or extramedullary, and primary tumors affecting the paravertebral area may spread and compress the cord, particularly within the intervertebral foramina (94). An enlarging cancerous lymph node can compress the cord, and cancer that metastasizes to the vertebrae or surrounding tissues may also cause spinal cord compression.

Pain-generating mediators are often released from certain tumors or from surrounding tissues involving invasion or metastasis, thereby producing pain itself.[5] Paradoxically, various cancer therapies may result in

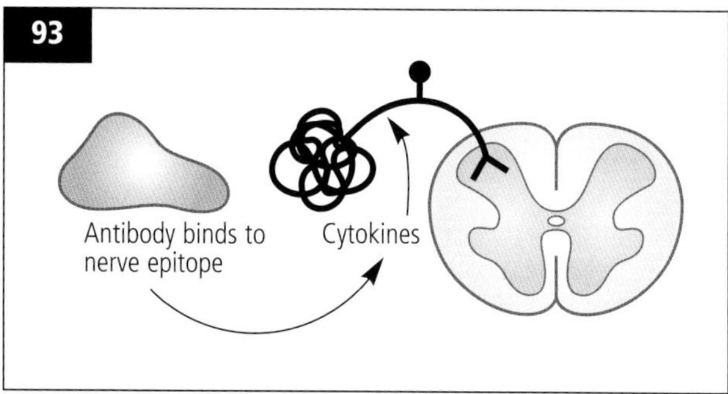

93 A paraneoplastic neuropathy can arise from tumors recognized as a foreign body.

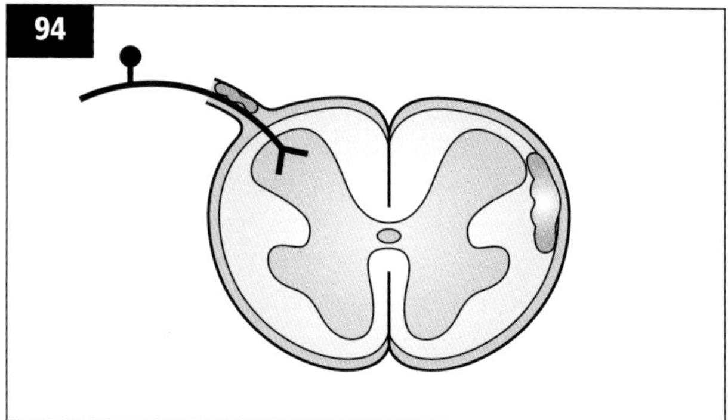

94 Spinal cord neoplasms may be intramedullary or extramedullary.

pain. Chemotherapeutic agents have been associated with peripheral neuropathies and acute pain in humans,[6] and radiation therapy may injure soft tissue or neuronal structures. Furthermore, immunosuppressive therapy may render some patients at increased risk for secondary infection and complications.

Although the inclusion of psychogenic pain in animals is controversial, nociceptive and neuropathic types of cancer pain are recognized. Stimulated afferent nociceptive pathways in visceral or somatic tissue lead to nociceptive pain. Neuropathic pain is caused by dysfunction of, or lesions involving, the PNS or CNS. Differentiating the two may influence the selection of a specific therapy. Nociceptive somatic cancer pain arises from soft tissue structures that are non-neurological and nonvisceral in origin, including skin, muscle, bone, and joints, and often correlates with the extent of tissue damage. Nociceptive visceral cancer pain arises from the deep organs of the abdomen, thorax or pelvis, and is often difficult to localize. Obstruction of hollow viscera, distension of organ walls, stretching of the pancreas or liver capsule, or extension of metastasis into mesentery may induce visceral pain.

Neuropathic cancer pain

Neuropathic pain affects the nervous system, and may have multiple etiologies, including nerve compression, deafferentation injury, and sympathetically induced origin.[7] Nerve compression has been identified as the most common cause of neuropathic pain in human cancer patients (79%), followed by nerve injury (16%) and sympathetically mediated pain (5%).[8] Neuropathic pain is considered to be relatively less responsive to opioids.[9] Nonopioid adjuncts such as antiepileptic, antidepressant, and antiarrhythmic agents or combinations of these should be considered.[10,11]

Noteworthy pain and neurological deficits result from tumor infiltration or compression of the PNS. This may include infiltration of spinal nerve roots, producing radicular symptoms, and invasion of neuronal plexuses. Such invasion or compression may involve a perineural inflammatory reaction that accentuates the nerve pain.[12] Degenerative changes and deafferentation are consequences of prolonged tumor infiltration or compression.[13] Resultant peripheral sensitization is associated with an increased density of sodium channels in the damaged axons and associated DRG.[14] Ectopic foci of electrical activity arise in injured axons and stimulus thresholds are decreased. Activated peripheral nociceptors release mediators for central sensitization, i.e. the amino acid glutamate and neuropeptides, such as sP and neurokinin A. In turn, these neurotransmitters cause an increase of intracellular calcium and upregulation of NMDA receptors. Associated with this increased intracellular calcium is activation of enzymatic reactions causing expression of genes that ultimately lower the excitatory threshold of dorsal horn neurons, exaggerate their response to noxious stimuli, and enlarge the size of their receptor fields (secondary peripheral sensitization).

Sympathetically dependent cancer pain

Sympathetically mediated cancer pain may result from direct or indirect involvement of the sympathetic chain. This pain is perceived in alignment with the pattern of sympathetic–vascular innervation, rather than localization to the area of distribution for a specific peripheral nerve or dermatome.[5] Although pathophysiological classification of cancer pain is informative for treatment insight, one study in humans has shown that 70% of patients showed two or more pathophysiological classes of pain in the advanced stages of cancer.[15]

Anatomically based cancer pain

Anatomic classification of cancer pain has limited applications since it lacks specificity as to the mechanism of pain; however, it does provide guidance for certain invasive therapies such as external radiation, neurolytic blocks, electrical stimulation, or perhaps, targeted drug delivery.

Severity-based cancer pain

Severity-based classification of cancer pain reflects the extent of tissue destruction, size of the tumor or its location. In human patients, metastatic bone lesions and injury to nerves are typically more painful than soft tissue tumors. The severity of cancer pain is dynamic, reflecting the course of the disease and different therapies administered, therefore, it is prudent to review the severity of the pain over time.

THE WHO CANCER PAIN LADDER

In 1986 the World Health Organization (WHO) developed a simple three-stage analgesic ladder for treatment of cancer pain that relies on widely available and inexpensive analgesic agents.[16]

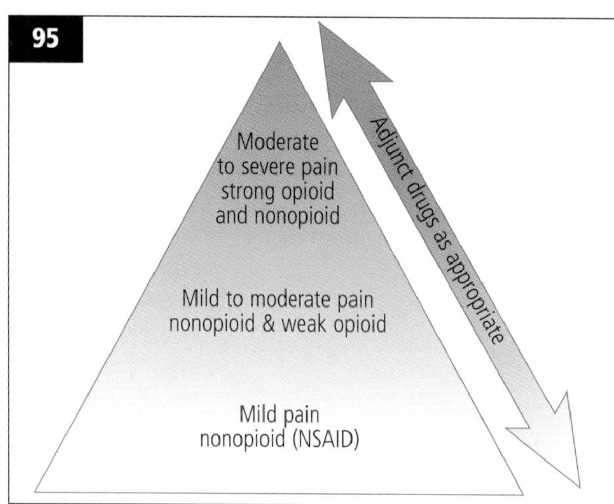

95 The World Health Organization (WHO) pain ladder was developed to give guidance for treating cancer pain in humans.

The WHO analgesic ladder provides clinical guidance from a severity-based pain classification system (95).

Although the quality of evidence for the WHO ladder approach has been challenged, it has been globally distributed and is considered the standard for cancer pain management in human patients. Contemporary thinking, however, is to use 'stronger' analgesics earlier.

MECHANISM-BASED TREATMENT

A mechanistic-based treatment strategy for managing cancer pain in humans has been studied,[15] i.e. neuropathic pain was treated with antidepressants and anticonvulsants, while opioids were integrated into the treatment protocol only after these drugs were considered ineffective. Interestingly, all human patients studied required concurrent therapy with a mean of three drug classes, including an opioid, to control their pain. This illustrates the heterogeneity of cancer pain mechanisms and the consequent value of a 'balanced or multimodal analgesia' approach to treatment.

PREVALENCE OF CANCER IN ANIMALS

The frequency of cancer pain in animals is difficult to identify as is the prevalence of cancer itself in the pet population. Not all cancers are painful, sensitivity to pain varies between individuals, and the degree of pain may vary during the course of the cancer. The most comprehensive effort to estimate cancer incidence rates was a survey of veterinary practices in Alameda and Contra Costa counties (California) from 1963–1966,[17] and remains as the seminal study for estimating the incidence of canine and feline cancers. See *Table 17*. This survey revealed an annual incidence rate of 381/100,000 among dogs living in households that used veterinary services, while the incidence rate for cancer in cats was 156/100,000.

Table 17 Annual crude incidence rates of cancer per 100,000 population for humans, dogs and cats, Alameda County, 1960–1966.[19]

Cancer site	Humans	Dogs	Cats
All sites	272.1	381.2	155.8
Skin, nonmelanoma	31.8	90.4	34.7
Malignant melanoma	8.3	25.0	ND
Digestive	74.5	25.2	11.2
Respiratory	32.9	8.5	5.0
Connective tissue	2.4	35.8	17.0
Mouth and pharynx	10.3	20.4	11.6
Breast	37.3	198.8	25.4
Lymphoid tumors	13.3	25.0	48.1
Bone	1.2	7.9	4.9
Testis	2.6	33.9	ND

Intuitively, these data are only estimates as not all cases of cancer are diagnosed equally, considering the many special procedures, diagnostic tests, and costs involved. In a study of 2002 dogs that underwent necropsy at the Angell Memorial Animal Hospital, cancer accounted for 20% of the deaths at 5 years and increased to over 40% in dogs 10 years of age.[18]

PREVALENCE OF ANIMAL CANCER PAIN

Currently, there are no estimates for the numbers of animals with cancer pain, and sparse data on the efficacy of various therapies. Cancer-related pain has been estimated to afflict 30–60% of human patients at the time of diagnosis and 55–95% of human patients during the advanced stages of disease.[20] Some authors have indicated that approximately 28% of human cancer patients die without adequate pain relief.[21] (Likely, this figure is less now than in 1984 when these data were published.) Several authors[22,23] have reported the under-use of perioperative analgesics, suggesting the likelihood that analgesic management of cancer pain in cats and dogs is quite low. Although inappropriate, under-treatment is not surprising since the medical profession (both human and veterinary) have historically been slow to administer analgesics. Reasons for this include:

- Under-utilization of clinical staff for assessing cancer pain during the course of the disease.
- Lack of good or validated methods for assessing animal pain.
- Failure to include the owner's input into their pet's ongoing assessment.
- Failure to appreciate the high frequency with which cancer patients experience pain.
- Lack of knowledge regarding analgesic therapies and the probable need to alter these therapies during the course of the cancer.

Considering that an overall average of about 70% of humans with advanced cancer suffer pain,[24] and that many biological systems are common between man and animals, a conservative estimate might be that 30% of animal cancers are painful.[25] As a rule, pain is more frequently associated with tumors arising in noncompliant tissue (e.g. bone) (*Table 18*).

Table 18 Tumors frequently associated with pain.

Tumor	Remarks
Bone	Noncompliant tissue tumors are typically painful
CNS	Tumors arising from neural tissue are not usually painful until late into the course of the disease. Extradural tumors are associated with pain
Cutaneous (invasive)	Ulcerative, invasive cutaneous tumors tend to be painful
Gastrointestinal	Distention of the esophagus, stomach, colon, and rectum are painful. Colonic and rectal pain often presents as perineal discomfort
Intranasal	Bone and turbinate destruction leads to pain
Intrathoracic and abdominal (e.g. mesothelioma, malignant histiocytosis)	Response to intracavity analgesics, such as local analgesics, suggests that these conditions are painful
Mammary carcinoma (inflammatory)	Dogs consistently show abnormal behavior considered to be pain-induced
Oral and pharyngeal	Soft tissue tumors of the pharynx and caudal oral cavity are particularly painful, perhaps due to constant irritation from eating. Soft tissue tumors of gingival origin are relatively nonpainful, but become very painful with invasion of bone
Prostate	Quite painful, particularly with bone metastasis
Surgery	Postoperative pain associated with tumor removal can be greater than anticipated, perhaps due to the presence of neuropathic pain

It should not be overlooked that some treatment therapies for cancer may create pain (*Table 19*).

CANCER PAIN ASSESSMENT IN ANIMALS

The assessment of cancer pain in animals is particularly challenging, and few reports have been made in this area. Yazbek and Fantoni[27] suggest that a simple questionnaire may be useful in assessing HRQL in dogs with pain secondary to cancer, in that dogs with cancer had significantly lower scores than did healthy dogs. A number of animal pain scales have been proposed (e.g. VAS, NRS, SDS, multifactorial pain scales (MFPS), and composite measure pain scales (CMPS)), however these are applied to the assessment of acute pain, where some are more valid than others. Physiological variables such as heart rate, respiratory rate, cortisol levels, temperature, and pupil size are unreliable measures for assessing acute pain[28,29] and behavioral changes are now considered the most reliable indicator of pain in animals.[30,31] Any change in an animal's normal behavior may be associated with pain. Herein lies the value of integrating the pet owner's observations into the patient's assessment on a continuum of follow-ups. In fact, some studies show that the owner was a better assessor of their animal's chronic pain than a veterinarian.

Certain behaviors are worth noting:

- Painful animals are less active.
- Animals in pain do not groom as frequently, especially cats.
- Dogs, in particular, may lick a painful area.

Table 19 Chemotherapy-induced dysfunction and pain syndromes (humans).[26]

Chemotherapeutic agent	Toxicity	Impact on pain
Vinca alkaloids (vincristin, vinblastin)	Neurological	Peripheral neuropathy, autonomic neuropathy
Paclitaxel/Docetaxel	Bone marrow depression, neurological	Neutropenia, mucositis
Platinum complexes (cisplatin, carboplatin)	Renal, bone marrow depression, neurological	Decrease creatinine clearance, peripheral neuropathy (cisplatin)
Ectoposide	Bone marrow depression	Leukopenia, thrombocytopenia, mucositis
Nitrogen mustards , (mechlorethamine, chlorambucil, cyclophosphamide, ifosfamide)	Bone marrow depression	Leukopenia, thrombocytopenia, hemorrhagic cystitis (cyclophosphamide)
Anthracycline antibiotics	Bone marrow suppression, cardiac	Leukopenia, thrombocytopenia/ anemia, stomatitis, cardiac arrhythmias, congestive heart failure
Mitoxanthrone	Bone marrow suppression	Mucositis
Cytarabine	Bone marrow suppression, neurological	Granulocytopenia/ thrombocytopenia, peripheral neuropathy
Methotrexate	Bone marrow suppression, renal	Pancytopenia, mucositis, chronic renal failure
Bleomycin	Pulmonary	Mucositis, lung fibrosis

- Both painful dogs and cats may show decreased appetites.
- Painful cats tend to seek seclusion.
- Dogs in pain tend not to yawn, stretch, or 'wet dog shake'.
- Animals in pain often posture differently.

One of the most reliable methods for identifying pain is the animal's response to analgesic intervention.

BONE CANCER MODEL

Periosteum, mineralized bone and bone marrow are highly innervated by Aβ, Aδ, and C fibers, all of which conduct sensory input from the periphery to the spinal cord (96). Recently, the first animal models of bone cancer pain have been developed. In the mouse femur model, bone cancer pain is induced by injecting murine osteocytic sarcoma cells into the intramedullary space of the femur. These tumor cells proliferate, and ongoing, movement-evoked, and mechanically evoked pain-related behaviors develop that increase in severity over time (97). These models have allowed elucidation of how cancer pain is generated and how the sensory information is processed when the molecular architecture of bone is changed by disease.

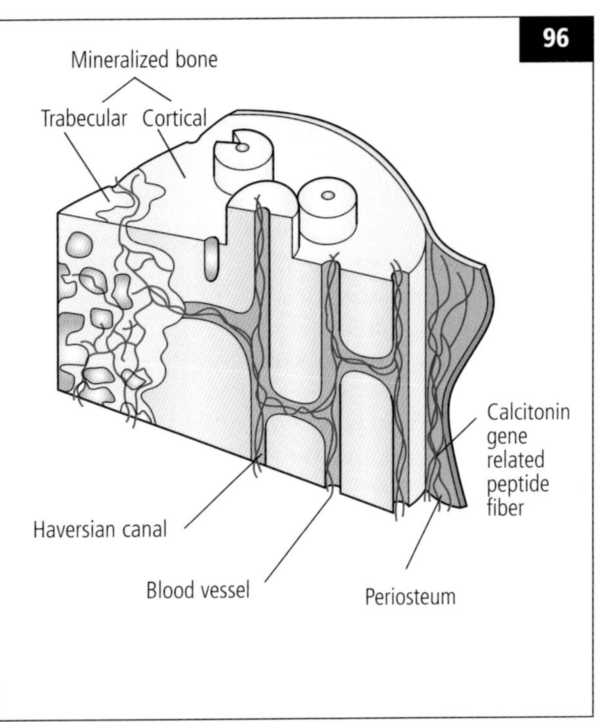

96 Bone marrow, mineralized bone, and periosteum are highly innervated, sending sensory input to the spinal cord.

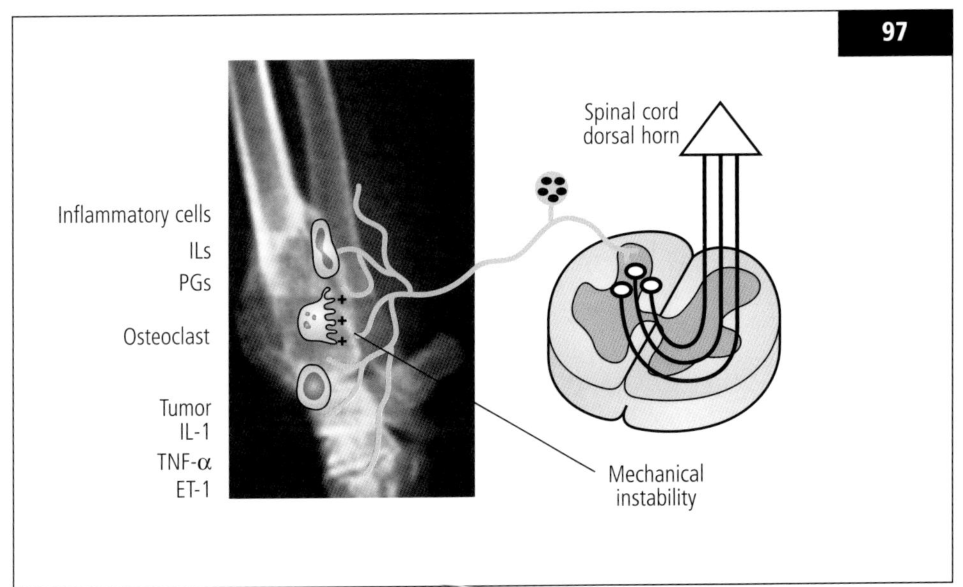

97 Bone cancer changes the molecular architecture and bioneurological status of the diseased bone. (ET-1 = endothelin-1)

AFFERENT SENSORY NEURONS

Primary afferent sensory neurons transfer sensory information to the spinal cord and brain. Most small diameter sensory fibers – unmyelinated C fibers and finely myelinated A fibers – are specialized sensory neurons called nociceptors that express a diverse repertoire of transduction molecules that sense different forms of noxious stimuli (thermal, mechanical, and chemical). To sense noxious chemical stimuli, nociceptors express an array of receptors capable of detecting inflammatory-related factors from damaged tissue, i.e. protons, endothelins, PGs, bradykinin, and NGF.

Sensory neurons are also highly 'plastic' – they can change their phenotype in response to a sustained peripheral injury. Altering patterns of signaling peptide and growth factor expression underlies peripheral sensitization, lowering the activation threshold and creating a state of hyperalgesia. Peripheral tissue damage also activates previously 'silent' nociceptors, which creates a state of hyperalgesia and allodynia.

In mice with bone cancer, normally nonpainful palpation of the affected femur induces the release of sP from primary afferent fibers that terminate in the spinal cord. sP in turn binds to and activates the neurokinin-1 receptor that is expressed by a subset of spinal cord neurons.[32] A similar activity is noted with *c-fos*.[33] Apparently, peripheral sensitization of nociceptors may be involved in the generation and maintenance of bone cancer pain.

NOCICEPTOR EXCITATION

Tumor and tumor-associated cells including macrophages, neutrophils, and T-lymphocytes secrete a wide variety of factors including PGs, endothelins, IL-1 and IL-6, epidermal growth factor, TGF, and platelet-derived growth factor, which directly excite primary afferent neurons. Each of these factors may play an important role in the generation of pain associated with various cancers. Pharmaceutical targeting of these factors provides opportunities for pain relief, while antiprostaglandin and antiendothelins are already commercially available.

Tumor-associated macrophages and several tumor cells express high levels of COX-2, producing large amounts of PGs.[34,35] Although all NSAIDs are antiprostaglandins, the new COX-2 inhibitors, or coxibs, preferentially inhibit COX-2 and avoid many of the COX-1 inhibition side-effects. Additionally, some experiments have suggested that COX-2 is involved in angiogenesis and tumor growth.[36,37] Although further research is required to characterize the effect of coxib-class NSAIDs on different types of cancer, in addition to blocking cancer pain, COX-2 inhibitors may have the added advantage of reducing the growth and metastasis of tumors.

A PubMed search for the terms NSAID and cancer conducted in February 2005 generated 7,513 abstracts. The same search conducted in December 2007 generated 9,624 abstracts. A similar search for the terms NSAID and COX-2 revealed 1,907 abstracts in February 2005, compared to 3,529 abstracts in December 2007. The role of NSAIDs, and particularly coxib-class NSAIDs, in cancer research is an area of intense interest.[38]

Canine patient tumors expressing COX-2 include:

- Transitional cell carcinoma.[39]
- Renal cell carcinoma.[40]
- Squamous cell carcinoma.[41]
- Prostate carcinoma.[42]
- Rectal polyps.[43]
- Nasal carcinoma.[44]
- Osteosarcoma.[45]
- Mammary carcinoma.[46]
- Intestinal adenocarcinoma.[43]
- Oral melanoma.[47]

In contrast to dogs, the absence of COX-2 expression in most feline neoplasms might suggest that COX-2 inhibitors would have a lower potential as anticancer agents in this species.[48]

The peptide endothelin-1 is another pharmacological target for treating cancer pain. A number of small unmyelinated primary afferents express receptors for endothelin,[49] and endothelins may well sensitize or excite nociceptors. Several tumors of humans, including prostate cancer, express high levels of endothelins,[50] and clinical studies have shown a correlation between the severity of the pain in human patients with prostate cancer and endothelin plasma levels.[51]

TUMOR-INDUCED LOCAL ACIDOSIS

Tumor burden often outgrows its vascular supply, becoming ischemic and undergoing apoptosis. Subsequently, an accumulation of acid metabolites prevails resulting in an acidotic local environment. This is relevant to cancer pain, in that subsets of sensory neurons have been shown to express different ASICs,[52] sensitive to protons or acidosis. Two major classes of ASICs expressed by nociceptors, both sensitive to decreases in pH, are TRPV1 and ASIC-3. As tumors grow and undergo apoptosis there is a local release of intracellular ions and inflammatory mediated protons that gives rise to a local acidic environment. This neurobiological mechanism is particularly relevant in bone cancer where there is a proliferation and hypertrophy of osteoclasts. Osteoclasts are multinucleated cells of the monocyte lineage that resorb bone by maintaining an extracellular microenvironment of acidic pH (4.0–5.0) at the interface between osteoclast and mineralized bone.[53] Experiments in mice have shown that osteoclasts contribute to the etiology of bone cancer pain,[54] and that osteoprotegerin[55] and a bisphosphonate,[55] both of which induce osteoclast apoptosis, are effective in decreasing osteoclast-induced cancer pain. TRPV1 or ASIC antagonists would act similarly, but by blocking excitation of acid-sensitive channels on sensory neurons.

GROWTH FACTORS FROM TUMOR CELLS

Different patients with the same cancer may have vastly different symptoms. Metastases to bone in the same individual may cause pain at one site, but not at a different site. Small cancer deposits in one location may be more painful than large cancers at an unrelated site. Why the variability? One explanation may be that changes in the periphery associated with inflammation, nerve injury, or tissue injury are reflected by changes in the phenotype of sensory neurons.[56] Such changes are, in part, caused by a change in tissue levels of several growth factors released from the local environment at the injury site, including NGFs[57] and GDNF.[58] Likely, the milieu of growth factors to which the sensory neuron is exposed will change as the developing tumor invades the tissue that the neuron innervates.

The murine sarcoma cell model has also demonstrated that growing tumor cells destroy both the hematopoietic cells of the marrow and the sensory fibers that normally innervate the marrow.[59] This neuronal damage can give rise to neuropathic pain. Gabapentin is a drug originally developed as an anticonvulsant, but is effective in treating several forms of neuropathic pain, and may be useful in treating cancer-induced neuropathic pain.[60]

Summarizing the contributors to bone cancer pain:

- Release of cytokines, PGs, and endothelins from hematopoietic, immune and tumor cells.
- Osteoclast activity $\Uparrow\Rightarrow$ lowered pH $\Rightarrow$ activation of TRPV1 and ASIC receptors.
- Bone erosion $\Rightarrow$ release of growth factors e.g. NGF.
- Tumor growth $\Rightarrow$ compression of afferent terminals.
- Neurochemical changes in DRG and spinal cord.

CENTRAL SENSITIZATION

If local neuropathic pain is a sequel to cancer, do the spinal cord and forebrain also undergo significant neurochemical changes? The murine cancer pain model revealed extensive neurochemical reorganization within the spinal cord segments receiving input from primary afferent neurons innervating cancerous bone.[61] Upregulation of the prohyperalgesic peptide, dynorphin, and astrocyte hypertrophy contribute to the state of central sensitization maintained by cancer pain.

THE MOVING TARGET OF CANCER PAIN

As the cancer progresses, changing factors may complicate the pain state. In the mouse model of bone cancer, as the tumor cells begin to proliferate, pain-related behaviors precede any noticeable bone destruction. This is attributed to prohyperalgesic factors, such as active nociceptor response in the marrow to PGs and endothelin released from growing tumor cells. At this point, pain might be attenuated by a coxib-class NSAID or endothelin antagonist. With continued tumor growth, sensory neurons innervating the marrow are compressed and destroyed, giving rise to neuropathic pain, possibly responsive to gabapentin. Once the tumor becomes invaded by osteoclastic activity, pain might be largely blocked by anti-osteoclastogenic drugs, such as bisphosphonates or osteoprotegerin. As the intramedullary space becomes filled with dying tumor cells, generating an acidic environment, TRPV1 or ASIC antagonists may attenuate the pain. In the later stages of bone destruction, antagonists to the mechanically gated channels and/or ATP receptors in the highly innervated periosteum may alleviate movement-evoked pain. This scenario illustrates how a mechanistic approach to designing more effective therapies for cancer pain should be created based on the understanding of how different stages of the disease impact on tumor cell influence on nociceptors, and how the phenotype of nociceptors and CNS neurons involved in nociceptive transmission changes during the course of advancing cancer.

Clearly, the mechanisms associated with cancer pain are complex. However, only through the understanding of these mechanisms can we best manage our patient's pain with evidence-based confidence. The murine bone cancer model has given us insights as to the progressing, dynamic neurobiological changes associated with cancer. These insights further lead us to the conclusion that effective treatment must be multimodal and dynamic.

VISCERAL CANCER PAIN

Many cancers involve internal organs and symptoms are silent until ischemia, compression, or obstruction reach a given stage, at which time visceral pain is manifest (98). Pain of visceral cancer origin can be divided into four groups:

- Acute mechanical stretch of visceral structures.
- Ischemia of visceral structures.
- Chemical stimuli from an infiltrating tumor or the body's reaction to infiltration.
- A compressive form of neuropathic pain that occurs due to direct invasion of nervous structures involving the viscera.

Visceral pain can also result from treatment damage of viscera and associated nerves from surgery, chemotherapy, or radiation.

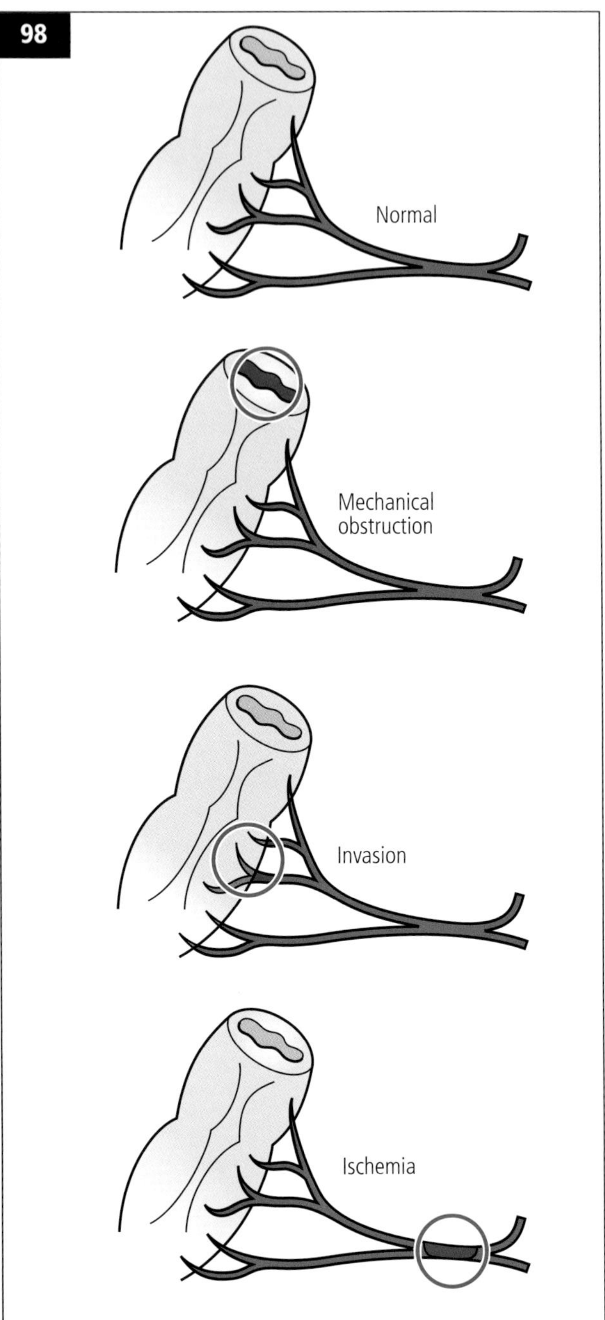

98 Cancer can disrupt normal visceral systems with resultant alterations that lead to pain.

CHEMOTHERAPY

Chemotherapy is a common treatment modality for cancer patients. Human cancer patients can complain of a wide range of cancer-related side-effects, such as pain, fatigue, depression, nausea, vomiting, diarrhea, constipation, cardiac arrhythmias, vascular and pulmonary toxicity, skin changes, mucositis, and sensory–motor disturbances.[62] Chemotherapy-induced peripheral neuropathy (CIPN) symptoms can present as pure sensory or motor disturbances, or as mixed sensory–motor neuropathy.[63] Cranial nerve neuropathy has been reported in humans treated with cisplatin or carboplatin.[64] Muscle pain is a symptom reported in human patients with CIPN, and is occasionally reported as muscle spasms. It is unclear if the cramps are a direct toxic effect of the antitumor agent on the muscle fiber or manifestations of a sensory neuropathy. To date there is no specific drug or method for prevention of CIPN.

CHEMOTHERAPEUTIC NEUROPATHIES

Several antitumor agents can lead to neuropathies.[63] Paclitaxel (taxol) has cytotoxic activity through its ability to interfere with microtubule function by inducing the polymerization of tubulin,[65] and induces peripheral neuropathy in a dose-dependent manner.[66] Platine-compound cytotoxic agents (e.g. cisplatin and carboplatin) also cause peripheral neuropathy in a dose-dependent manner in humans,[67] and apparently cisplatin is more neurotoxic than carboplatin.[68] The prevalence of platine-compound neuropathy is approximately 50% in human studies.[69] Vincristine is a microtubule-interfering agent that is administered to patients with hematological malignancies. The incidence of vincristine-induced peripheral neuropathy is between 50 and 100% in humans.[70] Ifosfamide is a cyclophosphamide-related drug with toxic effects on the CNS, and in humans these are manifest by hallucinations, confusion, and cranial nerve dysfunction.[71]

These are but a few of the cytotoxic drugs used to treat animals with cancer whose neuropathic toxic potential has been described in humans. Clinical manifestations of these drugs in veterinary patients may be more subtle or less severe since many animals undergo therapy for a shorter period of time than humans. Nevertheless, these neuropathic consequences from cytotoxic agents should be understood by the caregiver, and it should be appreciated that administration of two or more cytotoxic agents, which is a common practice, can aggravate or accelerate the induction of neuropathic manifestations.

RADIATION THERAPY

Radiation kills cells by causing irreversible DNA damage,[72] and there is a direct relationship between the amount of physical energy deposited, the degree of DNA damage, the number of cells killed, and the extent of tissue injury. Cell death by radiation is either by apoptosis or necrosis. With apoptosis, cells break down into apoptotic bodies and become resorbed by neighboring cells.[73] With necrosis, cells break down into fragments, release lysosomal enzymes, and generate inflammatory responses that can lead to fibrosis, atrophy and ulceration at the local tissue level. Adverse response to radiation can be divided into early and late effects. Early effects are most often seen in cell populations that have high turnover rates, e.g. gastrointestinal, oropharyngeal, and esophageal mucosa, bone marrow, and skin. Late radiation effects more often involves tissues that are nonproliferating or slowly proliferating, e.g. oligodendroglia, Schwann cells, kidney tubules, and vascular endothelium. Radiation-induced peripheral neuropathies result from late effects of radiation treatment. The actual axons of peripheral nerves are less likely to be affected, but supporting cells, such as Schwann cells, are vulnerable to ionizing radiation. Radiation can also affect tissues surrounding peripheral nerves leading to development of fibrosis around nerve trunks. This fibrosis with subsequent compression of nerve bundles is suspected to be the primary etiology of peripheral radiation neuropathies.[74]

Carsten *et al.*[75] have demonstrated that skin acute radiation score (ARS) in dogs with cancer of the forelimb undergoing curative intent radiation therapy was a highly statistically significant predictor of pain as reflected in VAS and the Glasgow composite measure of pain scale, short form (GCMPS). Skin ARSs increased prior to the increase in pain scores, but not simultaneously. The investigators concluded that it is optimal to combine daily ARSs with use of a pain scale to achieve optimal pain management in the radiation therapy patient.

Although cancer pain is associated with both tissue injury/inflammation and nerve injury, it is unlikely that the pain is just the sum of these two mechanisms, but rather, is a unique neurochemical pain state.

See *Table 20*.

Table 20 Effects of therapy and disease on tissue and nerve injury.

Iatrogenic	**Tissue injury**	**Nerve injury**
Chemotherapy		X
Radiation		X
Surgery	X	X
Disease		
Tumor compression		X
Release of active factors	X	
Immune response	X	X

ANALGESIA FOR CANCER PAIN

See *Table 21* and *Table 22*.

Table 21 Analgesics commonly used for cancer pain in the dog. (None have been assessed for dosage or efficacy in cancer, therefore empirical doses and efficacy reflect dose recommendations for osteoarthritic pain. Not all drugs are licensed in all countries.) * = empirical dose, based on personal experiences: pending further investigations.

Drug	Dose (dog)	Remarks
Amantadine	1.0–4.0 mg/kg orally sid* Caution use with selegiline or sertraline until interactions further elucidated	Available as tablet and elixir NMDA-antagonist Effective as adjunct with other drug classes Higher doses can produce gastrointestinal gas and loose stools
Amitriptyline	0.5–2.0 mg/kg orally sid*	Mode of action at (endogenous) descending serotonergic system Moderate to weak analgesic activity Often used as adjunct to NSAID Toxicity in the dog not evaluated
Aspirin	10 mg/kg orally bid	**NOT** approved for use in the dog Toxicities include: gastrointestinal, renal, and bleeding Better NSAID choices available
Butorphanol	0.2–0.5 mg/kg orally (sid–tid)	Poor bioavailability per os Weak analgesic Possible sedation at higher doses May be used as adjunct to NSAID
Codeine	0.5–2.0 mg/kg orally sid	Best bioavailability (~20%) among oral opioids Possible sedation at higher doses
Carprofen	2 mg/kg orally bid, or 4 mg/kg orally sid	COX-2 preferential Available as injectable, but with inferior pharmacokinetics to the tablet

– *Continued on facing page*

Table 21 Analgesics commonly used for cancer pain in the dog – *Continued.*

Drug	Dose (dog)	Remarks
Deracoxib	1–2 mg/kg orally sid (extended use)	COX-2 selective coxib-class NSAID May be effective in altering the course of certain types of COX-2 dependent cancer
Etodolac	5–15 mg/kg orally sid	COX-1 selective in the dog Associated with canine keratoconjunctivitis sicca (KCS)
Fentanyl (transdermal)	2–5 µg/kg/hr	Short-term use Variable absorption–systemic levels Expensive
Firocoxib	5.0 mg/kg sid	COX-2 selective coxib-class NSAID Questionable safety in dogs <7 months old No data in cancer dogs
Gabapentin	3–10 mg/kg orally sid–bid	No analgesic data in dogs Antiseizure effects Efficacy for neuropathic pain Rapidly metabolized in the dog Often used as adjunct with other analgesics
Glucosamine and chondroitin sulfate	Unestablished	Evidence base is weak Often used as adjunct with other analgesics Product quality is widely variable
Lidocaine (transdermal patch)	One (10 × 14 cm) patch per 20 lb (9.1 kg)	Clinical efficacy and toxicity not determined Duration of effect approximately 3 days Plasma steady state at 12–60 hours Ref:[76]
Meloxicam	0.2 mg/kg on day 1, then 0.1 mg/kg sid	Preferential COX-2 inhibitor Narrow safety profile Available as elixir and injectable only
Morphine (liquid)	0.2–0.5 mg/kg orally tid–qid	Poor bioavailability (<20%) Short duration of action Sedation and constipation may be seen at higher doses
Morphine (sustained release)	0.5–3.0 mg/kg orally tid–qid	Doses >0.5–1.0 mg/kg often reported to result in constipation
Pamidronate	1–1.5 mg/kg, diluted in 250 ml saline, slowly IV (once monthly)*	Inhibits osteoclast activity as a bisphosphonate Effective where osteolysis from bone tumor contributes to pain

– *Continued overleaf*

Table 21 Analgesics commonly used for cancer pain in the dog – *Continued.*

Drug	Dose (dog)	Remarks
Paracetamol (acetaminophen)	10–15 mg/kg orally tid for 5 days	Long-term: <10 mg/kg bid* Known as acetaminophen in US **Lethal in cats** Clinical toxicity not established in dogs Analgesic, but not anti-inflammatory
Piroxicam	0.3 mg/kg q48h*	Long-standing use as chemotherapeutic agent Narrow safety margin
Prednisolone	0.25–1 mg/kg orally sid–bid, taper to q48h after 14 days	**DO NOT use concurrently with NSAID** Most effective in cases with pronounced inflammation
Tepoxalin	10–20 mg/kg orally on day 1, then 10 mg/kg sid	COX and LOX 'dual pathway inhibitor' No data in cancer patients
Tramadol	2–4 mg/kg orally bid–qid*	Codeine analog Norepinephrine/serotonin reuptake inhibition No efficacy or toxicity data in dogs Often used as adjunct with other analgesics

Table 22 Analgesics commonly used for cancer pain in the cat. (None have been assessed for dosage or efficacy in cancer, therefore empirical doses and efficacy reflect dose recommendations for other painful conditions, and experience of the authors. Not all drugs are licensed in all countries.)

Drug	Dose (cat)	Remarks
Amantadine	3.0 mg/kg orally sid	Toxicity studies not available in cats 100 mg capsules require recompounding for cats Often used as adjunct with other analgesics
Amitriptyline	0.5–2.0 mg/kg orally sid	Apparently well tolerated for up to 12 months with daily dosing Occasional (<10%) drowsiness Often used as adjunct with other analgesics
Aspirin	10 mg/kg orally q48h	Associated with significant gastrointestinal ulcerations
Buprenorphine	0.02 mg/kg transbuccal q6–7h	Same dose IV provides similar analgesia Readily accepted by the cat, therefore acceptable for home administration Anorexia may occur after 2–3 days Ref:[77]

– *Continued on facing page*

Table 22 Analgesics commonly used for cancer pain in the cat – *Continued.*

Drug	Dose (cat)	Remarks
Butorphanol	0.2–1.0 mg/kg orally qid	Weak analgesic May be more effective in visceral pain Limited bioavailability and duration of effect when given orally Ref:[78,79]
Carprofen	Undetermined	Insufficient data on extended use
Etodolac	Undetermined	Insufficient data on extended use
Fentanyl (transdermal patch)	2–5 μg/kg/hr	Not suggested for cats <4.5 kg Do not cut or partially cover patches Ref:[80,81]
Flunixin meglamine	1mg/kg orally **as a single dose**	Insufficient data on extended use
Gabapentin	3–10 mg/kg orally sid–bid	No analgesic data in cats Anti-seizure effects Efficacy for neuropathic pain Rapidly metabolized in the cat Often used as adjunct with other analgesics
Glucosamine/chondroitin sulfate combinations	Unestablished: approximately 15 mg/kg CS orally sid–bid	Evidence base is weak Often used as adjunct with other analgesics Product quality is widely variable
Ketoprofen	1 mg/kg orally sid for a maximum of 5 days	Narrow safety range Possible use in 'pulse therapy' with a few 'rest' days between administrations
Lidocaine (transdermal patch)	One (10 × 14 cm) patch for 5–9.1 kg cat	Clinical efficacy and toxicity not determined Duration of effect approximately 3 days Plasma steady state at 12–60 hours Ref:[76]
Meloxicam	0.2 mg/kg orally on day 1, then 0.1 mg/kg orally sid for 4 days, then 0.05 mg/kg sid for 10 days, then 0.025 mg/kg sid	Extended use is off label Easy dosing as an elixir Honey base syrup is well accepted Ref:[82]
Morphine (oral, liquid)	0.2–0.5 mg/kg orally tid–qid	Limited bioavailability and duration of effect Poor palatability
Morphine (oral, sustained release)	Tablets too large for cats	

– *Continued overleaf*

Table 22 Analgesics commonly used for cancer pain in the cat – *Continued.*

Drug	Dose (cat)	Remarks
Paracetamol (acetaminophen)	**Contraindicated**	**Lethal in cats**
Piroxicam	0.3 mg/kg sid; however many use up to 1 mg/kg orally sid for up to 7 days. Every other day dosing suggested for long term	Decreased PCV in up to 30% of cats after 2–3 weeks of daily therapy Compounding may decrease drug activity
Prednisolone	0.25–0.5 mg/kg orally sid	**DO NOT use concurrently with NSAID** Most effective in cases with pronounced inflammation
Tolfenamic acid	4 mg/kg orally sid for a maximum of 3 days	Not licensed in many countries
Tramadol	4 mg/kg bid	Toxicity data not available in cats

NUTRITIONAL MANAGEMENT

Many types of cancer are influenced by nutrition, diet, and nutritional status of the patient. In humans cachexia is seen in 32–87% of cases, commonly associated with cancers of the upper gastrointestinal tract.[83] Weight loss can be detrimental to patient quality of life and prognosis, as well as dramatically impacting on the pharmacokinetics and pharmacodynamics of chemotherapeutics and contributing to increased treatment-related toxicity.[84] Malnutrition is arguably one of the most common causes of death in people with cancer. Association between documented metabolic abnormalities, actual weight loss, and poor prognosis in cats or dogs with cancer has not been convincingly demonstrated. One study from a referral oncology practice showed that only 4% of the dogs were cachectic and 15% of the dogs had detectable and clinically significant muscle wasting.[85] Nevertheless, nutritional assessment of the cancer patient should be part of every treatment plan focusing on history, physical examination, and routine hematological and biochemical parameters.

The following five steps have been proposed to define the nutritional requirements for dogs or cats with cancer:[86]

1. Estimate fluid requirements.
2. Estimate energy requirements.
3. Distribute calories (between protein, fat, and carbohydrates).
4. Evaluate remaining nutrients (i.e. vitamins, minerals, essential nutrients, etc.).
5. Select a method of feeding (voluntary intake being preferred).

END-OF-LIFE CONSIDERATIONS

Reflecting on Dr. Vertosick's insight that we are all born in another's pain and destined to die in our own, part of our moral obligation as veterinarians is to relieve pain and suffering in terminally ill cancer patients. Due to the strong human–animal bond built over the pet's lifetime, this obligation often involves assistance for both the pet and its owner. At this point a 'pawspice' end-of-life care program is a professional obligation. We can, with solidarity, offer pet owners supportive, palliative options for complete care and attention to their pet's special needs when death is imminent. Pet owners don't really care how much you know, they want to know how much you care.

Laurel Lagoni[87] (Colorado State University) states, 'In the new paradigm of veterinary medicine, and especially in veterinary oncology, providing comfort for both patients and clients is as much a priority as providing medical treatment.' Veterinary medicine is entrusted with the responsibility and option of euthanasia to help animals die in a humane and pain-free manner.

4 PHARMACOLOGICS (DRUG CLASSES)

OPIOIDS

The analgesic effects of opium have been known for over 5,000 years, but unfortunately, abuse has limited the use of opioids. Society has attempted to find a balance between licit and illicit use, therapeutic versus adverse effects, and medical needs with legal issues. Regardless of the legal, administrative, and social obstacles, no other class of drugs has remained in use for the treatment of pain as long as opioids.

OPIOID RECEPTORS

Knockout mice studies suggest that three opioid receptor types regulate distinct pain modalities:[1]

- Mu (μ) receptors (OP3) influence responses to mechanical, chemical, and supraspinal thermal nociception. (μ receptor densities are not identical among individuals, as shown by binding studies in human postmortem brain samples).[2]
- Kappa (κ) receptors (OP2) modify spinally mediated nociception and chemical visceral pain.
- Delta (δ) receptors (OP1) increase mechanical nociception and inflammatory pain. (To date there are no pure delta opiates commercially available.)

These receptors have several common properties:

- 370–400 amino acids; two to five glycosylation sites.
- Seven transmembrane spanning regions.
- All are negatively coupled through G_i protein to adenylate cyclase.

Opioid receptors are synthesized in the dorsal root ganglia and transported from the cell body to nerve terminals. Inflammation enhances the peripherally directed axonal transport of opioid receptors, leading to an increase in their number (upregulation) at peripheral nerve terminals. Further, pre-existing, but possibly inactive, neuronal opioid receptors may undergo changes in the inflammatory milieu (e.g. low pH), and become active. Ligands with a preference for μ receptors are generally most potent, but depending upon the circumstances, all three receptor types can be present and functionally active in subcutaneous tissue, viscera, or joints.

CHOLECYSTOKININ AND OPIOIDS

Cholecystokinin (CCK) is one of the most abundant of the neuropeptides present in brain and spinal cord small neurons. CCK and the opioids tend to have opposite effects, suggesting that the CCK system may represent an 'antiopioid' or 'antianalgesic' mechanism. CCK antagonists not only enhance opioid responses, they also reverse existing morphine tolerance.[3] Changes in the expression of the peptide CCK and its receptor (CCK-2) on primary afferent neurons may play a key role in the alterations of pain sensitivity and opioid responsiveness that occur in chronic pain conditions.

RESPONSE TO OPIOID RECEPTOR ACTIVATION

In common with spinal and supraspinal opioid receptors, the binding of opioid agonists results in potassium-channel-mediated neuronal hyperpolarization, attenuation of calcium entry through voltage-gated calcium channels and reduced cAMP

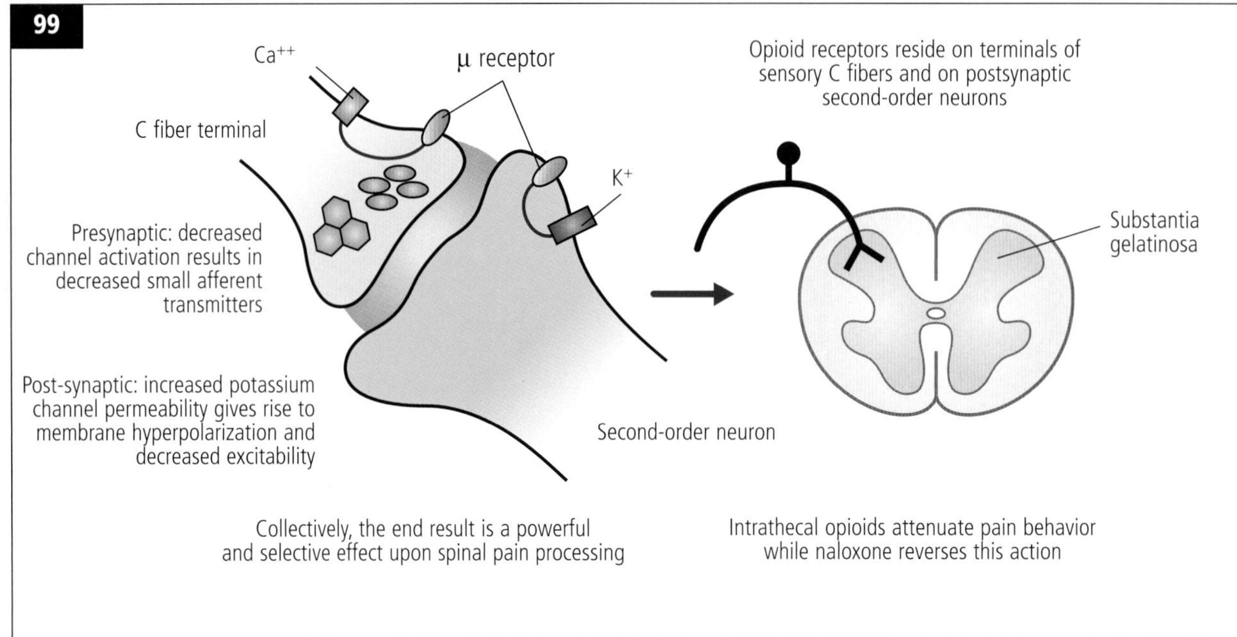

99 Activity of spinal opiate analgesia.

availability, with resultant reduction in nociceptor activity (99):[4]

- μ and δ (and to some degree κ) agonists induce a membrane hyperpolarization through the activation of an inwardly rectifying potassium channel.
- Inhibition of the opening of voltage-sensitive calcium channels, that will subsequently depress the terminal release of neurotransmitter from the cell. Occupancy of the presynaptic μ and δ sites reduces the release of sP and or CGRP in part by an inhibition of the opening of voltage-sensitive calcium channels.

That said, research over the last decade suggests that morphine and other opioids do not have fixed actions, but operate on receptor mechanisms that are subject to alterations by other transmitters and receptors.

Supraspinal activity of opioids occurs at several locations:

- Diencephalons: with active regions within the basolateral amygdala.
- Mesencephalon: with active sites within the substantia nigra.
- Mesencephalon: lateral regions of the mesencephalic reticular formation and medial region of the periaqueductal gray.
- Medulla: rostral ventral medulla within the midline structure corresponding to the raphe magnus.
- Spino/medullary: substantia gelatinosa regions of the spinal and medullary dorsal horn.

The tenet that opioids are centrally acting is long-standing. Yet, direct application of opioids to the peripheral nerve can produce a local anesthetic-like action at high concentrations, but this is not naloxone reversible. Models in which peripheral opioids appear to work are those that possess a significant degree of inflammation and are characterized by a hyperalgesic component. Mechanisms for this antihyperalgesic effect are currently unexplained, but injection of morphine into the knee joint of humans after surgery has shown a powerful sparing effect upon subsequent analgesic use.

Although controversial, studies suggest neuropathic pain secondary to peripheral nerve damage, more often than not, shows reduced sensitivity to opioids.[5] This is attributable to a reduction in spinal opioid receptors, nonopioid receptor-expressing Aβ fiber-mediated allodynia, increased cholecystokinin antagonism of opioid actions, and NMDA-mediated dorsal horn neuronal hyperexcitability, likely requiring a greater opioid inhibitory counter-effect.

OPIOID CLASSIFICATION

Opioids may be the best drugs available for pain control, and one might argue that 'serious pain control' cannot be implemented without them.

Table 23 Classification of opioids based upon binding activity.

A pure opioid *agonist* binds to one or more types of receptor and causes certain effects, such as analgesia or respiratory depression (e.g. morphine)	An opioid *antagonist* binds to one or more types of receptor, but causes no effect at those receptors. By competitive displacement, an antagonist reverses the effect of an agonist (e.g. naloxone reverses morphine)
A *partial agonist* binds at a given receptor causing an effect less pronounced than that of a pure agonist (e.g. buprenorphine is less effective than morphine, it is considered a partial agonist at the μ receptor and an antagonist at the κ receptor)	An *agonist–antagonist* binds to more than one type of receptor, causing an effect at one receptor, but no or a lesser effect at another receptor (e.g. butorphanol is considered a κ agonist and a μ antagonist, with minimal effect at the μ receptor)

Morphine, oxymorphone, fentanyl, hydromorphone, and meperidine are opioid agonists acting mainly at the μ receptor, where they have a high affinity. The agonist–antagonists (butorphanol, nalbuphine, pentazocine) are able to reverse some effects of the pure agonists, but can produce analgesia. Buprenorphine is a κ antagonist, with high affinity for μ receptors, classified as a partial agonist, while butorphanol acts at the κ receptor and acts as a μ antagonist. Opioid antagonists including naloxone, naltrexone, and nalmefene, reverse the actions of both μ and κ agonists. See *Table 23*.

The reported 'potency' of different opioids can be misleading in that relative ranking is based upon affinity of the specific drug for binding to the receptor. The most common side-effects seen with opioids include respiratory depression, nausea and vomiting, histamine release, constipation, and central excitement. Urine production may be decreased for several hours following morphine administration, however this does not appear to be related to arginine vasopressin (previously known as antidiuretic hormone or vasopressin) concentrations in the dog.[6]

OPIOID-ENHANCED PAIN

The chronic nature of cancer pain often requires prolonged opioid administration by various routes, and doses are often escalated over time, as the disease progresses. Clinical studies with humans report that opioids can unexpectedly produce hyperalgesia and allodynia, particularly during rapid opioid dose escalation.[7,8] Preclinical human studies have unexpectedly demonstrated that opioids can paradoxically enhance pain.[9,10] In a murine model of bone cancer, King *et al.*[11] showed that in a dose-dependent manner, morphine enhanced, rather than diminished, spontaneous and evoked pain. Additionally, morphine increased osteoclast activity and upregulated IL-1β within the femurs of sarcoma-treated mice, suggesting enhancement of sarcoma-induced osteolysis. The authors proposed that sustained morphine increases pain, osteolysis, bone loss, and spontaneous fracture, as well as markers of neuronal damage in DRG cells and expression of proinflammatory cytokines. The observed osteoclastogenesis was attributed, in part, to intraosseous IL-1β levels. Although these data raise concern, their relevance must be considered in perspective. Subject mice in this study were given high doses of morphine delivered with minipumps. Bolus opioid administration has been shown to effectively alleviate bone cancer pain in humans as well as in animals, and all opioids are not the same. Additionally, morphine is infrequently used alone for cancer pain. In adherence to the WHO's cancer pain ladder, the patient should be started on a NSAID and progress to the *addition* of an opioid, and then other drug class agents, as appropriate. Nevertheless, sustained opioid delivery through patches and controlled-release delivery systems is becoming more commonly used for pain management, and these data demonstrate that prolonged morphine treatment may have unexpected antianalgesic effects.

ORALLY ADMINISTERED OPIOIDS

Oral administration yields low (<30%; morphine 5%) bioavailability[12,13] because opioids are metabolized in the liver. Codeine has the highest bioavailability, approaching 60%,[14] and is often administered in combination with acetaminophen

Table 24 Available oral/rectal preparations of morphine (for human use) in the US.

Duration of action	Preparation	Dosage formulation
Immediate release	Tablet/capsule	1.5 mg, 30 mg
	Soluble/sublingual	10 mg
	Solution	10 mg/5 ml; 10 mg/ 2.5 ml; 20 mg/5 ml;
	Concentrate	20 mg/ml
	Suppository	5, 10, 20, 30 mg
Controlled/sustained release	MS Contin	15, 30, 60, 100, 200 mg
	Oramorph SR	15, 30, 60, 100 mg
	Kadian (food sprinkles)	20, 30, 50, 60, 100 mg
	Avinza (food sprinkles)	30, 60, 90, 120 mg

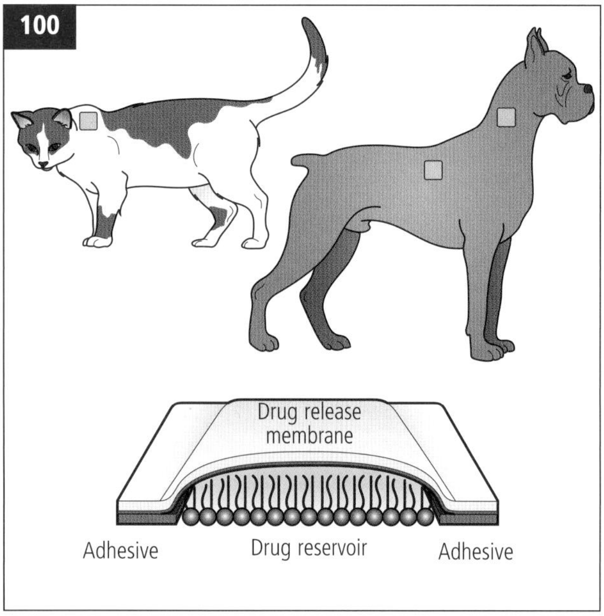

100 The fentanyl 'patch' provides transdermal delivery.

(*acetaminophen is lethal in cats*). Although morphine and hydromorphone are available as suppositories, there appears to be little difference in efficacy or bioavailability (~20%) from oral administration;[15] however, this delivery form is an option if oral administration is unavailable. See *Table 24*.

OPIOID PATCH DELIVERY

The highly lipid-soluble opioid fentanyl lends itself to transdermal delivery and is available in a patch containing a drug reservoir (Duragesic®: Janssen Pharmaceutica, Inc.). An ethylene–vinyl acetate copolymer membrane controls the rate of delivery to the skin (100). (A recent development is the Matrix® adhesive delivery patch from Noven Pharmaceutical Inc.)

Due in part to the differences in dermal vascularization, drug uptake varies between the dog and cat. Studies suggest it takes 12–24 hr to reach peak effect in the dog,[16,17] whereas peak values in the cat are reached sooner (2–18 hours).[18,19] Fentanyl patches certainly have their place, however they are not without concerns, which include: Class II Drug Enforcement Agency accountability; expense; difficulty with maintaining placement; variable absorption; possible skin reaction; the need to shave the hair; and choosing an optimal location. Following discharge, if a pet at home shows hyperexcitability the pet owner cannot differentiate if the behavior is due to uncontrolled pain or excessive opioid absorption. Patches may have their optimal use in chronic conditions such as cancer. For postoperative pain, one might consider a patient requiring opioid administration as an in-house hospital patient where it can be closely monitored and treated with cost-efficient morphine, then discharging the patient only when appropriate pain management can be provided by oral medication, i.e. an NSAID and/or an adjunct.

INTRA-ARTICULAR OPIOID DELIVERY

Morphine is also used for intra-articular analgesia, and several investigators suggest that in combination with bupivacaine, morphine works best.[20]

Because opioid receptors are found in the spinal

cord, opioids can be applied directly to these receptors by epidural or intrathecal administration. This takes advantage of smaller doses and central administration to minimize systemic uptake and possible side-effects associated with higher dose recommendations.

TRAMADOL

Tramadol has become a very popular analgesic adjunct over the past decade, having gained a worldwide reputation as an effective, safe, and well tolerated drug for inhibition of moderate pain in humans. It has come to fill the gap on the WHO analgesic ladder between the 'weak analgesics' (NSAIDs) and the strong opioids of the morphine type. The original compound comprised S- and R-enantiomers that could easily be separated by solubility differences of their compounds with an optically active compound. Pharmacological testing of the individual enantiomers showed the R-enantiomer to be the stronger analgesic and erroneously this was further presumed to come from the *trans*-configuration, therefore the compound was named *tra*madol. Both enantiomers are required for full analgesic activity. The S-enantiomer inhibits serotonin reuptake and has weak affinity for opioid receptors, while the R-enantiomer inhibits NE reuptake. Each enantiomer independently produces centrally mediated analgesia and the combination of enantiomers produces a greater effect than the additive effect of each enantiomer alone, i.e. they are synergistic.

Tramadol is not approved for dogs or cats, and only preparations for oral administration are available in the US. There are no safety or efficacy data in dogs or cats. Metabolism of tramadol through hepatic demethylation to O-desmethyl-tramadol (M1 demethylated metabolite) is reported in several species (including dog, where levels are quite low, and cat), and O-desmethyl-tramadol has been shown to bind to the μ-opioid receptor with a much higher affinity than the parent drug, likely providing noteworthy analgesic effect to tramadol. Metabolic clearance is probably through hepatic metabolism and renal excretion of unchanged drug. The lower clearance in cats compared to dogs may reflect the cat's lower capacity of the liver to biotransform tramadol.

The unique characteristics of tramadol were identified by incomplete inhibition of intraperitoneal tramadol-induced antinociception by subcutaneous naloxone, compared with the complete inhibition of antinociception induced by codeine and morphine in the mouse abdominal constriction test (**101, 102**).[21]

Tramadol does not inhibit COX activity. Seizure risk is cautioned in human patients receiving CNS drugs that reduce seizure threshold, such as tricyclic antidepressants, selective serotonin-reuptake inhibitors, monoamine oxidase inhibitors or neuroleptics. Tramadol may also be associated with gastrointestinal bleeding, exacerbated by the concurrent use with an NSAID.

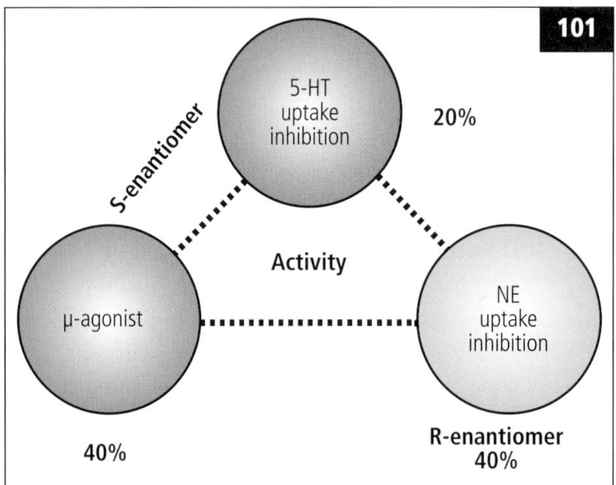

101 40% of the activity of tramadol is 'opioid-like' with activity at the μ receptor, while 60% of its activity is associated with serotonergic and noradrenergic functions.

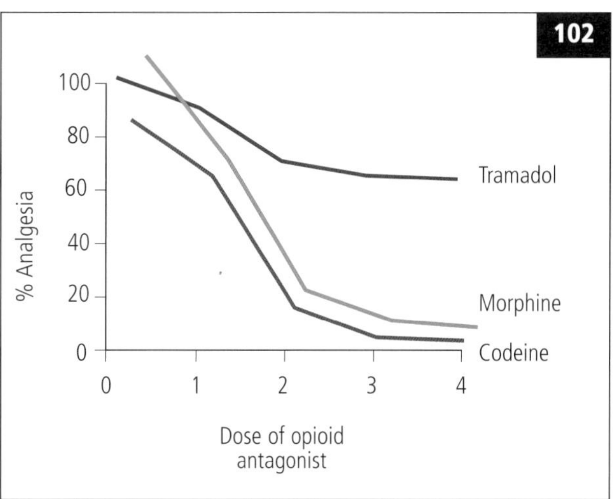

102 While traditional μ receptor agonists (morphine and codeine) show pronounced analgesic reversal with the opioid-antagonist naloxone, tramadol does not – confirming that it is not a 'pure' opioid.

One study[22] in human patients demonstrated that both tramadol and its M1 demethylated metabolite penetrate into synovial fluid, significantly reducing synovial fluid concentrations of sP. IL-6 synovial fluid concentrations were not significantly decreased. In dogs the systemic clearance of orally administered tramadol is almost five times faster than in humans, with at least 32 metabolites identified.[23] In a different study,[24] simulated oral dosing regimens at 5 mg/kg every 6 hours and 2.5 mg/kg every 4 hours were predicted to produce tramadol and M1 levels consistent with analgesia in humans, noting that pharmacodynamic studies are lacking to confirm the plasma concentrations needed to provide analgesia in dogs. In cats, tramadol is rapidly absorbed after oral administration and eliminated relatively slowly.[25] See *Table 25*.

Arguably, it is concerning how commonly this drug is being used with virtually no evidence base for its safety or efficacy in veterinary patients

Most analgesic combination products currently marketed for moderate-to-severe pain are mixtures of codeine, hydrocodone, oxycodone, or propoxyphene with aspirin, acetaminophen, or ibuprofen.

OPIOID OVERVIEW

Opioids are relatively safe. Potential side-effects include:

- Sedation or CNS depression.
- Excitement or dysphoria.
- Bradycardia.
- Respiratory depression.
- Panting.
- Laryngeal reflex depression.
- Histamine release (particularly with intravenous administration).
- Vomition and defecation (nausea).
- Constipation (longer-term use).
- Urinary retention (more common with epidural administration).
- Hyperthermia (especially in cats (with hydromorphone)).

Mechanistic summary of opioids:

- Act at μ, δ, and κ opioid receptors.
- Hyperpolarize by increased K^+ conductance; block transmitter release by blocking calcium conductance. Act in brain, spinal cord, and at peripheral afferent terminals.
- Brainstem: periaqueductal gray–activate several mechanisms including increased activity in descending/ascending pathways.
- Spinal cord: act in the substantia gelatinosa to block C fiber release and hyperpolarize dorsal horn nociceptive neurons.
- Periphery: act to alter the excitability in terminals located in an inflammatory milieu; only block hyperalgesia.
- Central: raise nociceptive thresholds.

Table 25 Pharmacokinetic parameters for orally administered tramadol.

	Tramadol		O-desmethyl-tramadol	
	Dog	Cat	Dog	Cat
Availability	65±38%	93±7%		
$T_{½}$ Elimination			2.18±0.55 hr	4.82±0.32 hr
$T_{½}$	≤1.7 hr	3.4 hr		
C_{max}	1402.75±696 ng/ml	914±232 ng/ml		
T_{max}	1.04±0.51 hr	0.42 hr		

OPIOIDS AT A GLANCE

See *Table 26*.

Meperidine (pethidine, Demerol)

- Less sedation than morphine.
- More likely to cause histamine release; intravenous administration can cause excitement in animals.
- Anticholinergic effects associated with structural similarity to atropine.
- In humans, the metabolite normeperidine is a neurotoxic CNS stimulant associated with adverse reactions.[26]
- Very short acting (<2 hours in cats).

Oxymorphone

- Does not cause histamine release.
- May induce panting.

Methadone

- Does not cause histamine release.
- NMDA and serotonin reuptake inhibitor activity.

Hydromorphone

- More sedation than oxymorphone, but shorter duration.
- No histamine release with intravenous administration.
- Hyperthermia in cats.

Fentanyl

- Rapid onset of action (2–3 minutes).
- Short duration of action (thermal threshold testing revealed that 10 μg/kg IV lasts approximately 2 hours in cats).

Butorphanol

- Agonist–antagonist.
- Weak analgesic, with analgesic ceiling effect.
- Short duration of analgesia (~40 minutes in the dog; approximately 90 minutes after intravenous dosing in cats).

Buprenorphine

- Agonist (strong for μ receptor)–antagonist (κ receptor).
- Slow onset (30–60 minutes), long acting (8–12 hours).
- Affinity for μ receptor makes reversal more difficult.
- Most popular opioid used in small animal practice in the UK, Australia, New Zealand, and South Africa.
- Oral transmucosal administration very effective in the cat.
- Considered by some to be the best opioid investigated in the cat.[27]

Table 26 World Health Organization's opioid classification.

Strength	Functional
Weak opioids	**Full agonists**
Codeine	Morphine
Dihydrocodeine	Fentanyl
Dextropropoxyphene	Hydromorphone
Tramadol	Codeine
	Methadone
Strong opioids	Tramadol
Morphine	Meperidine (pethidine)
Methadone	
Fentanyl	**Partial agonists**
Hydromorphone	Buprenorphine
Meperidine (pethidine)	Pentazocine
Oxycodone	Butorphanol
Buprenorphine	
Levorphanol Dextromoramide	**Agonists–antagonists**
	Nalbuphine
	Nalorphine
	Full antagonists
	Naloxone
	Naltrexone
	Alvimopan

Codeine

- 'International standard' weak opioid.
- Approximately 9% of Caucasians lack enzyme to provide analgesia[28]–relevance in animals unknown.
- Substantially improves analgesia of nonopioids (e.g. NSAIDs).

Tramadol

- 40% activity at the μ receptor, 60% as serotonin and NE neuronal reuptake inhibitor (monoaminergic).
- Reduces synovial fluid concentrations of sP and IL-6 in human patients with knee OA.[22]
- Augments analgesia of opioids[29] and NSAIDs.[30]
- Bioavailability is about 65%, with a short half-life (≤1.7 hr) in dogs; bioavailability is 93% with a half-life of 3.4 hr in the cat.
- Simulated oral dosing regimens at 5 mg/kg q6h and 2.5 mg/kg q4h in the dog are predicted to produce tramadol and M1 levels consistent with analgesia in humans.[24]
- Effective in neuropathic pain.[31]
- Very low abuse potential.
- Possible potentiation of bleeding, especially when combined with a NSAID.
- No efficacy or safety data in dog or cat.

ALPHA$_2$ AGONISTS

The prototypical α_2-adrenergic agonist used in veterinary medicine has been xylazine. Since its introduction in 1962, xylazine has been used, mostly in horses and ruminants, as a sedative–analgesic or anesthetic adjuvant (it is *not* an anesthetic). The newer α_2-adrenergic agonist, medetomidine, has gained acceptance in companion animal practice. Medetomidine is an equal mixture of two optical enantiomers, of which dextromedetomidine is a potent α_2 agonist, while levomedetomidine is pharmacologically inactive. Medetomidine has a high affinity for the α_2 receptor, with an α_2/α_1 binding ratio of 1620, compared with ratios of 260, 220, and 160 for detomidine, clonidine, and xylazine, respectively.[32] Currently, it is uncommon practice to administer large doses of an α_2 agonist as a single agent, but it is commonly accepted that low doses are very useful when used as adjuncts in a balanced analgesic protocol.

Bulbospinal noradrenergic pathways can regulate dorsal horn nociceptive processing by the release of NE and the subsequent activation of α_2-adrenergic receptors. Epidural delivery of α_2 agonists can produce potent analgesia in humans and animals.[33] Although the receptor is distinct, spinal action of an α_2 agonist is mediated by a mechanism similar to that of spinal opioids: (1) α_2 binding is presynaptic on C fibers and postsynaptic on dorsal horn neurons, (2) α_2 receptors can depress the release of C fiber transmitters, and (3) α_2 agonists can hyperpolarize dorsal horn neurons through a G_i-coupled potassium channel (**103**).

Alpha$_2$-mediated analgesia (in neuropathic pain) involves spinal muscarinic and cholinergic receptor activation with NO mechanisms; supporting that α_2 receptors may be primarily located on spinal cholinergic interneurons.[34] Spinal α_2 receptors, in conjunction with periaqueductal gray opioid receptors, mediate the analgesic actions of NO. Sedative effects are presumed to be mediated at the level of the brainstem. It is generally accepted that effects of spinal α_2 adrenoreceptor agonists are not naloxone reversible and show no cross-tolerance to opioids.

One mechanism of α_2 agonist action is the inhibition of adenylate cyclase. Decreased availability of intracellular cAMP attenuates the stimulation of cAMP-dependent protein kinase, and hence, the phosphorylation of target regulatory proteins.[35] In addition α_2 adrenoreceptor activation of G-protein-gated potassium channels results in membrane hyperpolarization, causing a decrease in the firing rate of excitable cells in the CNS.[36]

Presynaptic α_2 adrenoreceptors secrete NE, which binds with postsynaptic adrenoreceptors to stimulate target cell response governing autonomic functions. Medetomidine produces rapid sedation by selectively binding to α_2 adrenoreceptors in the neuron, inhibiting release of NE necessary for neurotransmission (**104**).

Dense populations of α_2 adrenoreceptors are concentrated in the mammalian spinal cord dorsal horn, both pre- and postsynaptically, on non-noradrenergic nociceptive neurons. On presynaptic α_2 adrenoreceptors, when G_0 proteins are activated, a decrease in calcium influx is mediated, leading to decreased release of neurotransmitters and/or neuropeptides, including glutamate, vasoactive intestinal peptide, CGRP, sP, and neurotensin. At postsynaptic α_2 adrenoreceptors, G_i protein-coupled potassium channels produce neuronal hyperpolarization that dampens ascending nociceptive transmission, thereby producing postsynaptically mediated spinal analgesia. The sedative–hypnotic effects are apparently mediated by activation of supraspinal α_2 adrenoreceptors located in the brainstem, where there is a relatively high density of α_2 agonist binding sites.

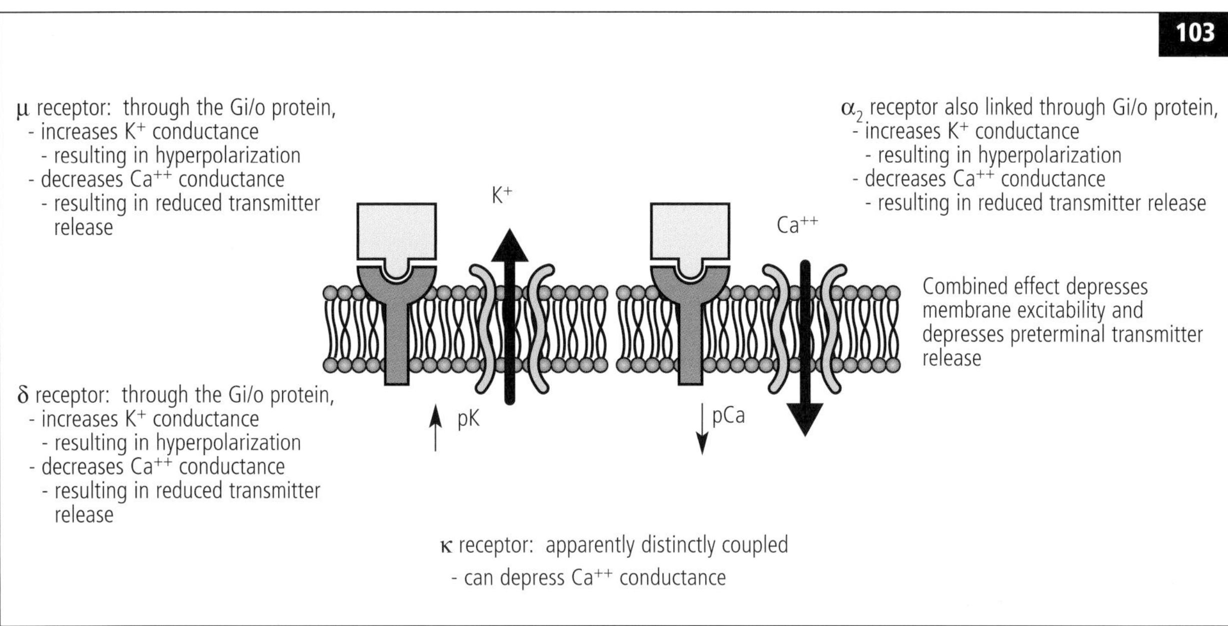

103 Summary of opiate and α_2 receptor action.

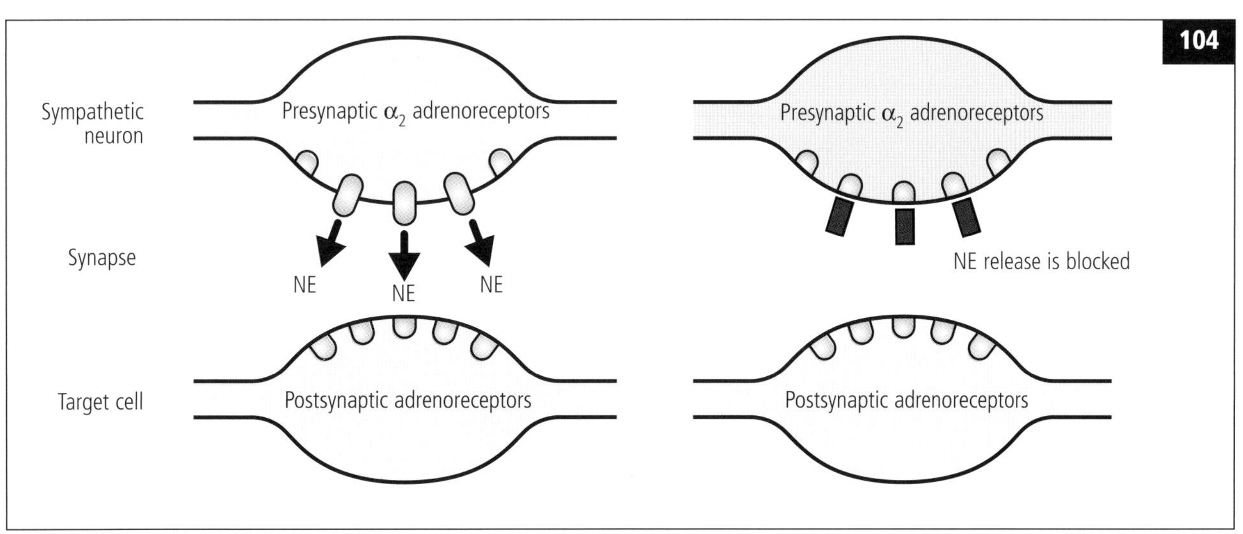

104 The release of NE is blocked by the administration of an α_2 agonist.

Potential features include:

- Sedation, muscle relaxation, and anxiolysis.
- Short-duration hypertension accompanied by a compensatory baroreceptor-mediated reflex bradycardia.
- Decreased respiratory rate, but with pH, PaO_2, and $PaCO_2$ maintained within normal limits.
- Both cats and dogs may vomit: cats (90%) > dogs (20%).
- Gastrointestinal atony with possible gas accumulation.
- Increased urinary output.
- Transient hypoinsulinemia and hyperglycemia have been reported in dogs.
  See *Table 27*.

ALPHA$_2$ MECHANISTIC SUMMARY

- Act at α_2 adrenergic receptor.
- Hyperpolarize by increased potassium conductance; block transmitter release by blocking calcium conductance.
- Act in the brain to produce sedation and depress arousal.
- In the spinal cord, produce analgesia and depress sympathetic outflow.
- In the spinal cord, act in the substantia gelatinosa to block C fiber release and hyperpolarize dorsal horn nociceptive neurons, producing analgesia.
- Effects on neuropathic pain may reflect mild sympatholytic action.

ALPHA$_2$ AGONISTS AT A GLANCE

- Not first-line analgesic agents, but excellent analgesic adjuncts.
- At low doses, both sedation and analgesia are dose dependent.
- Ceiling effect at higher dosages.
- Co-administration with anticholinergics is controversial.
- Inclusion in a premedication protocol markedly reduces the required dose of induction and maintenance anesthetic agents.
- Up to 20% of dogs and 90% of cats will vomit after administration.
- Increased urine output is reported in both dogs and cats.
- Transient hypoinsulinemia and hyperglycemia are reported in dogs.
- α_2 agonists are sedative–analgesics, *not* anesthetics. Therefore, under their influence, the animal is still arousable and may still bite in response to a noxious stimulus.
- Reflex bradycardia and bradyarrhythmias are common. Heart rates may decrease by 50%.[37]

Table 27 The following data were taken from an educational demonstration in a live dog, demonstrating the physiological responses to the α_2-agonist (medetomidine); anticholinergic (atropine); and reversal agent (antipamezol). Drs. WJ Tranquilli and KA Grimm; University of Illinois (data come from a demonstration given to Pfizer Animal Health veterinarians).

Parameters [normal]	Heart rate (beats/min) [70–110]	Mean BP (mmHg) [60–100]	Cardiac output (L/min) [2.5–6]	O_2 sat (%) [95–100]	Mucous membrane color [pink, 1–3 s]	PaO_2 (mmHg) [500–600]	$PaCO_2$ (mmHg) [40–55]	Resp rate (breaths/min) [6–20]
Baseline (1.1% isoflurane)								
	91	76	2.95	98	Pink, fast	575	52	20
(10 µg/kg; IM) medetomine admin								
+ 5 min	49	96	1.33	93	Pale, slow	630	55	24
+ 15 min	50	90	1.36	95	Pinker, slow	563	54	18
(0.04 mg/kg, IV) anticholinergic admin								
+ 3 min	77	125	1.45	100	Pink, faster	602	59	13
(50 µg/kg; IM) antipamezol admin								
+ 1 min	86	147	1.56	99	Pink, fast	X	X	15
+ 5 min	89	96	2.3	98	Pink, fast	597	54	12

- Blood pressure may fall by one-quarter to one-third and cardiac output may decrease by one-third to one-half of baseline value.
- Should be avoided in animals with compromising cardiopulmonary disease.

MEMBRANE STABILIZERS

Neuropathic pain is often a result of many underlying mechanisms, yet there may be a dominant mechanism that, when treated, reduces pain to a tolerable level. For example, if it can be demonstrated that ectopic impulse generators, due to abnormal sodium channel activity, located in injured or abnormally functioning primary afferent fibers, are generating increased traffic entering CNS pathways, treatment with a sodium channel-blocking agent that reduces ectopic firing may dramatically reduce pain. Mechanism-based pain management is an area of intense research.[38] This includes reducing transmitter release in pronociceptive neurons by opioids or α2δ calcium channel-binding drugs, by inhibiting postsynaptic excitatory receptors such as the NMDA or AMPA-kainate receptors, by potentiating inhibitory transmitters through reduced transmitter uptake or by agonist administration, and by use-dependent sodium channel blockers.

Trafficking, up- and downregulation, and even functional modulation of sodium channels, are the primary players in neuropathic membrane remodeling and hyperexcitability, with potassium channels playing an important role. Many drugs that block sodium channels are available for clinical use. Local anesthetics are the most widely used: lidocaine and bupivacaine. When applied at high concentrations to a nerve, impulse conduction and pain stop when the impulse originates distal to the application site. This is effective for both nociceptive and neuropathic pain. Low concentrations of lidocaine, two to three orders of magnitude lower than those required to block normal impulse propagation, selectively suppress subthreshold oscillations, and ectopic neuroma and DRG discharge, with similar CNS activity. Such sensitivity to sodium channel blockage is the basis for these drugs being given systemically without serious toxicity from failure of normal neuronal conduction within the cardiovascular and nervous systems.

Systemic local anesthetics have long been used for analgesia, particularly in humans for neuropathic pain. The primary mode of action of intravenous lidocaine is a dose-dependent blockade of spontaneous ectopic activity in peripheral nerves and DRG cells.[39] Importantly, these effects occur at plasma concentrations that are lower than those required to produce a frank block of nerve conduction (5–10 µg/ml): for lidocaine, effective concentrations may be in the order of 1–3 µg/ml. Neuropathic pain relief could be explained, in part, by their actions on the CNS, such as postsynaptic modification of NMDA-receptor activity.[40]

Long-term use of systemic (parenteral) local anesthetics (e.g. lidocaine) in humans is often precluded by tachyphylaxis and dose-related toxic effects. Orally administered lidocaine-like antiarrhythmics, such as mexiletine, have been used as an alternative with favorable results.[41] The topical application of lidocaine (e.g. lidocaine patch) is reported to be effective for some forms of nerve injury pain (e.g. PHN), offering the advantage of fewer side-effects because plasma concentrations are well below toxic levels.

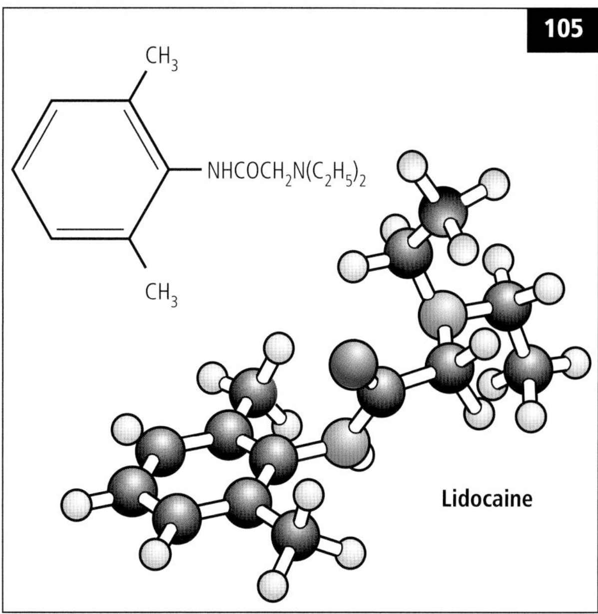

105 Lidocaine. Systemic sodium channel blocking is provided (in humans) by plasma lidocaine (1–3 µg/ml), thereby providing anti-hyperpathia by blocking ectopic activity from a neuroma/DRG. See also *Table 28*.

MECHANISTIC SUMMARY OF INTRAVENOUS LIDOCAINE

- Intravenous lidocaine is *not* recommended for cats due to cardiovascular depression.
- Lidocaine is a sodium channel blocker (**105**).
- Sodium channels appear to be responsible for spontaneous activity in nerve terminals after local tissue and nerve injury.
- Intravenous sodium channel blockers at concentrations that do not block enough sodium channels to suppress conduction will block the ectopic generators.
- Low-dose intravenous sodium channel block is antihyperalgesic and antiallodynic, and may have little effect upon high-intensity stimulus-induced acute nociceptor-mediated pain.
  See *Table 28*.

A problem with systemic lidocaine is its short duration of action and the need to administer intravenously. This first issue is solved by anticonvulsants, whose mode of action is sodium channel blockade (e.g. phenytoin, lamotrigine, carbamazepine, oxcarbazepine, and zonisamide).[58] TCAs circumvent the requirement for intravenous administration.

LOCAL ANESTHETICS

As previously stated, local anesthetics act by blocking VGSCs, which are responsible for the transient increase in the permeability of excitable membranes to sodium that is normally produced by depolarization of the membrane. This anesthetic effect elevates the threshold and slows the rate of rise of the action potential; at lower concentrations it slows conduction velocity. Aδ and C fibers are more susceptible to local anesthetics than large fibers; they are blocked earlier and to a greater degree–apparently related to the shorter internodal distances of smaller nerve fibers.

The functional blockade density and duration of action of a local anesthetic for a peripheral nerve block are dependent on both the concentration of local anesthetic used (sufficient to inhibit sodium channels) and the use of a critical drug volume to achieve a sustained critical exposure length. Raymond *et al.*[59] interpreted three nodes of Ranvier as the minimal nerve length exposure necessary to block effective nerve transmission (corresponding to a nerve length of approximately 3.4 mm). Campoy *et al.*[60] reported that in the dog, volumes of 0.3 and 0.05 ml/kg produced sufficient distribution for performing brachial plexus and sciatic nerve blocks, respectively.

Topical local anesthetics for neuropathic pain could depend on peripheral factors such as ectopic discharges from sensitized cutaneous nerves bombarding the dorsal horn of the spinal cord. Damaged or regenerating sensitized fibers undergo changes in the number and location of sodium channels, and ectopic impulses from injured peripheral nerves may be sensitive to lower concentrations of local anesthetics than are required for blocking normal impulse conduction.[61] A topical lidocaine patch (Lidoderm®: Endo Laboratories) holds promise for treatment of neuropathic pain conditions, as it has shown benefit for several human neuropathic pain states including incisional neuralgia, painful diabetic neuropathy, complex regional pain syndrome, and postamputation stump pain.[62]

Local anesthetics at a glance

- The amide link (lidocaine, bupivacaine) or ester link (procaine, benzocaine) for the different local anesthetics determines the drug disposition within

Table 28 Intravenous lidocaine efficacy in humans. See also 105.

Clinical state	Efficacy	Reference
Postoperative		
Abdominal – opiate sparing	–	42
Cardiac – opiate sparing	–	43
Abdominal hysterectomy	–	44
Cholecystectomy	+	45
Cancer		
Bony metastases	+	46
Neuropathy	–	47
	+	48
	+	49
Nerve injury		
Nerve injury – VAS	+	50
Nerve injury – allodynia	+	51
Nerve injury – VAS	+	52
Nerve injury – VAS	+	53
Stroke – stroke pain	+	54
Postherpetic neuropathy	+	55
	+	56
Fibromyalgia	+	57
Diabetic neuropathy	+	58
	+	59

the body.

Metabolism of ester linked local anesthetics is primarily by nonspecific pseudocholinesterase enzymatic hydrolysis in the plasma.

Amide local anesthetics are metabolized primarily in the liver.

- Local anesthetics are weak bases, and the predominant form of the compound in solution at physiological pH is the ionized or cationic form.
- At clinical doses, vasodilation is present, whereas at low concentrations, local anesthetics tend to cause vasoconstriction.
- Adding a vasoconstrictor to the local anesthetic decreases local perfusion, delays the rate of vascular absorption, and prolongs anesthetic action. Epinephrine (5 μg/ml or 1:200,000) is commonly used for such a response.
- There is presently no data to enlighten the concept of mixing local anesthetics, e.g. short onset and duration agent with a different agent of long onset and duration.
- Harmful side-effects are usually associated with accidental intravenous administration of vascular absorption or large amounts of anesthetic after aggressive regional administration. *Always aspirate before injecting. Bupivacaine can cause cardiac dysrhythmias and ventricular fibrillation if injected intravenously.*
- Clinical applications:

  Local infiltration–soaker catheters.

  Topical anesthesia.

  Intravenous administration *NOT* recommended for cats.

  Epidural block.

  Spinal (supra-arachnoid) block.

  Peripheral nerve block.

  Intra-articular administration.

TRICYCLIC ANTIDEPRESSANTS

For many years drugs with a characteristic tricyclic structure have been used to treat depression in humans (**106**).

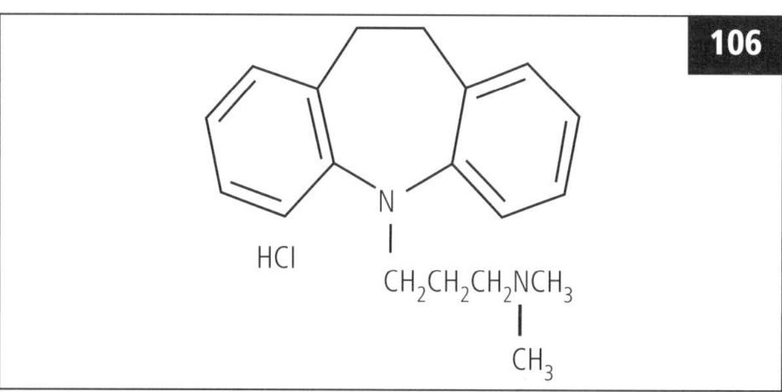

106 Imipramine: one of the first tricyclic antidepressants.

Table 29 Tricyclic antidepressant exploration for human use over the decades.[64]

Clinical development	Pharmacological discoveries
1958: Report of antidepressant effect	
1960: First suggestion of analgesic effect	1960–1980: Presynaptic reuptake inhibition (NE and serotonin) Postsynaptic receptor blockage (α-adrenergic, cholinergic, histaminergic)
1970–1980: Observations of analgesic effect in painful diabetic neuropathy	1980: μ opioid receptor interaction
1980: First controlled trial in painful diabetic neuropathy	1988: NMDA-antagonist-like effect
1984– : Numerous controlled trials in neuropathic pain	1992: Calcium channel blockade
1990– : Systematic reviews	1998: Sodium channel blockade

Imipramine was among the first drugs in its class, and only a few years after its introduction in 1958, its analgesic properties were identified (*Table 29*).[63] For a number of years, TCAs were the mainstay for treatment of neuropathic pain in humans (having been replaced by gabapentin and pregabalin). And, although treatment of neuropathic pain with TCAs in humans is evidence-based, it is not clear how these drugs actually relieve pain. Most research is based on their ability to inhibit presynaptic reuptake of NE and serotonin, but these drugs also act as NMDA-receptor antagonists and apparently block ion channels.

TCA MODE OF ACTION

TCAs are characterized by their multiple modes of action, with a particular ability to inhibit reuptake of monoamines (serotonin and NE) from presynaptic terminals. Additionally, TCAs block several receptors (cholinergic, adrenergic, histaminergic) and ion channels, including sodium channels. Mechanism of TCA action might best be identified as five drugs in one: serotonin reuptake inhibitors, NE reuptake inhibitors, anticholinergic–antimuscarinic drugs, α_1-adrenergic antagonists, and antihistamines. NE is an inhibitory transmitter that activates descending inhibitory pathways and has been associated with hyperalgesia in patients. Serotonin can activate the primary afferent nerve fibers via 5-HT_3 receptors. In addition, serotonin can cause mechanical hyperalgesia, most likely by effects on the 5-HT_{1A} receptor subtype. Opioids can be displaced from their binding sites with initial administration of antidepressants. With chronic administration, antidepressants can lead to modifications in opioid receptor densities leading to increased endogenous opioid levels. Additionally, antidepressant medications can bind to the NMDA receptor complex, which reduces intracellular calcium accumulations acutely. Longer-term administration alters the receptor binding of NMDA. Additionally, antidepressants can inhibit potassium, calcium, and sodium channel activity.

Opioid activity of TCAs may have the same effect as inhibition of NE and serotonin reuptake–enhancing activity of neurons in the network comprising diffuse noxious inhibitory controls, although TCAs have low affinity for the μ opioid receptor.[65] Therefore, their opioid effect is likely minimal. Tricyclic–NMDA activity is likely analgesic via its inhibition of neuronal hyperexcitability.[66] Alpha-adrenergic receptor blockade in peripheral neuropathy may be relieving pain generated or maintained by noradrenergic stimulation of highly sensitive receptors such as those identified on sprouts from diseased peripheral nerves.[67] Antihistamines have been shown to relieve pain, and TCAs may play a role in analgesia through their antihistaminergic action. TCAs may actually stabilize both diseased peripheral nerves and hyperexcitable neurons of the CNS by blocking sodium channels.[68] Only a few studies have shown calcium channel blockade with tricyclics. Selective serotonin reuptake inhibitors (SSRIs), lacking NE reuptake, having weaker ion channel blocking effects, and having no postsynaptic effects are rendered less effective than the TCAs.

TCAs express many modes of action which could contribute to pain relief, and because of their multimodal mechanisms of action, their efficacy may be greater than other agents which demonstrate a more selective pharmacological effect. The NNT for TCAs is quite similar across different human neuropathic pain conditions, with values of two to three, meaning that every second or third patient with neuropathic pain treated with a TCA will experience more than 50% pain relief.[69] Genetic polymorphism of different drug metabolizing enzymes likely explains pharmacokinetic variability of these drugs.

TCAs were the first evidence-based neuropathic pain treatments to be studied, and it is now understood that pain relief and relief of depression are independent effects.[70,71] Amitriptyline is best known as an inhibitor of catecholamine reuptake, although it is also a strong local anesthetic as well,[72] and is likely to relieve neuropathic pain by suppressing ectopic discharge. The newer non-TCAs, such as SSRIs, antidepressants that alter both serotonergic and noradrenergic neurotransmission, and NE-selective antidepressants, have preferential use in human medicine because of better tolerability, however their efficacy for neuropathic pain relief are not yet as convincing (*Table 30*).

Tricyclic antidepressants (TCAs) (amitriptyline, imipramine):

- Block the reuptake of serotonin and NE in the CNS. They also have antihistamine effects.
- Are used for the treatment of chronic and neuropathic pain in humans at lower doses than required for depression.

Antidepressant summary

- May be 5-HT selective or NE/5-HT selective.
- Most reliable efficacy is noted with mixed

inhibitors, but possibly NE alone.

- Hypothesized to augment tone in bulbospinal monoamine pathways and in ascending pathways to the forebrain.
- Some antidepressants also have NMDA and sodium channel blocking properties, which may account for some side-effects.

SEROTONIN

The idea that combined blockade of serotonin, otherwise known as (5-HT) and NE uptake might be useful in the treatment of pain has gained recognition from recent data on antidepressants and utilization of tramadol. There are at least seven major subtypes of

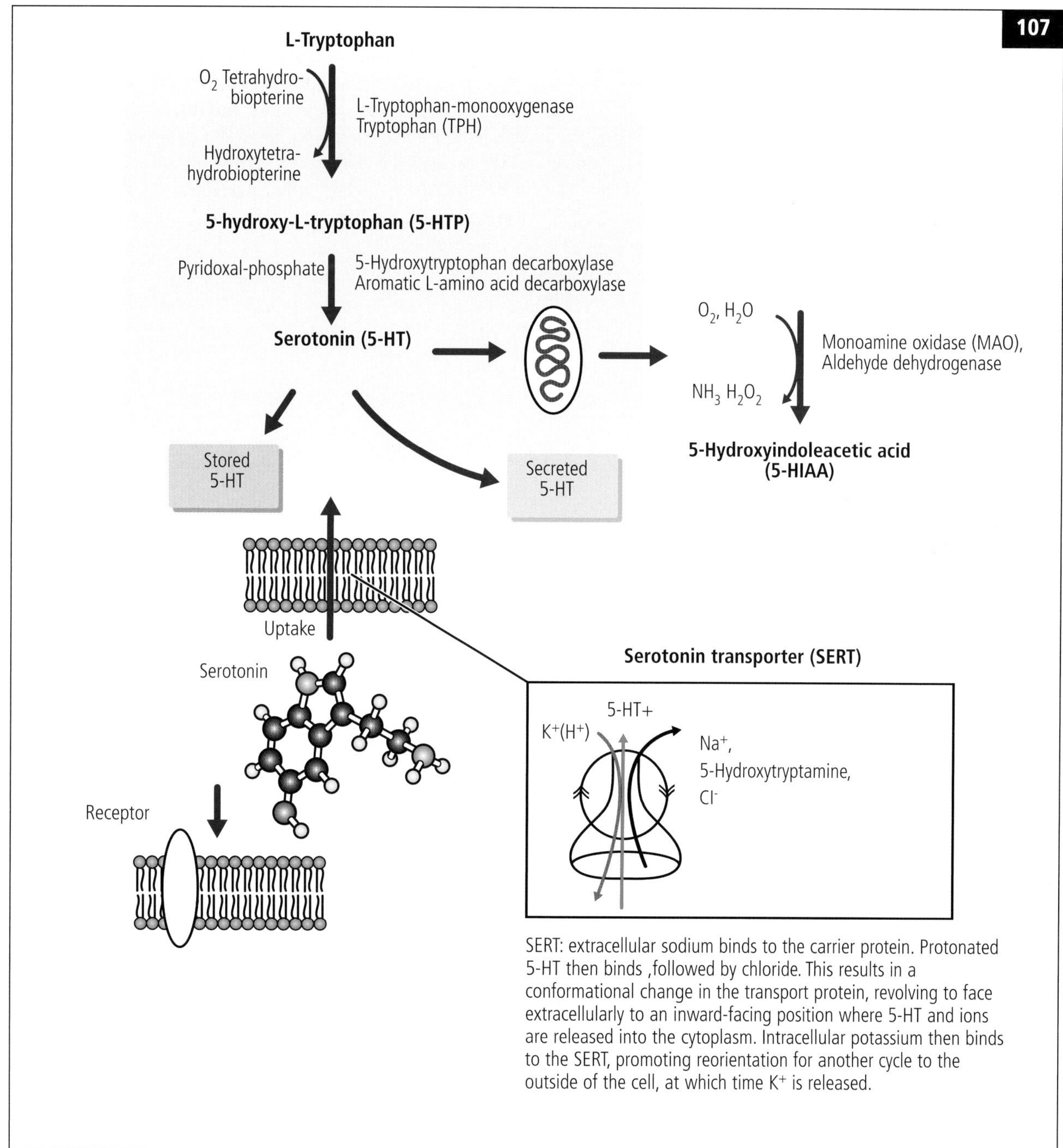

107 Serotonergic synapse and movement of 5-HT from synthesis, storage, release, and uptake via SERT and metabolism.

serotonin receptors, several of which have been identified in the spinal cord.[73] The serotonin transporter (SERT) is best recognized as the site of action of the SSRIs, which increase availability of serotonin at the synaptic junction for receptor binding (**107**).

Although metabolism occurs very rapidly, storage protects serotonin against metabolism. It is synthesized and stored in presynaptic neurons (serotonergic neurons, pineal gland, and catecholaminergic neurons). Outside the CNS, serotonin synthesis is limited to enterochromaffin cells of the gastrointestinal tract, and platelets, where 90–95% of the body's serotonin is stored. Platelets are unable to synthesize serotonin, yet they avidly take up the amine from plasma, using the same transporter used by neurons.[73] Although serotonin is a relatively weak platelet activator, in the presence of proaggregatory factors, such as ADP, epinephrine, and collagen, serotonin significantly potentiates aggregation.[74] Accordingly, any intervention that affects platelet serotonin content or its release from dense granules may theoretically have an impact on hemostasis and thrombosis. In studies performed in humans, all SSRIs have consistently shown a drastic decrease in platelet serotonin content after several weeks of treatment, reaching levels around or below 10% of the pretreatment serotonin levels.[75] A similar effect has been shown with clomipramine.[76] This potential for gastrointestinal bleeding associated with the administration of antidepressants is particularly noteworthy in recognition of the increased veterinary use of tramadol with NSAIDs. Sixty percent of the activity of tramadol is associated with the monoamine pathway, and De Abajo *et al.*[75] have documented the synergistic effect of NSAIDs together with SSRIs for causing upper gastrointestinal bleeding in the human population.

See *Table 30.*

Table 30 Antidepressants and mechanisms of action in producing analgesic effects.[64]

	Reuptake inhibition		**Receptor blockade**				
	Serotonin	**Norepinephrine**	**α-adrenergic**	**H1-histaminergic**	**Muscarinic cholinergic**	**Opioid receptor interaction**	**Quinidine-like effect**
Classic TCAs							
Imipramine	+	+	+	+	+	+	+
Clomipramine	+	+	+	+	+	+	+
Amitriptyline	+	+	+	+	+	+	+
Desipramine	–	+	+	+	+	+	+
Nortriptyline	–	+	+	+	+	+	+
SSRIs							
Paroxetine	+	–	–	–	+	?	–
Citalopram	+	–	–	–	–	?	–
Fluoxetine	+	–	–	–	–	+	–
S-NRIs							
Venlafaxine	+	+	–	–	–	?	–
Tetracyclines							
Mianserin	–	+	+	+	–	+	–

ANTICONVULSANTS

Even before peripheral and central sensitization had been defined in detail, the first controlled clinical trials in humans with the anticonvulsant carbamazeprine established its efficacy in relieving the pain of trigeminal neuralgia and diabetic neuropathy. Only carbamazepine, phenytoin, gabapentin, and lamotrigine have been studied in randomized human clinical trials for relief of pain in neuropathic pain disorders. Currently, only carbamazeprine and gabapentin have proved effective in humans.

Carbamazeprine blocks ionic conductance by suppressing spontaneous Aδ and C fiber activity without affecting normal nerve conduction.[77] However, carbamazeprine has not been widely embraced in human medicine because of side-effects, interaction with other drugs metabolized in the liver, and erratic pain relief.

Anticonvulsants are a category of medications grouped together based only on their ability to suppress epileptic seizures. Anticonvulsants, together with antiarrhythmic drugs, can be looked at as sodium channel or other channel neuronal activity regulators. Evidence firmly supports that anticonvulsants and local anesthetic drugs relieve neuropathic pain.[78,79] Based on NNT calculations, gabapentin is comparable with TCAs for neuropathic pain and is currently used more frequently than any anticonvulsant for human chronic pain.

Gabapentin was developed as an analog of the neurotransmitter GABA, but it has since been shown not to interact with either $GABA_A$ or $GABA_B$ receptors (**108**). Although not a sodium channel blocker, gabapentin depresses ectopic discharge by suppression of calcium ion conductance. Its mode of action is associated with binding to a highly specific [^{3}H]gabapentin-binding site in the brain – the α_2-δ site on voltage-gated calcium channels (**109**).[80]

Its mechanism of action is, therefore, likely associated with modulation of certain types of calcium ion currents. Gabapentin is unlike other antiepileptic drugs in that it does not affect voltage-dependent sodium channels.[81]

NMDA ANTAGONISTS

A single brief noxious stimulus results first in a pricking pain sensation by the afferent high-frequency, brief-latency, myelinated Aδ fibers. A moment later, afferent long-latency unmyelinated C fibers convey a burning, throbbing, aching pain. Both of these impulses are received in sequence by the same second-order neuron. Repetition of the brief noxious stimulus at less than 3 s intervals will result in magnification of the secondary burning component conveyed by the C fibers: termed temporal summation or 'windup'. NMDA receptor antagonists block prolonged depolarization and temporal summation of electrically stimulated C afferent fibers without abolishing Aδ activation.

The channel associated with the NMDA receptor is blocked by normal resting physiological levels of magnesium, and no change in excitability of the neurons possessing NMDA receptors can occur until this is removed.

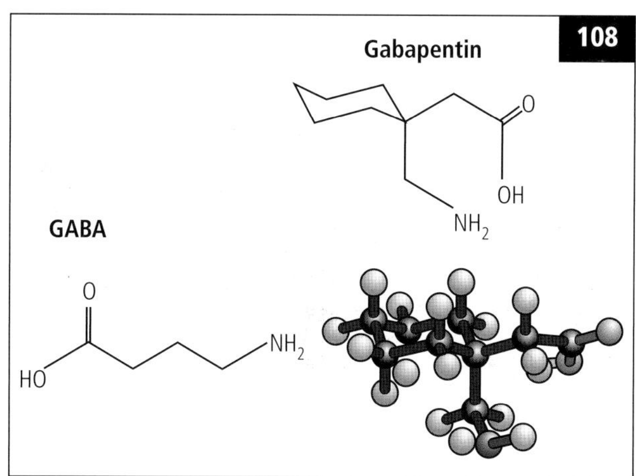

108 Gabapentin (1-(aminomethyl) cyclohexane acetic acid) was developed as a GABA analog, but does not interact with the GABA receptor. It has anticonvulsant activity.

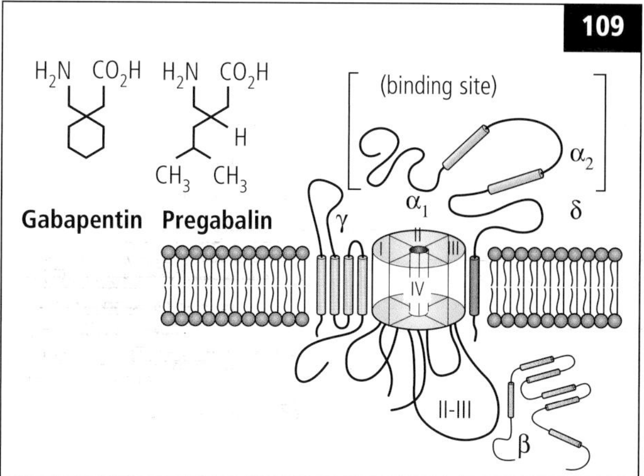

109 Gabapentin is the most frequently used anticonvulsant for chronic pain in humans. Both gabapentin and pregabalin bind at the α_2-δ subunit of voltage-dependent calcium channels.

The magnesium block is removed only by a shift in the membrane voltage towards depolarization. Binding of glutamate to the receptor alone is insufficient to activate the channel. Further, glycine is a required co-agonist with glutamate for activation of the receptor: the release and binding of glycine and glutamate are needed together with a non-NMDA-induced depolarization to remove the magnesium block.

Gabapentin is an anticonvulsant, but also a 'classic' NMDA antagonist in its mode of action. Gabapentin was originally synthesized to treat human spasticity, however it has been found to be effective in chronic pain and anxiety disorders. Gabapentin has no effect on the nocifensive behaviors observed during the acute phase of the formalin test, but does block the development of the late phase, demonstrating a selective antihyperalgesic action.[82,83] It is an effective antihyperalgesic agent in a knee joint model of acute arthritis induced by administration of kaolin and carrageenan.[84,85] Gabapentin has demonstrated analgesic efficacy for human patients with PDN and PHN: NNT of 3.8 and 3.2, respectively.

Importantly, NMDA antagonists are not only effective in preventing the development of pro-nociceptive changes, but may also reduce hyperalgesia, even when the changes have already developed.[86] Some preclinical studies report a synergistic interaction between opioids and NMDA antagonists. This synergism is found in acute pain models, in which NMDA antagonists are normally rather inactive.[87]

Gabapentin has also been observed to possess pre-emptive analgesic activity in a rat surgical pain model.[88] A single pre-emptive administration dose-dependently blocked the development of both static allodynia and thermal hyperalgesia for over 48 hours. Functional disruption of the α_2-δ subunit by gabapentin may result in an inhibition of excitatory neurotransmitter release that leads to a decrease in mechanosensitivity during mechanical manipulation of a joint,[89] collaborating in its peripheral effect.[90] Gabapentin has been shown to modulate the effect of sP by inhibiting its facilitation mechanism in the rat,[91] while Boileau *et al.* showed that a compound chemically related to pregabalin and gabapentin (PD-0200347) reduced the production of several catabolic factors, including MMPs and iNOS in a canine anterior cruciate ligament sectioning model.[92]

Apparently, anticonvulsants that act synaptically, such as barbiturates, are nonanalgesic, while membrane-stabilizing anticonvulsants are analgesic. Corticosteroids also have membrane-stabilizing properties, which may be a major mechanism of pain control when depot-form corticosteroids are injected. Topical forms of the TCA doxepin, gabapentin, lidocaine,[93] and bupivacaine, as well as ketamine are now available for use in humans.

GABAPENTIN OVERVIEW

- Originally introduced as an antiepileptic drug.
- Apparently, has no analgesic effect at GABA receptors.
- Well suited for neuropathic pain.
- Gabapentin is highly bioavailable in dogs.
- Gabapentin is metabolized by the liver and excreted almost exclusively by the kidneys. Half-life is approximately 3–4 hr.
- As an NMDA-antagonist, gabapentin does not alter nociceptive thresholds; therefore does not produce analgesia, but assists other drugs' analgesic response (**110**).
- Appears effective only against hypersensitivity induced by tissue damage or neuropathy, and may well be referred to as an antihypersensitive agent.
- Gabapentin does not interact with any known antiepileptic drug receptor sites.
- It does not exhibit affinity for common CNS receptors, including adrenergic (α_1, α_2 or β_1), cholinergic (muscarinic or nicotinic), dopaminergic (D_1 or D_2), histamine, serotonin (S_1 or S_2), or opiate (μ, δ, or κ) receptors.[94]
- No data on efficacy or safety in the dog or cat.

KETAMINE

Ketamine was synthesized in 1963, deriving its name from being a 'keto' derivative of an amine. It has a chiral center in the cyclohexanone ring, thereby existing as optical isomers (**111**). The S(+) isomer has a fourfold greater affinity for the NMDA receptor compared to the R(-) isomer, has twice the analgesic potency, and presents fewer psychomimetic effects.[95] (S-ketamine is now available commercially: Ketanest S®.) Ketamine binds to many sites in the CNS and PNS including nicotinic, muscarinic, opioid, AMPA, kainite, and $GABA_A$ receptors.[96] Ketamine also inhibits serotonin and dopamine reuptake and downregulates voltage-gated sodium and potassium channel function.[97] It preserves sympathetic reflexes that help support blood pressure. In human clinical studies, low-dose ketamine given before surgical incision in combination with opioids produced a 60% reduction in morphine use in postoperative patient-controlled analgesia.[98] In a study of dogs undergoing ovariohysterectomy, Slingsby and

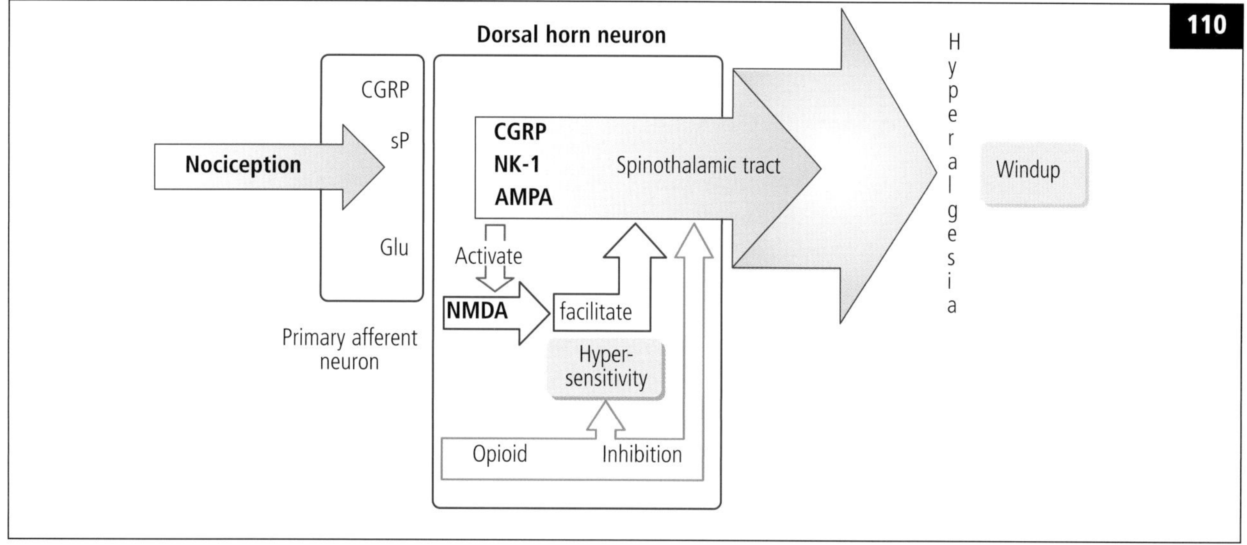

110 It is important to note that NMDA activation facilitates the nociceptive process to a state of windup. Therefore, NMDA antagonists, such as gabapentin and ketamine, act as analgesic adjuncts that address this facilitation, while etiology of the 'baseline' pain must be addressed with other agents. (CGRP = calcitonin gene related peptide; sP = substance P; GLU = glutamate; NK-1 = neurokinin 1; AMPA = alpha-amino-3-hydroxy-5-methyl-4-isoxazolepropionic acid).

Waterman-Pearson demonstrated that ketamine was effective, but short acting.[99]

At high doses, ketamine causes dissociative anesthesia, whereby subjects are awake but dissociated from the environment. Dorsal horn windup is inhibited by low-dose ketamine, whereas it is enhanced by low-dose morphine: differentiating the analgesic role of NMDA blockade versus opiate agonism.[100] Additionally, NMDA blockade does not alter tactile or thermal sensory threshold.

An important field of ketamine application is for neuropathic pain in humans. Studies report a relief of both spontaneous and evoked pain by prolonged treatment with ketamine for neuropathic pain syndromes of either peripheral or central origin.[101] Some report effectiveness of ketamine in neuropathic pain after chronic subcutaneous infusion[102] or oral administration.[103] Dysphoric and psychotomimetic effects are the major limiting problems with the clinical use of ketamine (and dextromethorphan) in the treatment of pain.

The analgesic action of low, subanesthetic doses of ketamine acts predominantly from blockade of the NMDA receptor. In its resting state, the NMDA receptor is inactive and does not participate in synaptic modulation because its ion channel is plugged by magnesium. The magnesium plug is dislodged by postsynaptic depolarization or when serine residues on the channel protein are phosphorylated following activation of calcium-dependent intracellular protein kinases. The NMDA receptor's ion channel must be open or 'active' before ketamine can bind to or dissociate from its binding site within the channel. Binding of ketamine to phencyclidine sites within the ion channel decreases the channel's opening time and frequency, thus reducing calcium ion influx and dampening secondary intracellular signaling cascades.

The NMDA receptor–channel complex is activated only by intense synaptic transmission across the second-order neuron and not by routine physiological transmission.

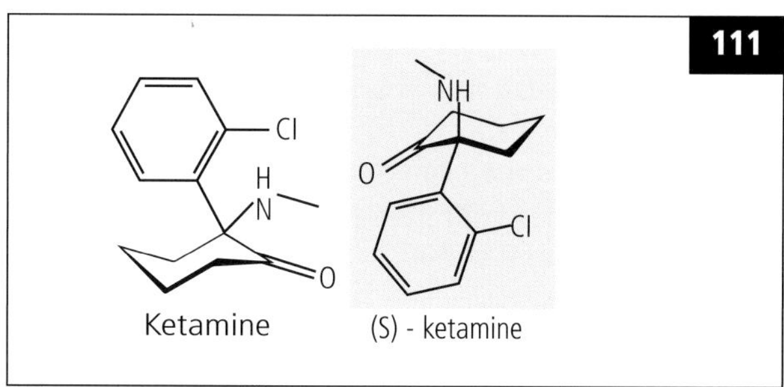

111 Ketamine has a chiral center, and thereby exists as optical isomers.

Accordingly, meta-analyses of human clinical trials indicate that ketamine supplementation of opioids for acute postoperative pain does not significantly improve analgesia; however, ketamine does benefit 'pathological' pain as a 'central sensitization modulator' (antiallodynic, antihyperalgesic, and opioid tolerance-reversing) in pain states of neuropathic or cancer pain (*Table 31*).

AMANTADINE

Amantadine is an orally available NMDA-antagonist, first recognized as an antiviral agent and later found to be useful in the treatment of Parkinson's disease. Administered intravenously, amantadine abolished or reduced pathological pain in humans with chronic neuropathic pain[104] and surgical neuropathic pain in cancer patients.[105] Oral amantadine reduced experimental sensitization and pain in human patients with chronic back pain.[106] Lascelles *et al.*[107,108] reported that the administration of amantadine might be a useful adjunct therapy for clinical management of osteoarthritic and cancer pain in dogs refractory to a NSAID.

NMDA ANTAGONISTS AT A GLANCE

(Ketamine, tiletamine, amantadine, methadone, dextromethorphan, gabapentin)

- Ketamine acts both centrally and peripherally at multiple receptor sites, including NMDA, opioid, AMPA, kainate, and $GABA_A$ receptors.
- Oral administration of ketamine produces few adverse effects and may be more effective than subcutaneous administration.[109]
- Microdoses of ketamine have few if any side-effects, and its best use is with an analgesic such as an opioid.
- Amantadine was originally developed as an antiviral drug for use in humans, and is available as an oral preparation. It is well absorbed in the gastrointestinal tract and excreted relatively unchanged in urine.
- The pharmacology of amantadine in dogs and cats has not been well established.
- In humans, amantadine has been used for neuropathic pain.
- Amantadine is used in veterinary patients for allodynia and opioid tolerance, allowing lower opioid doses and complementing the opioid analgesia.
- Amantadine is available in 100 mg capsules and 10 mg/ml elixir.
- The feline toxic dose of amantidine is 30 mg/kg.[104]
- Behavioral side-effects from amantadine in dogs and cats begin at 15 mg/kg orally.[105]
- Methadone and dextromethorphan (the active ingredient in many over-the-counter cough syrups) are opioid derivatives. Both are weak, noncompetitive NMDA-antagonists.
- Methadone also functions as an NE reuptake inhibitor.
- Methadone is commonly used for cancer pain in human patients because of its high oral bioavailability, rapid onset, and time to peak analgesic effect as well as the relatively long duration of activity.
- In contrast to its pharmacokinetics in humans, methadone has a short elimination half-life, rapid clearance, and low bioavailability in dogs,[12] accounting for its infrequent use.
- Erratic absorption, short elimination half-life, rapid clearance, and adverse effects limit the usefulness of dextromethorphan for therapeutic purposes in dogs.[110]
- Parenteral formulations of dextromethorphan are currently unavailable.

SUMMARY

Opioid analgesics have provided the most consistent and effective analgesia for many years and are still the best drugs available for both acute and severe pain control in small animals. It is frequently said that one cannot implement 'serious' pain management without the availability of opioids. Opioids are the cornerstone of perioperative pain management, where they are commonly supplemented with other classes of drugs such as α_2 agonists, NSAIDs, and local anesthetics. The actual agents administered within these classes of drugs are patient-dependent, and include selection criteria of: the patient's physiological status, pain syndrome treated, concurrent drug administration, delivery form, duration of effect, potential for side-effects, drug familiarity of the prescriber, and cost.

Whereas opioids are the cornerstone for 'severe' and perioperative pain, NSAIDs are the cornerstone for 'lesser' pain states treated longer term. This is because of the NSAID characteristics as anti-inflammatories, analgesics, and antipyretics. Further, administration is easier and side-effects of NSAIDs are fewer than with extended-use opioids. Accordingly, the World Health Organization suggests the management of pain by the analgesic ladder (**95**).

As veterinary medicine becomes more sophisticated in delivering pain therapy, drug profiles from human medicine are being considered (and often implemented) for veterinary application. Consequently, a number of

Table 31 A summary of evidence for ketamine analgesia in humans. Adapted from: National Health and Medical Research Council. How to use the evidence: assessment and application of scientific evidence. Ausinfo, Canberra, Australia, 2000, p.8.

Level 1	**Evidence obtained from a systematic review (or meta-analysis) of all the relevant randomized clinical trials**
	Low-dose perioperative ketamine is opioid-sparing, reduces nausea and vomiting, and has minimal side-effects Ketamine added to opioid patient-controlled administration provides no additional analgesic benefit Ketamine is most effective as a continuous low-dose infusion for acute pain management Ketamine has 'preventive' but not 'pre-emptive' analgesic effects Ketamine is a safe and effective sedative/analgesic for painful procedures, particularly in children
Level II	**Evidence obtained from at least one properly designed randomized clinical trial**
	Ketamine is most effective as an 'antihyperalgesic', 'antiallodynic', or 'tolerance-protective' treatment Ketamine is effective as a 'rescue analgesic' for acute pain unresponsive to opioids Ketamine reduces acute wound hyperalgesia and allodynia Ketamine may reduce the incidence of chronic postsurgical pain following laparotomy, thoracotomy, and mastectomy Ketamine reduces lower-limb ischemic rest pain, peripheral neuropathic pain, and spinal cord injury pain Ketamine improves fibromyalgia symptoms, including tender point count and aerobic endurance Intranasal ketamine reduces breakthrough pain of cancer-related and noncancer origin Ketamine reduces migraine severity in both acute and prophylactic therapy Ketamine does not improve analgesia when used alone or in combination with local anesthetic for peripheral nerve blocks, intra-articular injection, or wound infiltration
Level III	**Evidence obtained from nonrandomized controlled trials**
	Ketamine may be effective for refractory cancer pain in terminal stage disease Ketamine may reduce severe chronic phantom limb pain
Level IV	**Evidence obtained from case series**
	Ketamine improves analgesia in opioid-tolerant patients Intranasal ketamine may relieve migraine aura Ketamine may be effective in visceral pain based on human experimental models and limited case reports At least 50% of patients fail to respond to oral ketamine and experience side-effects in the treatment of chronic neuropathic pain Long-term ketamine use may be associated with impairment of memory, attention, and judgement

drugs administered in human medicine are being used in veterinary medicine based on an anthropomorphic approach and empirical or anecdotal support. However, considering that veterinary clinical trials with many of these drugs (such as tramadol, amantadine, and gabapentin) are currently nonexistent, the use of such drugs may have its place in veterinary medicine, provided: (1) the drug's mode of action is understood, (2) that the pharmacokinetics have been studied in the target species, and (3) that physiology as well as pathophysiology between man and the veterinary target species is similar.

Neuropathic pain can be thought of as the 'maladaptive pain state', potentially resultant from any significant noxious insult. And, it is much easier to identify in man than in nonverbal animals. Although not evidence-based, **112** suggests a logical approach to managing the progressive pain state, wherein pain management utilizes a multimodal scheme, where drug classes are added rather than substituted. The doses are empirical, and one could debate the order of implementation from bottom to top. The merit of this approach is the addition of agents from different drug classes, attempting to block as many of the 'pain pathways' (transduction, transmission, modulation, and perception) as possible.

There exist a plethora of potential sites of analgesic action that may be exploited with the development of agents directed toward both peripheral and spinal targets. See *Table 32* and *Table 33*.

IDEALIZED CRITERIA FOR NEW ANALGESIC THERAPY IN CHRONIC PAIN

- Analgesic properties:
  - Moderate–strong analgesic activity.
  - Delayed onset of action is acceptable for treating chronic pain; fast onset of action is required for treating acute or breakthrough pain.
  - No or low analgesic tolerance profile.
  - Not cross-tolerant to morphine.
- Side-effect profile compatible with chronic use:
  - Non-sedating.
  - No or minimal respiratory depression.
  - Minimal gastrointestinal, cardiovascular, renal effects.
  - No or minimal physical drug dependence.
  - Minimal mood-altering activity.
  - Not immunosuppressant.
- Pharmaceutics considerations:
  - Acceptable bioavailability for oral use preferred; alternatives include nasal, rectal, oral transmucosal, transdermal, or injectable use.

Table 32 Various drug classes, mechanism of action and effective application.

Drug class	Mechanism	Acute	Tissue injury	Nerve injury
Opioid (morphine)	Opioid receptors on high threshold C fibers	X	X	X
NMDA antagonist (ketamine)	Blocks glutamate-spinal facilitation	0	X	X
NSAID	Inhibits PG synthesis at injury site and spinal cord	0	X	0
IV lidocaine	Blocks sodium channels	0	0	X
Anticonvulsant (gabapentin)	Reduces spontaneously active neurons	0	0	X
TCA (amitryptyline)	Increases catecholamine levels	0	0	X

Table 33 Summary of peripheral pain mechanisms and potential targets for new analgesics. (TTX-s = tetrodotoxin-sensitive ion channel; TTX-r = tetrodotoxin-resistant ion channel; VR = vanilloid receptor)

Peripheral mechanism	Peripheral target	Type of drug
Nociceptor activation	Sodium channels	TTX-s channel blocker
Ectopic activity (neuroma, DRG)		TTX-r channel blocker
Nociceptor sensitization	Calcium channels	N-channel blocker
		L-channel blocker
	Acid-sensitive ion channel	Channel blocker
	P 2 X 3 receptor	Receptor antagonist
	VR1 receptor	Receptor agonist or antagonist
	Opioid receptors	μ, δ, and κ receptor agonists
	Cannabinoid receptors	CBI and CB2 agonists
	Nicotinic receptors	Receptor agonist
	Adrenergic receptors	α_2 agonist
		α_1 antagonist
	Prostanoid receptors	EP antagonist
	Prostanoid production	COX I/II inhibitors
	Serotonin receptors	5-HT_1D agonist
		5-HT_2 antagonist
	Kinin receptors	B1 antagonist
		B2 antagonists
	Glutamate receptors	NMDA antagonists
	Nerve Growth Factor	Trk A receptor antagonist
	Cytokines	IL-1β receptor antagonist
		Interleukin-converting enzyme inhibitor
	Protein kinase	TNF-α receptor antagonist
		Kinase isotype inhibitor

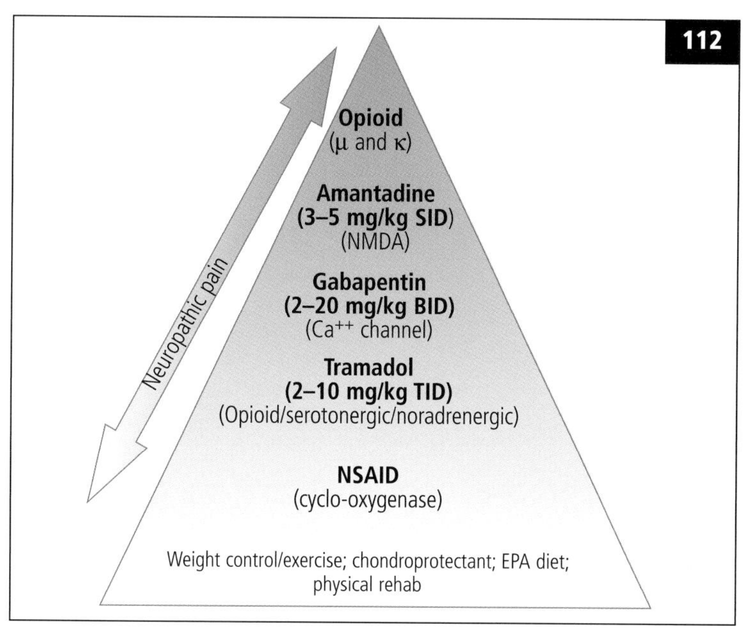

112 A multimodal drug scheme would be a logical approach to managing progressive neuropathic pain. Logic resides in each drug's independent efficacy, and each drug's different mode of action/site of action.

- Half-life and duration of action consistent with chronic use; once per day dosing.
  - No drug accumulation with chronic use.
  - Nontoxic metabolite(s).
  - Known and acceptable drug interactions; compatible use with opioids, NSAIDs.
  - Acceptable for use in senior populations.
- Mechanism of action considerations:
  - Nonopioid mechanisms of action preferred.
  - Agonists at non-μ opioid receptors may have advantages.
  - Indirect opioid agonists/peptide releasers, opioid potentiators, and opioid tolerance inhibitors may be useful.
  - Drugs with novel or 'unknown' mechanisms of action are good.
  - Analgesics that also treat the emotive aspects of chronic pain, stress, or depression are useful.

MAJOR THEMES IN ANALGESIC PRODUCT DEVELOPMENT

- Opioid combination products:
  - Increased analgesic potency.
  - Increased analgesic efficacy.
  - Reduced side-effects.
  - Reduced tolerance/dependency potential.
- Central opioid receptor analgesics:
  - Opioid-active partial μ agonist.
  - Morphine metabolite (M6G).
  - μ-δ opioid analgesic.
  - κ agonist analgesic.
  - Controlled-release drug delivery systems.
- Peripheral opioid receptor analgesics:
  - Peripheral μ agonist.
  - Peripheral κ agonist.
- Anti-inflammatory analgesics:
  - COX-2 inhibitors.
  - COX–LOX inhibitors.
  - COX–NO releasing compounds.
  - Disease-modifying compounds.
- Novel mechanism of action:
  - Ion channel blocking drugs.
  - Cannabinoid analgesics.
  - Muscarinic/nicotinic/α_2 agonist drugs.
  - Special-use products (e.g. unique efficacy for one disease condition or one species: e.g. OA in cats).

MARKET DATA (US)

The 2008/2009 US dog and cat pain management project (C.F. Grass Consulting, St. Louis MO (February 2009)) data provide insight as to trends in the use of various pain management drug classes. In the US a total of 26.7 million dogs were treated for pain in 2008 – down from 27.5 million in 2007. A total of 6.1 million cats were treated for pain – down from 8.3 million in 2007. By product class, NSAIDs account for the vast majority of the pain market, followed by opioids (**113**).

Of the total 2008 US market value, 44.6% was accounted for by the treatment of OA, 24.1% for postoperative use, and 11.0% for nonsurgical soft tissue trauma (**114**). Growth is observed in all types of managed pain (*Table 34*). More than 94.3% of clinics use two or more pain products (*Table 35*).

The 6-year growth curve for pain market pharmaceuticals has been positive, however this trend is predicted to fall by approximately 10% due to a flattened economy. (**115**, *Table 36*).

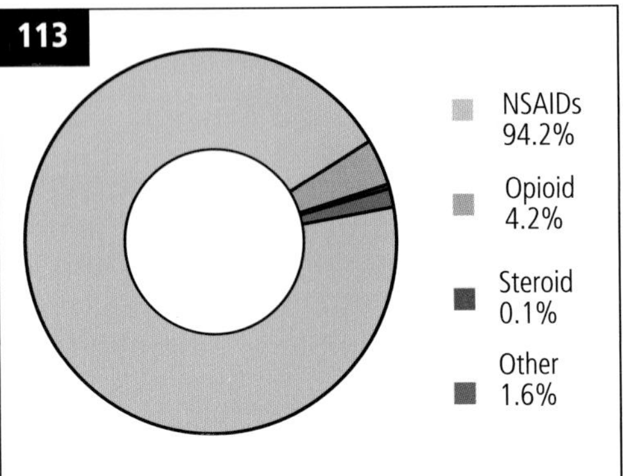

113 2008 market by product class. Total sales $207.8 million.

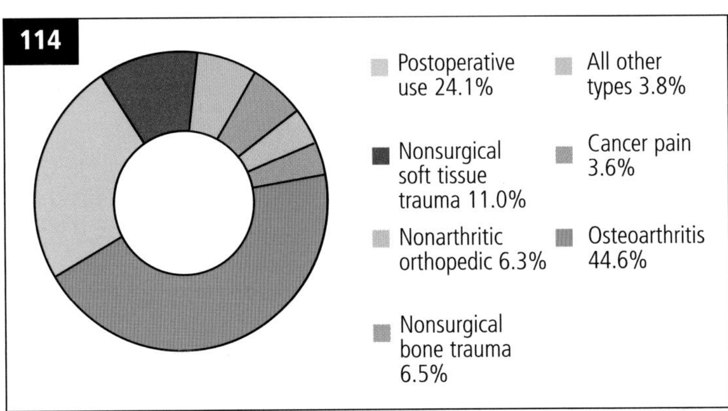

114 2008 market by type of pain treated.

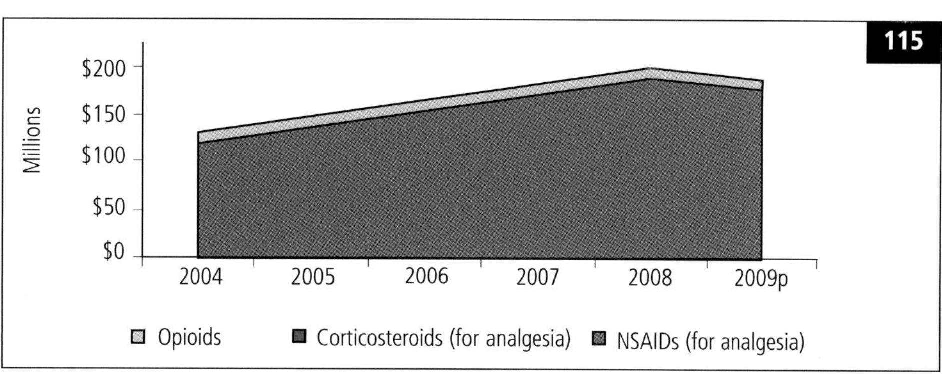

115 Pain product sales trend 2004–2009p. (p = prediction in early 2009).

Table 34 Growth in management of pain.

Type of pain	2008 value	Growth
Osteoarthritis	$103,119,966	5.0%
Postoperative use	$55,881,752	11.0%
Nonsurgical soft tissue trauma	$25,461,610	23.2%
Nonsurgical bone trauma	$15,123,896	31.2%
Nonarthritic orthopedic	$14,584,676	5.2%
Cancer pain	$8,422,485	21.8%
All other types	$8,826,407	28.6%

Table 35 Number of pain products used in clinics in 2008.

Number of pain products used	% of clinics in 2008	% of clinics in 2007
1	0.4%	3.1%
2	5.3%	18.7%
3	17.8%	28.0%
4	25.0%	19.5%
5	20.1%	13.2%
6	9.1%	7.8%
7	9.7%	9.7%

Table 36 Pain products sales trend, 2004–2009p (dollars). (p = prediction in early 2009).

	2004	2005	2006	2007	2008	2009p
Opioids	5,721,439	6,963,277	10,588,891	10,256,220	8,717,506	8,558,857
Corticosteroids (for analgesia)	806,895	908,264	663,408	685,929	105,969	100,512
NSAIDs (for analgesia)	124,998,342	145,021,959	161,351,595	175,986,872	195,774,224	185,040,699

5 NONSTEROIDAL ANTI-INFLAMMATORY DRUGS

INTRODUCTION

NSAIDs are the fastest growing class of drugs in both human and veterinary medicine. This reflects their broad use as anti-inflammatories, analgesics and antipyretics. As with antibiotics, NSAIDs can be considered to have been introduced in successive generations to date:

- First-generation, i.e. aspirin, phenylbutazone, meclofenamic acid.
- Second-generation, i.e. carprofen, etodolac, meloxicam.
- Third-generation, i.e. tepoxalin, deracoxib, firocoxib, mavacoxib, robenacoxib.

However, unlike the logic of 'saving the big gun

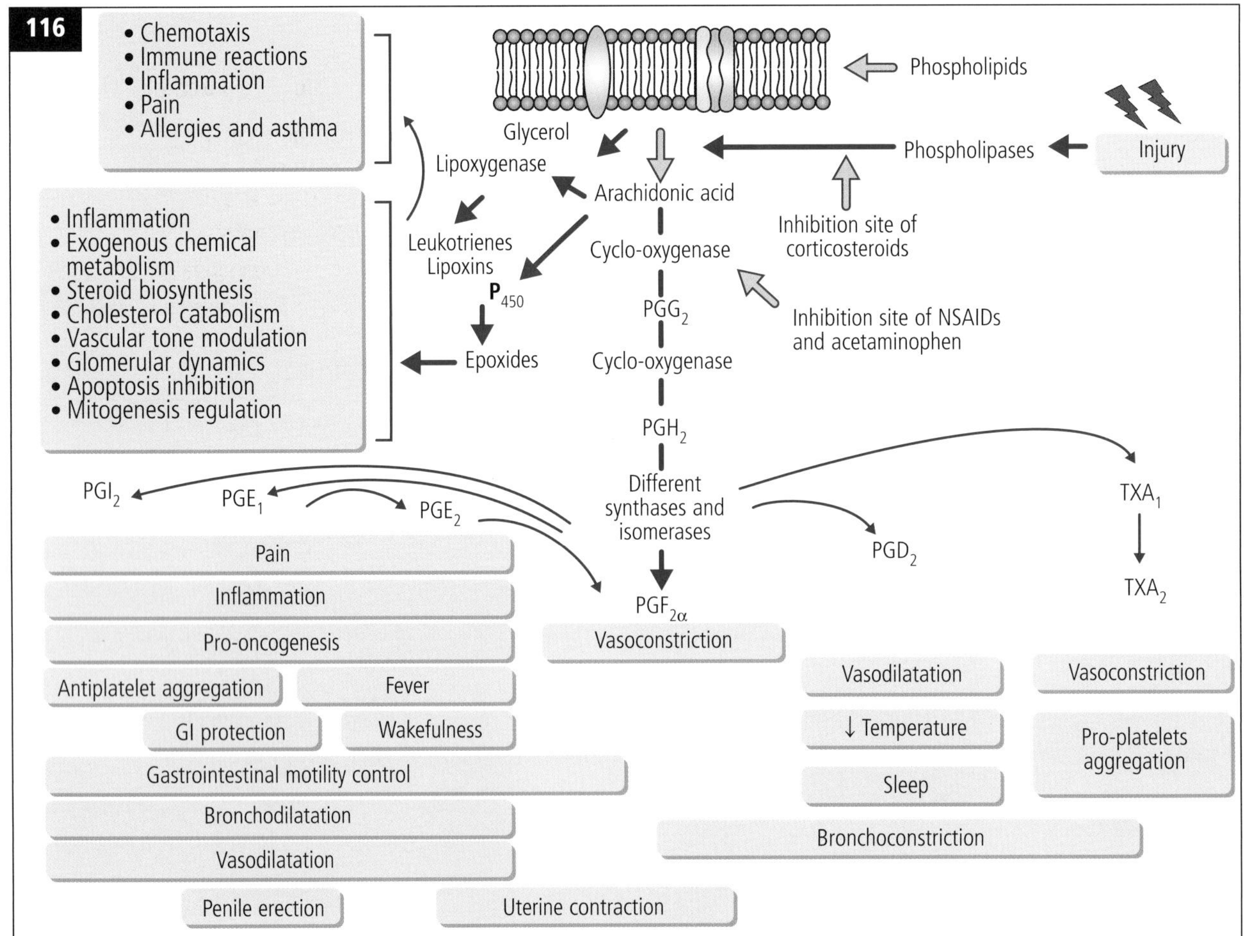

116 The AA pathway generates a variety of eicosanoids that influence various physiological functions.

antibiotic' for last, so as to avoid microbial suprainfections, logic would dictate using the optimal NSAID at the earliest opportunity, so as to avoid the physiological complication of windup.

Currently, several NSAIDs (aspirin, carprofen, cinchophen, deracoxib, etodolac, firocoxib, flunixin, ketoprofen, mavacoxib, meloxicam, phenylbutazone, robenacoxib, tepoxalin, tolfenamic acid, and vedaprofen) have approval for the control of canine perioperative and/or chronic pain in various countries. NSAIDs approved for feline use are far more limited (meloxicam, tolfenamic acid, ketoprofen, robenacoxib, carprofen, and aspirin in various countries for short-term administration).

ARACHIDONIC ACID PATHWAY

In most respects NSAIDs can be characterized as a class, although there are molecule-specific characteristics among individual drugs. NSAIDs manifest their mode of action in the AA cascade (**116**).

AA is an ubiquitous substrate derived from the continual degradation of cell membranes. Corticosteroids express their activity in the early stages of this course. AA is thereafter metabolized to various eicosanoids via the COX pathway to PGs or via the LOX pathway to LTs. Under the influence of local tissues, these end-product prostanoids can be proinflammatory and enhance disease processes and pain (*Table 37*).

It is important to note that the function of many prostanoids is tissue-dependent, e.g. PGs may contribute to pain and inflammation in the arthritic joint, while they enhance normal homeostatic functions of vascularization, and bicarbonate and mucous secretion in the gastrointestinal tract.

At one time it was believed that blocking the COX pathway led to a build-up of the substrate AA, which would then lead to increased production of LTs.

Table 37 Major prostanoids and their functions.

Prostanoid	Primarily found in	Major biological action
TXA_2	Platelets Monocytes	Platelet aggregation Vasoconstriction Bronchoconstriction Cellular proliferation
PGI_2 (prostacyclin)	Vascular endothelium Vascular subendothelium	Inhibition of inappropriate platelet aggregation Vasodilatation Vascular permeability Bronchodilatation Inflammation Cholesterol efflux from arteries
PGE_2	Renal medulla Gastric lining Platelets Microvascular endothelium	Vasodilatation Inflammation Fever Na^+-K^+ excretion/reabsorption Bronchodilatation Presynaptic adrenergic activity Cardioprotection
$PGF_{2\alpha}$	Brain Uterus	Vasoconstriction Bronchoconstriction Uterine constriction
PGD_2	Mast cells Brain	Sleep regulation Bronchoconstriction Temperature control Vasodilatation

This has been refuted by some,[1] while supported by others.[2] Because corticosteroids have their mode of action at a location higher in the arachidonic cascade than do NSAIDs, it is redundant to use them concurrently, and doing so markedly increases the severity of adverse reactions.[3–5] Data from humans show that the risk of NSAID-induced gastrointestinal complications is doubled when an NSAID is used concurrently with a corticosteroid.[6]

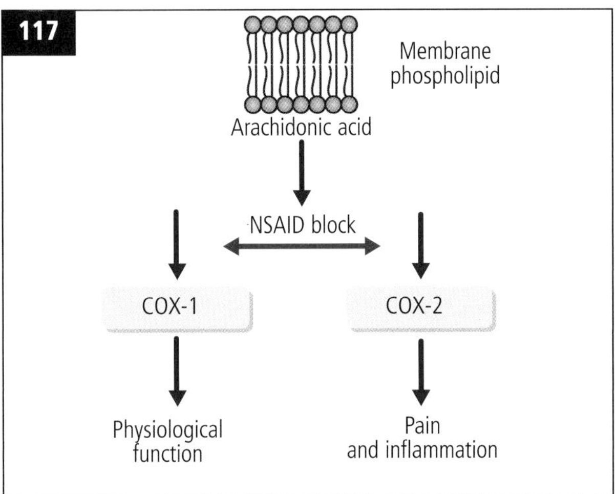

117 COX-1-mediated PGs tend to be more associated with constitutive physiological functions, while COX-2-mediated PGs tend to be more associated with pain and inflammation.

COX ISOZYMES

Approximately 20 years following discovery of the AA pathway as the mode of action for NSAIDs, it was discovered that the COX enzyme exists as at least two isoenzymes: COX-1 and COX-2.[7,8] These two distinct COX isoforms have been identified as products of two separate genes.[9] Early thinking was that COX-1-mediated PGs were constitutive physiologically, and should be retained, while COX-2-mediated PGs were pathological and should be eliminated for the control of inflammation and pain (**117**). COX-2-selective NSAIDs were designed for this purpose: the selective suppression of COX-2-mediated PGs (**118–120**).

In contrast to COX-1, COX-2 is not widely expressed under normal physiological conditions, but is upregulated in cells such as synoviocytes, fibroblasts, monocytes, and macrophages under the influence of proinflammatory mediators. Both isoforms are membrane-bound glycoproteins found in the endoplasmic reticulum and, particularly COX-2, in the nuclear envelope of the cell. The overall amino acid sequences of COX-1 and COX-2 are similar, the only difference in humans between the two isoforms being in the active site region that occurs at residue 523, where the isoleucine residue in COX-1 is replaced by a valine residue in COX-2. This single difference has been shown to have a marked effect on the overall size and shape of the binding site, apparently the basis for COX-2-inhibitor selectivity (**121**).

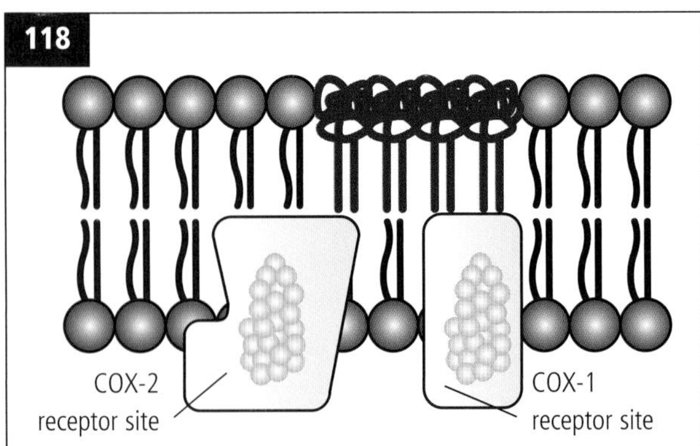

118 The COX-1 receptor site differs from the COX-2 receptor site by only a single amino acid, however the COX-2 site has a larger entry port and a characteristic side pocket. Small, traditional NSAIDs fit into both sites, blocking both COX-1- and COX-2-mediated PG production from AA, hence the term *nonselective NSAID*.

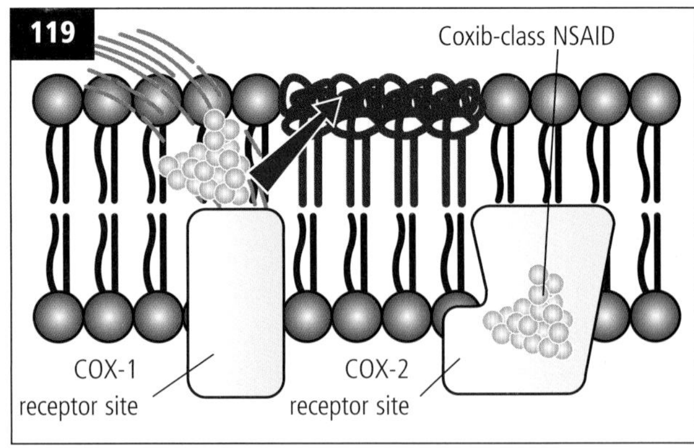

119 Coxib-class NSAIDs were designed to be too large for the COX-1 receptor site (at labeled dose); however, they fit hand-in-glove within the COX-2 receptor site. These drugs spare COX-1-mediated PG production and block COX-2-mediated PG production, i.e. they are COX-1 *sparing* and COX-2 *selective*.

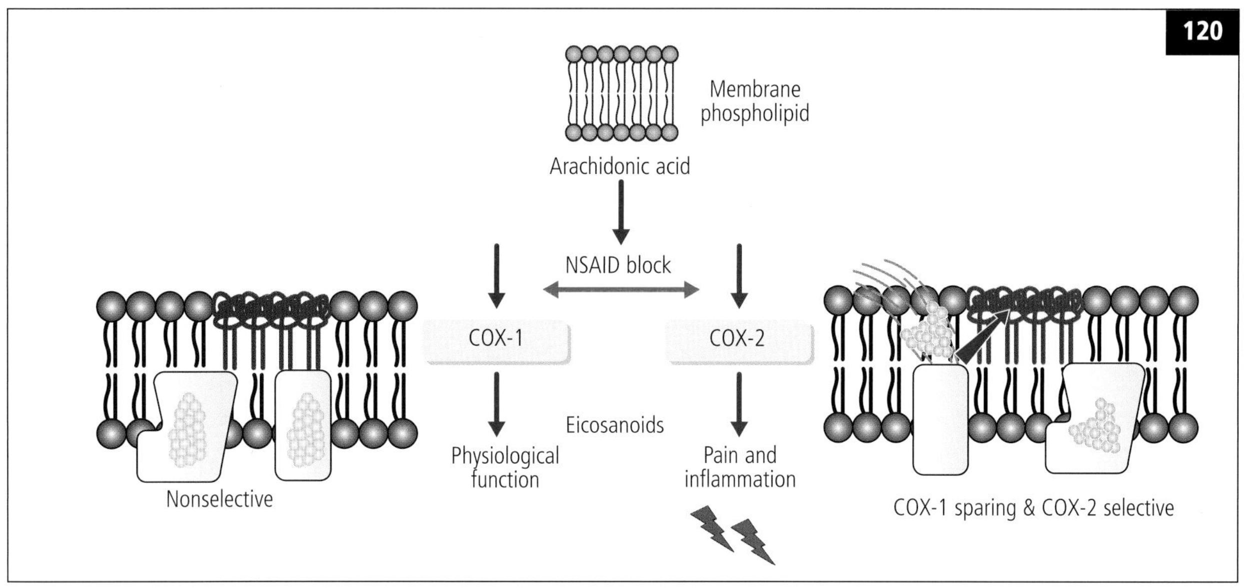

120 Overview of COX-1 and COX-2 nomenclature and clinical relevance.

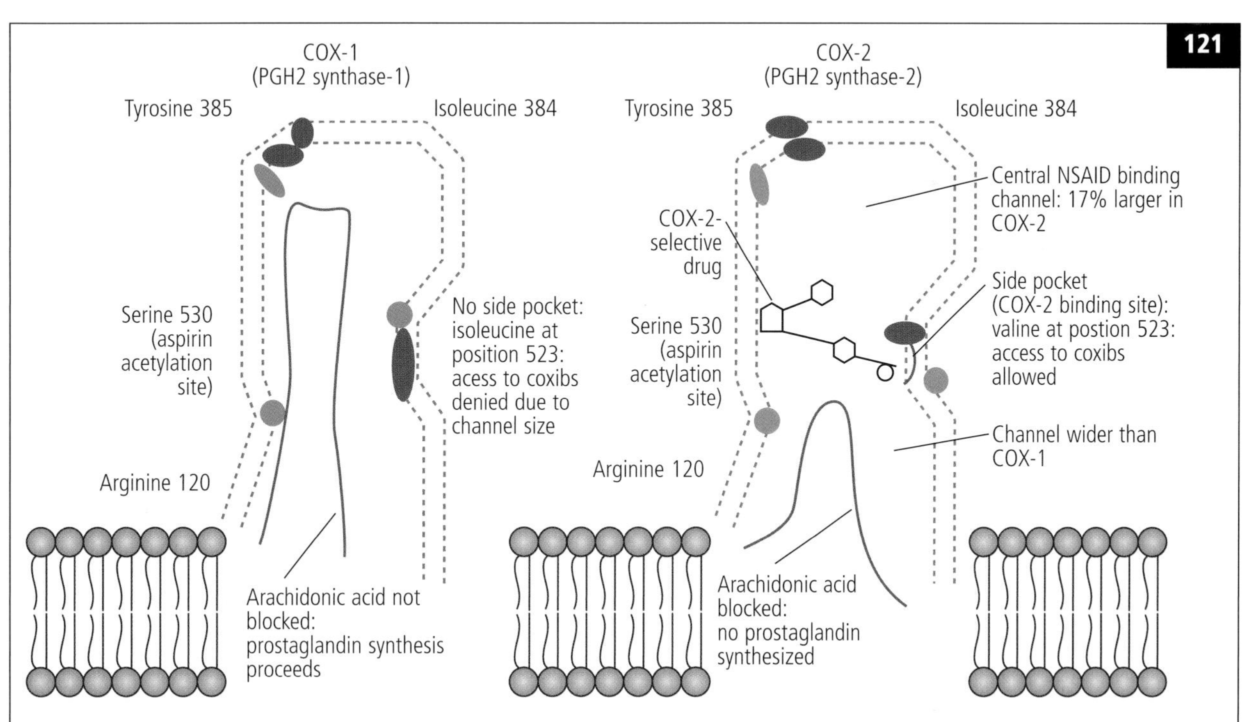

121 In humans, the two COX isoforms differ by a single amino acid, however, this single difference influences COX-2 inhibitor selectivity.

The IC_{50} is defined as the concentration of drug (NSAID) needed to inhibit the activity of the enzyme (COX) by 50%. In keeping with the above rationale, one would like to have a high concentration of NSAID before causing 50% inhibition of COX-1 ('good guy') and a low concentration of NSAID to reach the IC_{50} for COX-2 ('bad guy'):

$$\frac{IC_{50} \text{ of COX-1 (good) HIGH}}{IC_{50} \text{ of COX-2 (bad) LOW}}$$

The higher the numerator and lower the denominator, the higher the absolute value. Therefore, a greater COX-1/COX-2 ratio suggests (theoretically) the more optimal performing NSAID. With this in mind, pharmaceutical companies began designing NSAIDs for which it takes a low concentration to inhibit COX-2, but a high concentration to inhibit COX-1. Many factors such as species, incubation time, and enzyme source can influence the data obtained from enzyme preparations. Additionally, particularly when measuring COX-2 potency, the kinetics of inhibition are very complex and time dependent. Consequently, different values have been reported for the same drug. Although COX-1:COX-2 ratios vary by investigators, relative ratio standings provide insight as to a drug's expected species-specific COX activity (*Table 38*). Complicating this issue, some report ratios of COX-2:COX-1 rather than the more conventional COX-1:COX-2.

It has been suggested that a COX-1:COX-2 ratio of <1 would be considered COX-1-*selective*, a ratio >1 as COX-2-*preferential*, a ratio >100 as COX-2-*selective* and a ratio >1,000 as COX-2 *specific*. Selectivity nomenclature is used loosely and such comparative ranking has not been associated with clinical correlation. Hence, almost all discussions of COX data presented by pharmaceutical manufacturers include the disclaimer, 'clinical relevance undetermined', because the data are sourced *in vitro*.

We now know that the 'good-guy-COX-1', 'bad guy COX-2' approach is naïve, recognizing that COX-2 is needed constitutively for reproduction, CNS nociception, renal function, and gastrointestinal lesion repair. In fact, the physiological functions associated with COX activity overlap (**122**).

Accordingly, there is likely a limit as to how COX-2-selective an NSAID can be without causing problems, e.g. inhibiting endogenous repair of a gastric lesion. This limit is not known. More important than how COX-2-selective an NSAID might be, is whether or not the NSAID is COX-1-sparing, i.e. preserving homeostatic physiology. Further, it is logical to avoid a COX-1-selective NSAID (ratio <1) perioperatively, so as not to enhance bleeding. The coxib-class NSAIDs, with their high COX ratio and COX-1-sparing feature, have been shown to be associated with less risk for gastrointestinal complications in human studies.[15]

Table 38 Canine COX-1:COX-2 ratios of contemporary veterinary NSAIDs reported by different investigators.

Investigator	Drug	Ratio of IC_{50} Cox-1:COX-2
Kay-Mungerford *et al.*[10]	Meloxicam	12.2
	Carprofen	1.8
	Ketoprofen	0.4
Brideau *et al.*[11]	Meloxicam	10
	Carprofen	9
	Ketoprofen	6.5
Streppa *et al.*[12]	Meloxicam	2.7
	Carprofen	16.8
	Ketoprofen	0.2
	Aspirin	0.4
Li *et al.*[13]	Carprofen	5
	Celecoxib	6.2
	Deracoxib	36.5
	Firocoxib	155

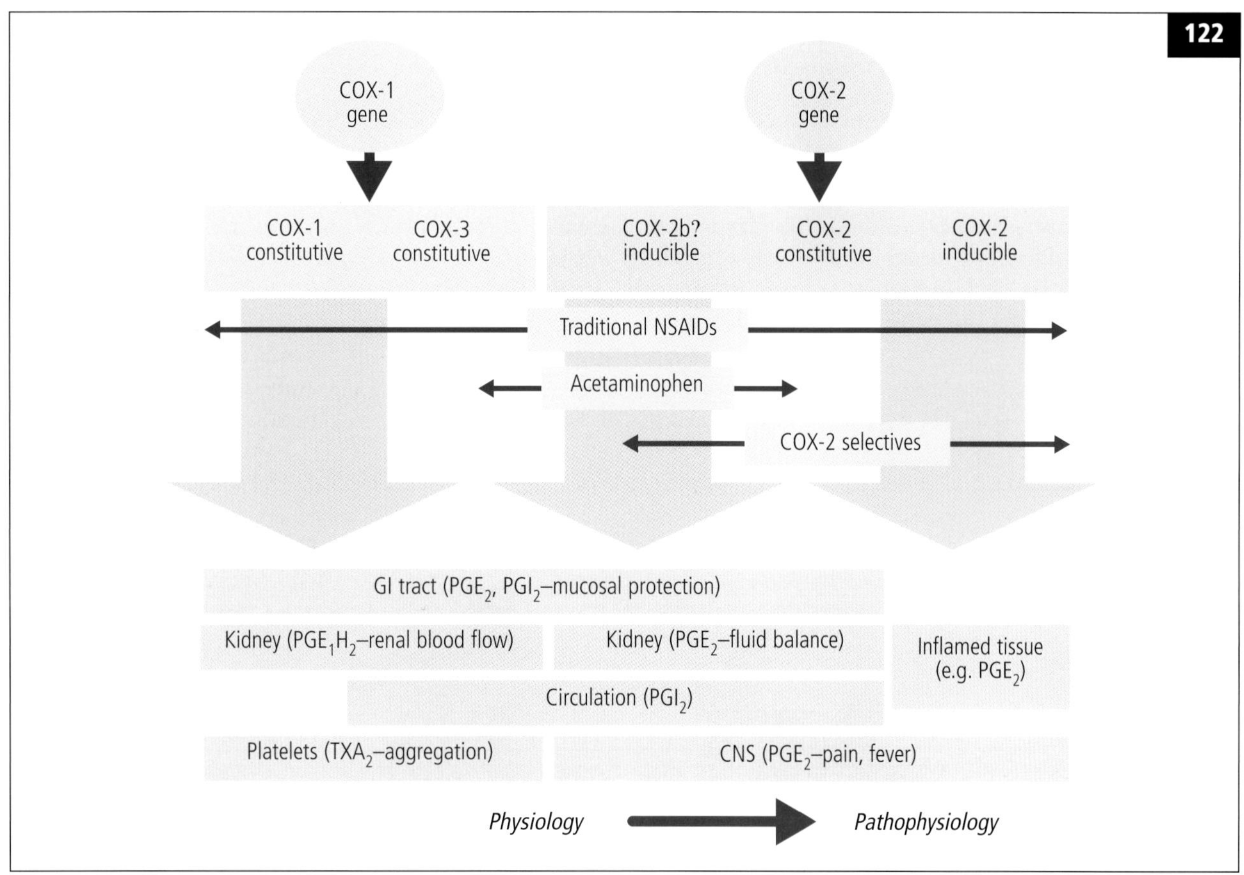

122 The clinical relevance of COX activity overlaps.[14]

COXIB-CLASS NSAIDs

Human coxib-class NSAIDs were designed to be more safe for the gastrointestinal tract, although any NSAID can be at risk for adverse reactions (adverse drug event (ADE)). Analogous safety profiles have not been extensively investigated in the canine. Coxib-class NSAIDs were not designed to be more safe for renal or hepatic function and they have been associated with potential cardiovascular risks in humans. Fortunately, companion animals are not at risk for coxib-class NSAID cardiovascular problems (atherosclerosis)[16] as are humans, and it may well be that the canine is an optimal target species for this class of drugs. The label precaution regarding potential sulfonamide hypersensitivity is likely theoretical. Trepanier[17] reported that 'sulfur drugs' other than the antimicrobial sulfonamides do not produce a similar pathogenesis for the same hypersensitivity.

NUCLEAR FACTOR κB

The most commonly accepted theory accounting for the inhibitory effects of NSAIDs on the inflammatory response suggests inhibition of COX, thus preventing PG synthesis. Yet, some suggest that additional mechanisms are involved in the actions of these agents. Several studies have demonstrated unequivocally that NSAIDs such as sulindac, ibuprofen, and flurbiprofen cause anti-inflammatory and antiproliferative effects independently of COX activity and PG inhibition, and can inhibit nuclear factor κB (NF-κB) activation by decreasing serine/threonine κ beta (IKκβ) kinase activity (IKK plays a role in the translocation of NF-κB from the cytoplasm to the nucleus).[18] In 1994 Kopp and Ghosh reported that aspirin and salycilates block NF-κB.[19]

NF-κB is a transcription factor that plays a critical role in the coordination of both innate and adaptive immune responses in sepsis by regulating the gene expression of many cellular mediators.[20] Activation allows NF-κB to translocate into the nucleus, where it regulates the expression of hundreds of genes that are important in immune and inflammatory responses (**123**). Additionally, NF-κB stimulates the expression of enzymes whose products contribute to the pathogenesis of the inflammatory process in sepsis, including COX-2, the inducible form of NOS, and a variety of proinflammatory cytokines. Several of these mediators can, in turn, further activate this transcription factor, which creates a self-maintaining inflammatory cycle that increases the severity and the duration of the inflammatory response, as well as regulate a negative-feedback control by inducing the transcription of its own inhibitor.[21] In addition to their mechanism of action on glucocorticoid receptors, glucocorticoids also antagonize the activation of the NF-κB pathway.[21]

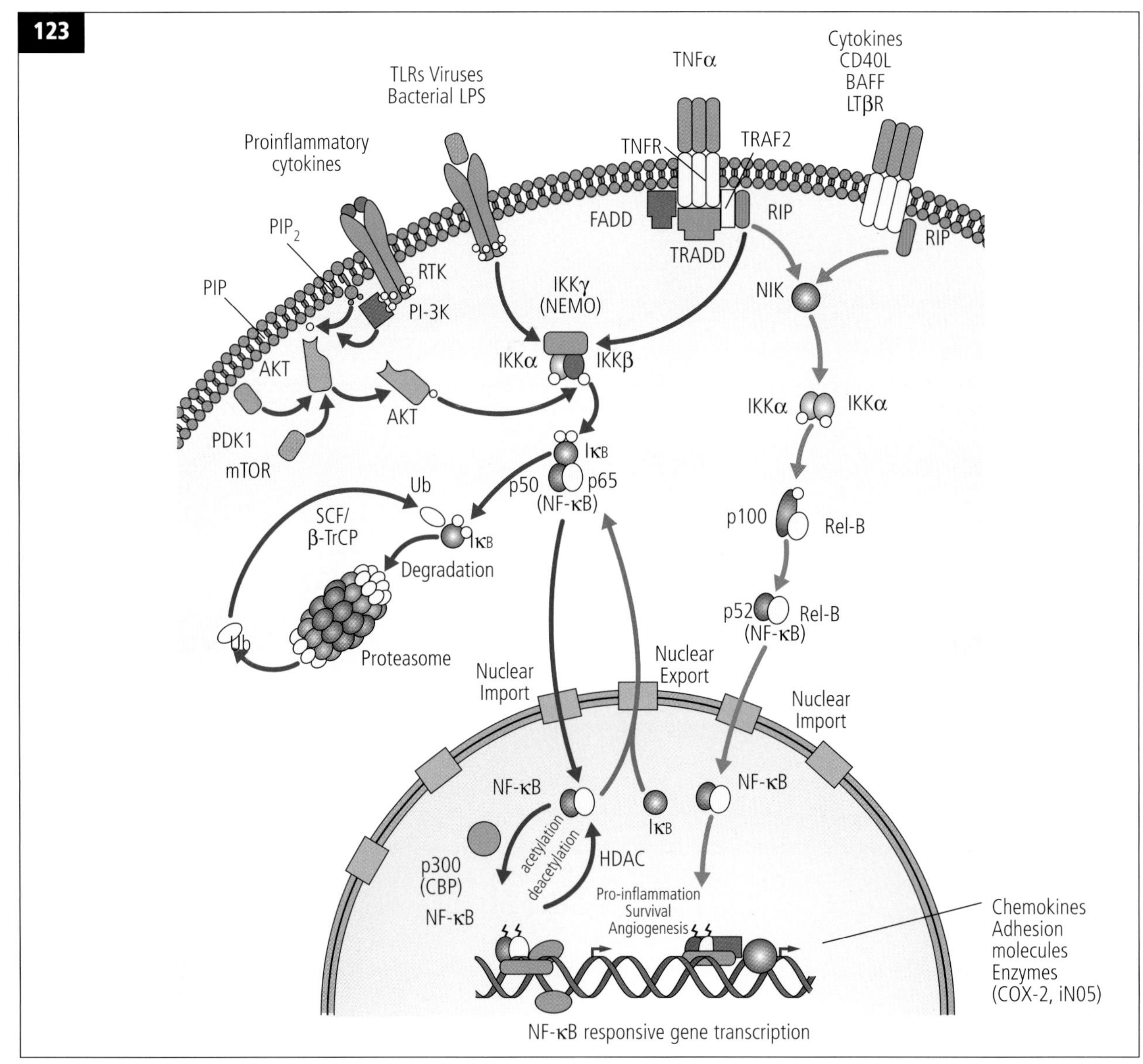

123 NF-κB activity (pathway).

The inhibitory effects on the NF-κB pathway are not shared by all NSAIDs (indomethacin and ketoprofen are inactive[18]); however coxib-class NSAIDs appear effective. NF-κB activity of veterinary NSAIDs has only recently been investigated.[22]

NSAID SAFETY

Comparative safety of different NSAIDs in dogs is difficult to determine. Such a query compares the incidence of problems with one NSAID to that of a second NSAID. Incidence would then be a ratio consisting of the number of dogs with problems (numerator) over the number of dogs treated with that drug at a given point in time (denominator). Not all adverse drug events are reported and not all reported events are directly causal, therefore the numerator is unknown. The denominator is also unknown, because it is impossible to determine the number of dogs on a drug at any given time. For these reasons, accurate comparative data are unobtainable. Accordingly, most NSAID manufacturers can state with credibility, 'no NSAID has been proved safer than (*fill in the blank*)'. Nevertheless, all ADEs should be reported to the appropriate authority and drug manufacturer so that general trends can be tracked and documented.

Adverse drug event reports at the United States Food and Drug Administration Center for Veterinary Medicine provide some insights as to why ADEs from NSAID use might be so high:[23]

- 23% of pet owners state that veterinarians never discuss adverse effects of the medication.
- 22% of pet owners state they are not given client information sheets about the prescribed drugs which are provided by pharmaceutical companies for the purpose of pet owner education.
- 14% of prescribed NSAIDs are dispensed in other than original packaging, thereby denying pet owners drug information provided on the label.
- Only 4% of pet patients prescribed drugs are given preadministration blood analyses.

As a class of drug, NSAIDs are most commonly associated with adverse reactions to the gastrointestinal tract (64%), renal system (21%), and liver (14%), respectively.[23] There is no published information relating to similar feline adverse drug events. Gastrointestinal problems associated with NSAIDs can be as benign as regurgitation or as serious as gastric ulceration and perforation (*Table 39*). Vomiting has been identified as the most frequent clinical sign associated with gastric perforation.[3] Pet owners should be informed that while taking an NSAID, if their pet experiences vomiting, the drug should be stopped and the patient should promptly be examined. This is a conservative approach since dogs are considered a 'vomiting species' and some NSAIDs are associated with more vomiting than others.

NSAID-ASSOCIATED GASTROINTESTINAL ULCERATION

Gastric perforations are most frequently found near the pyloric antrum of the stomach and have a poor prognosis if not discovered early and treated aggressively.[3]

Table 39 Gastrointestinal adverse events reported in clinical trials. Values represent mean of test article (placebo). Data sourced from drug inserts. Caution should be used in comparing adverse events among different drugs because of differences in study populations, data collection methods, and reporting methods.

Drug	Vomiting	Diarrhea
Carprofen	3.1% (3.8%)	3.1% (3.8%)
Etodolac	4.3% (1.7%)	2.6% (1.7%)
Deracoxib	2.9% (3.8%)	2.9% (1.9%)
Tepoxalin	2.0% (4.8%) at 7 days	4.0% (0) at 7 days
	19.6% at 28 days	21.5% at 28 days
Meloxicam	25.5% (15.4%)	12.1% (7.4%)
Firocoxib	3.9% (6.6%)	0.8% (8.3%)

Risk factors identified with NSAID associated gastric ulceration are most commonly seen with inappropriate use: (1) overdosing, (2) concurrent use of multiple NSAIDs, and (3) concurrent use of NSAIDs with corticosteroids.[3] For nearly 50 years 'steroid ulceration' has been recognized with the sole use of corticosteroids, attributed to a steroid-induced gastric hypersecretion of acid together with a decreased rate of mucus secretion.[24]

Lascelles *et al.*[3] observed that 23/29 gastrointestinal perforations in an NSAID retrospective review occurred in the area of the pyloric antrum (**124**). Possible reasons for this anatomical focus being at higher risk include that it is subject to recurrent bathing by irritable bile reflux through the pylorus. Apart from a few studies that have examined the effect of NSAIDs on gastric mucosal production of prostanoids,[25–27] COX-selectivity has largely been determined using *in vitro* assays, and assumptions have been made about gastrointestinal effects based on these *in vitro* data. Given the variability in results from *in vitro* assays, and the lack of understanding of COX physiology in the canine proximal gastrointestinal tract, making assumptions about the clinical effects of various NSAIDs based on *in vitro* data may lead to erroneous conclusions.

Wooten *et al.*[28] reported an assessment of the *in vivo* action of NSAIDs in the region of the gastrointestinal tract which appears to be at greatest risk for ulceration in the dog. Purpose-bred mongrel dogs were given a COX-1-selective NSAID (aspirin at 10 mg/kg bid PO), a COX-2-preferential NSAID (carprofen at 4.4 mg/kg sid PO), and a COX-2-selective NSAID (deracoxib at 2 mg/kg sid PO), or placebo for 3 days, with a 4-week washout period between treatments. Endoscopic mucosal biopsies were obtained from the pyloric and duodenal mucosa, and evaluated histologically, measuring COX-1 and COX-2 protein expression with Western blotting and prostanoids via enzyme-linked immunosorbent assay (ELISA). This investigation can be considered clinically relevant as it reflects the effect of a drug treatment on the actual tissue levels of prostanoids, not the drug effect on the total *possible* production of prostanoids by a tissue, as has previously been inferred from *in vitro* sourced COX ratios.

PG levels were found to be significantly higher in the pylorus than in the duodenum, which may be explained by differences in COX expression in the pylorus versus the duodenum, where the need for protection from refluxed bile is high. The 'more traditional' NSAIDs (aspirin and carprofen) decreased the total concentration of PGs in the gastric mucosa, while PG levels were not altered by the coxib-class NSAID (deracoxib) (**125**).

Thromboxane (TX) has been shown to be indicative of COX-1 activity in the gastrointestinal tract of several species;[29] however the linkage of TXB_2 to COX-1 activity in the canine gastrointestinal tract is speculated, but not confirmed. Carprofen administration also significantly reduced TXB_2 concentrations compared to deracoxib, suggesting that carprofen inhibits COX-1 in the gastric mucosa, whereas deracoxib had no effect on TXB_2 (COX-1) concentrations (**125**).

This is in keeping with the findings of Brainard, et. al., who reported that carprofen decreased clot strength and platelet aggregation (a COX-1-related phenomena), while the coxib-class NSAID deracoxib actually increased clot strength. Changes in platelet function, hemostasis, and prostaglandin expression after treatment with nonsteroidal anti-inflammatory drugs with various cyclooxygenase selectivities in dogs.[29]

124

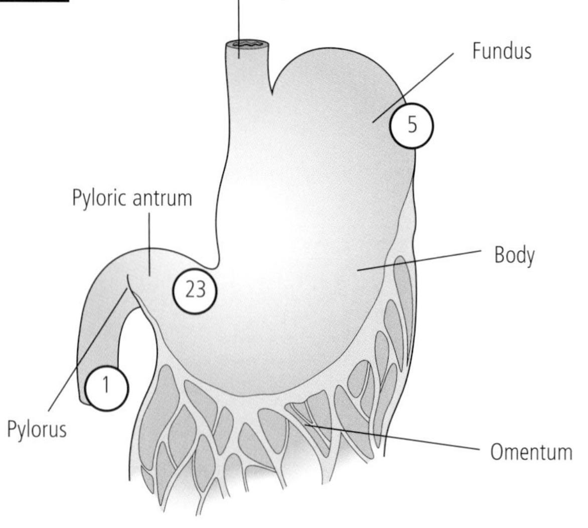

124 In a retrospective NSAID-associated gastrointestinal perforations study, 23/29 perforations were identified in the pyloric antrum.

Other investigators have reported *in vivo* findings for commonly used NSAIDs. Sessions *et al.*[25] reported that carprofen and deracoxib were both COX-1-sparing, while Punke *et al.*[31] reported that firocoxib and meloxicam were COX-1-sparing, while tepoxalin was not.

A novel finding of the Wooten study[28] was the intestinal mucosal presence of COX-2 in the healthy research dogs. Heretofore, the presence of COX-2 was believed to be upregulated by disease. This finding might suggest that COX-2 serves some unknown constitutive role in the intestinal mucosa. If this is true, the premise can be validated that an NSAID can be 'too' COX-2 selective.

Findings from these studies demonstrate that different NSAIDs reduce prostanoid production to a different degree in the canine pylorus and duodenum, and this appears to be related to their COX selectivity. Which begs the question as to why NSAIDs that appear to be highly selective for COX-2 have been shown to be apparently associated with perforating ulcers in the pylorus and duodenum in the dog. To date, the only study assessing the association between a selective COX-2 inhibitor (deracoxib) and gastroduodenal perforation revealed that in almost all cases (26/29) of ulceration in dogs receiving the coxib-class NSAID, an inappropriately high dose, or concurrent administration with other NSAIDs or corticosteroid, or rapid switching (<24 hr) from one NSAID to another was identified.[3] This suggests that when gastrointestinal perforation occurs following administration of a selective COX-2 inhibitor, other factors such as overdosing, concurrent administration of drugs inhibiting prostanoid production, rapid change from one NSAID to another, or hitherto unrecognized factors, play a major role in the production of ulceration. This is corroborated by documentation that 75–80% of all ADE reports with deracoxib use are associated with inappropriate use.[32]

NSAIDs AND RENAL FUNCTION

Through regulation of vascular tone, blood flow, ion and water balance, and renin, PGs are important for normal renal function.[33] In situations of decreased systemic blood pressure or circulating blood volume,

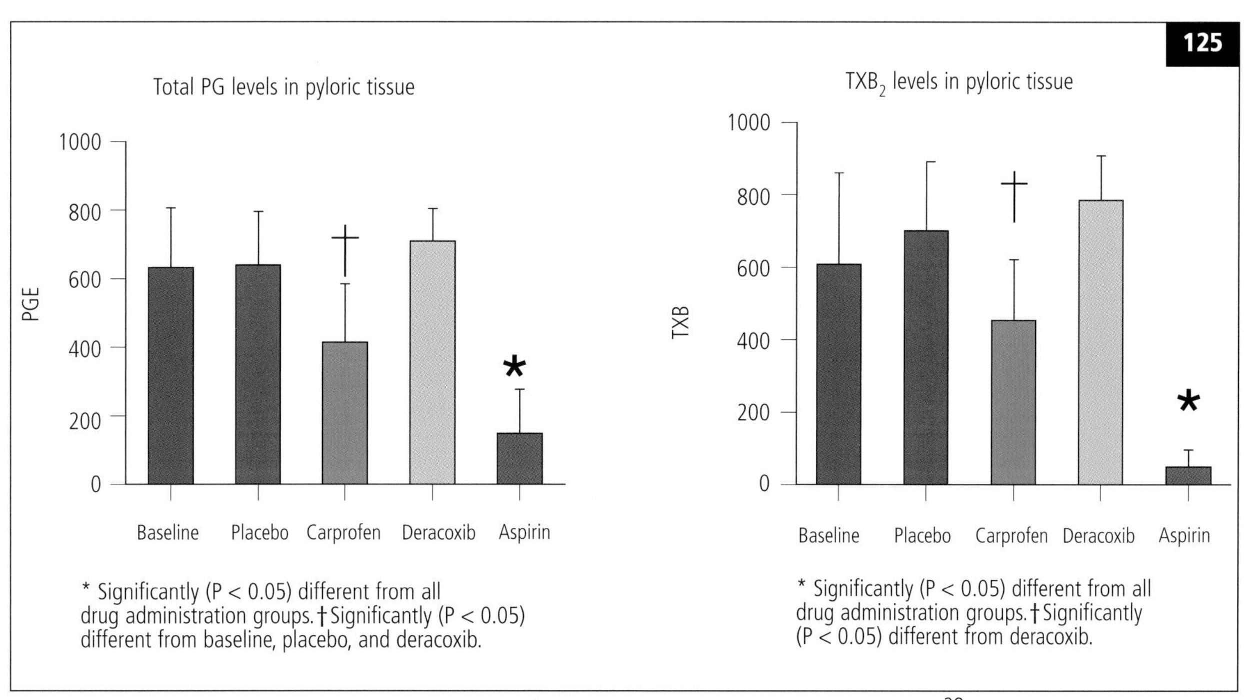

125 Total PG and TXB_2 pyloric tissue levels in an *in vivo* study of traditional vs coxib-class NSAID.[28]

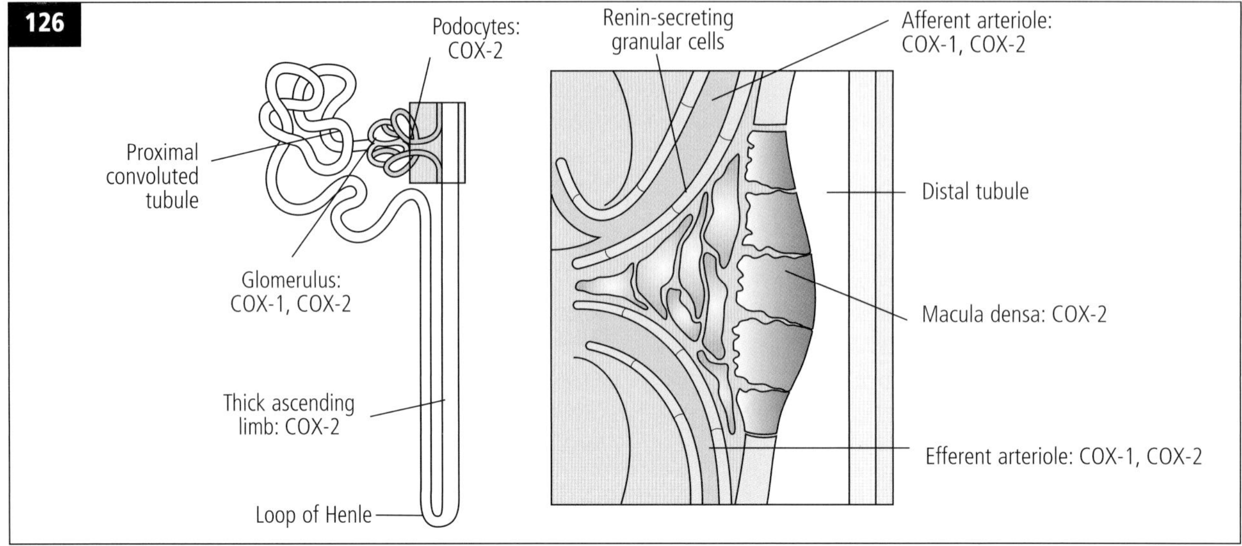

126 Cyclooxygenase presence in the kidney.[35, 36]

PGs assist in regulating and maintaining renal blood flow to maintain a mean arterial pressure ranging from 60–150 mmHg.[34] Both the COX-1 and the COX-2 isoforms are expressed in the kidneys of dogs, rats, monkeys, and humans where they both play constitutive roles (**126**).

Therefore, at recommended dosing, no one NSAID is more safe than another on renal function in these species. NSAID drug complications of hypovolemia and hypotension have led to acute renal failure and death in both dogs and cats.[37] Information regarding COX-1 and COX-2 distribution or expression under varying conditions of the feline kidney is unknown. Meloxicam is, perhaps, the most frequently administered NSAID in cats, and repeated use (off-label) has been associated with acute renal failure in cats. The manufacturer cautions against such repeated use.

Blood urea nitrogen (BUN) and creatinine elevations occur relatively late in renal disease, therefore screening urine for protein has been suggested for early disease detection. Any positive screening result should be followed by measurement of urine protein:creatinine ratio for a more complete assessment. Any patient with compromised renal function is at risk with any NSAID administration, particularly when under-hydrated.

Table 40 Approximate plasma half-life of hepatic enzymes in the dog and cat.

Enzyme	Dog	Cat
Alanine aminotransferase (ALT)	40–61 hr	3.5 hr
Aspartate aminotransferase (AST)	12 hr	1.5 hr
Glutamate dehydrogenase (GLDH)	18 hr	-----
Alkaline phosphatase (ALP)		
Hepatobiliary isoenzyme	66 hr	6 hr
Corticosteroid isoenzyme	74 hr	-----
Intestinal isoenzyme	6 min	2 min

NSAIDs AND HEPATIC FUNCTION

Serious liver injury can occur from acetaminophen (paracetamol) overdose in humans and dogs. (Technically, acetaminophen is not a true NSAID since it is considered analgesic but not anti-inflammatory.) Acetaminophen toxicity in cats presents primarily as methemoglobinemia and Heinz body anemia, likely from enhanced susceptibility of feline erythrocytes to oxidative injury.[38]

Drug-induced *hepatopathy* (defined as an elevation of liver enzyme values) is a rare, but potentially serious adverse consequence of several drug classes including NSAIDs, volatile anesthetics, antibiotics, antihypertensives, and anticonvulsants. This can occur with all NSAIDs. In comparison idiosyncratic *hepatotoxicosis* has become associated with the rare (estimated 0.02% incidence[39]) lethal liver toxicity of carprofen. All dogs with hepatotoxicosis have a hepatopathy; however, not all cases of hepatopathy are lethal. This hepatotoxicosis does not appear to be associated with dose or duration of administration, and no epidemiological study has shown the hepatotoxicosis to be breed related. A hypothesis for carprofen-related hepatotoxicosis is that reactive acyl glucuronide metabolites are generated that can covalently bind and hepatize hepatocyte proteins, thereby promoting an immunological response in the liver.[40–42]

It is good advice to characterize liver enzymes before and during NSAID administration, especially when an NSAID is being administered long term. However, an increase in liver enzymes is difficult to interpret, as any chronic drug administration can cause an elevation, and liver enzymes are not a good measure of hepatic function. When liver enzymes are elevated and concern for liver function is present, liver function tests should be performed. Mere elevation of liver enzymes may not be cause for discontinuing an NSAID. See *Table 40*, **127**, **128**.

ASPIRIN

Aspirin presents unique risk factors to the canine patient. Aspirin is both topically and systemically toxic (even at low doses of 5–10 mg/kg sid), chondrodestructive, causes irreversible platelet acetylation, and is associated with gastrointestinal bleeding of approximately 3 ml/day.[43,44]

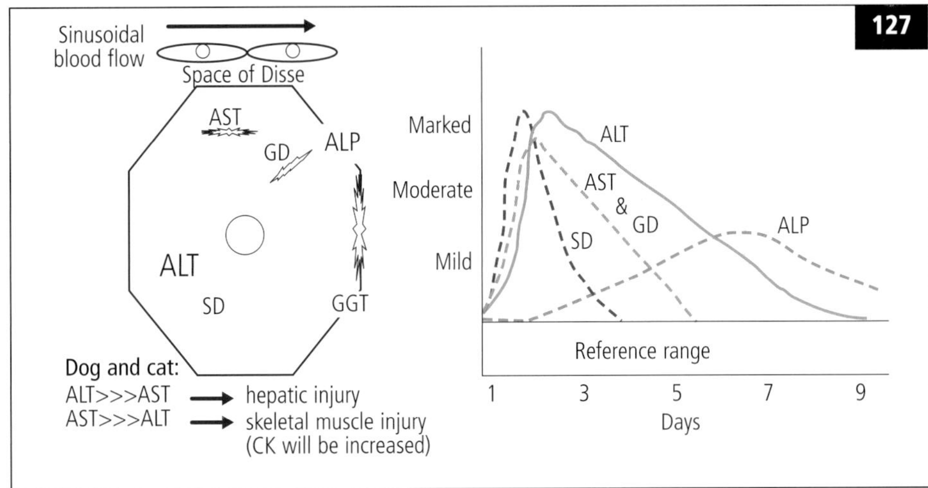

127 Subcellular location of hepatobiliary enzymes and relative magnitude and duration of increase of plasma activities following acute, severe, diffuse injury to the liver.

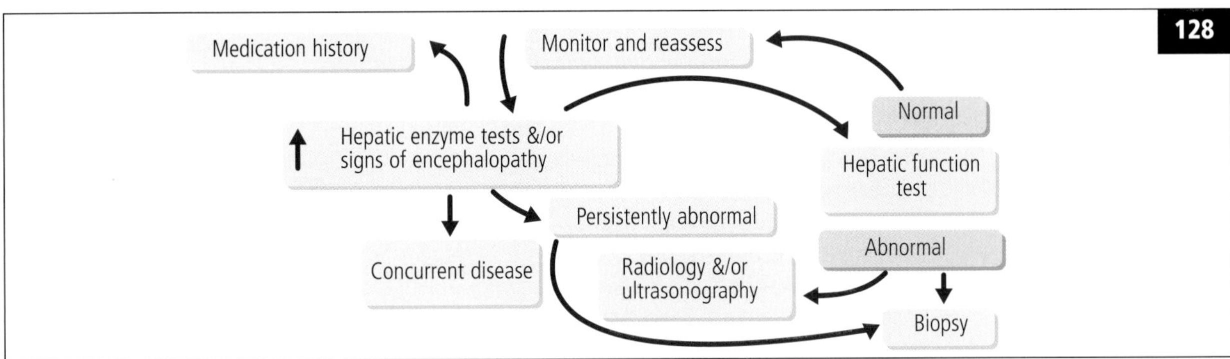

128 Simplified algorithm for investigation of abnormal hepatic tests in an animal without severe anemia. Concurrent extrahepatic diseases such as lymphocytic–plasmacytic enteritis, pancreatitis, heart failure, and endocrinopathies can cause hepatic tests to be abnormal.

The American Medical Association (AMA) reports that 16,500 people die each year associated with NSAID toxicity,[45] yet with an over-representation of aspirin; pet owners often consider aspirin benign because it is available over-the-counter and the media suggest it is safe. Even low-dose aspirin has consistently been associated with gastrointestinal petechiation and hemorrhage. Aspirin does not have a US Food and Drug Administration (FDA) license for use in the dog, and the plasma concentrations regarded as being therapeutic are relatively close to the toxic levels.[46] In theory, since aspirin causes gastrointestinal lesions, it would be inappropriate to sequentially progress from aspirin to a strongly COX-2-selective NSAID (which might restrict the COX-2 necessary for repair) without an adequate washout period following the aspirin. It is also perilous to use aspirin together with another NSAID or corticosteroid.

Development of gastric mucosal hemorrhage, erosion, and ulceration associated with administration of NSAIDs is largely attributed to reduction of PGE synthesis in the gastric mucosa. PGs play a key role in protection of the gastrointestinal mucosal barrier by: (1) increasing mucus and bicarbonate secretion, (2) enhancing mucosal blood flow, (3) stimulating epithelial cell growth, and (4) suppressing acid secretion.

In addition, aspirin can cause direct cellular toxicosis, independent of the inhibition of PG synthesis. Aspirin may cause gastric mucosal injury via two mechanisms: (1) direct damage to the gastric epithelial cell, and (2) indirect damage caused by its antiprostaglandin effects.[46] The erosive effects of aspirin on the canine stomach have been known since 1909, when Christoni and Lapressa administered 150–200 mg of aspirin to dogs and noted gastric lesions.[47] Interestingly, the discovery of aspirin's ulcerogenic properties resulted in its use in the study of gastroduodenal ulcer disease in animal models.[48,49] Topical irritation and physical damage to the gastric mucosa barrier may result from a pH-mediated effect of mucosal hydrophobicity and from direct contact between aspirin and gastric epithelium. In the highly acidic gastric lumen, aspirin is mostly nonionized and lipid soluble. In this form, it can freely diffuse into mucosal cells where, at neutral pH, aspirin becomes ionized and water soluble. The water-soluble form cannot penetrate lipid cell membranes and consequently becomes trapped in mucosal cells. The presence of intracellular aspirin causes increased membrane permeability, leading to an influx of hydrogen ions from the gastric lumen or an increased 'back-diffusion' of acid across the gastric mucosal barrier. This increased acid back-diffusion is crucial in initiating and perpetuating mucosal injury. The result is edema, inflammation, hemorrhage, erosions and ulceration, and submucosal capillary damage.

Standard formulations of buffered aspirin have been shown not to provide sufficient buffering to neutralize gastric acid or to prevent mucosal injury.[51]

Enteric-coated aspirin causes less gastric injury in humans, compared with that from administration of nonbuffered or buffered aspirin, but absorption is quite variable,[52,53] with coated tablets having been observed to pass in the feces. See *Table 41*, **129**, **130**.

ANTIULCER AGENTS

One goal of antiulcer treatment is to lower intragastric acidity so as to prevent further destruction of the gastrointestinal tract mucosa. Cimetadine, a histamine (H_2)-receptor blocker, is

Table 41 Risk factors for NSAID-induced gastrointestinal complications (human).[53]

	Risk factor	Estimated increased risk
Established	Prior clinical GI event (ulcer/complication)	2.4–4×
	Advanced age (65+)	2–3.5×
	Concomitant anticoagulation therapy	3×
	Concurrent corticosteroid use	2×
	High-dose NSAID or multiple NSAID use	2–4×
	Major comorbidity (e.g. heart disease, etc.)	Variable
Probable	Long-term NSAID use	
	Coexisting *H. pylori* infection	
	Dyspepsia caused by an NSAID	

commonly used. Cimetidine requires dosing three to four times daily, however it is not effective in preventing NSAID-induced gastric ulceration. Omeprazole is a substituted benzimidazole that acts by inhibiting the hydrogen–potassium ATPase (proton pump inhibitor) that is responsible for production of hydrogen ions in the parietal cell. It is five to ten times more potent than cimetadine for inhibiting gastric acid secretion and has a long duration of action, requiring once-a-day administration. It may be useful in decreasing gastric hyperacidity, but has minimal effect on ulcer healing. Misoprostol is a synthetic PGE_1 analog used to prevent gastric ulceration. It decreases gastric acid secretion, increases bicarbonate and mucus secretion, increases epithelial cell turnover, and increases mucosal blood flow. Both cimetidine and misoprostol require dosing three to four times daily and adverse reactions mimic those of gastritis and ulcerations. See *Table 42*.

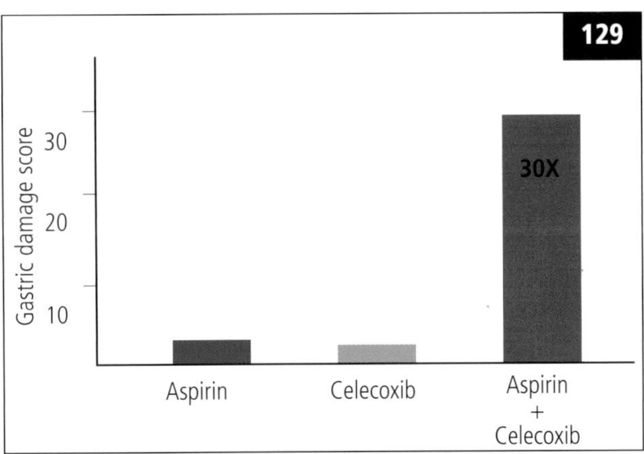

129 Some human patients take high-dose aspirin for their cardiac condition and a 'third-generation' NSAID for their musculoskeletal discomfort, thereby increasing their potential for gastric damage.[55]

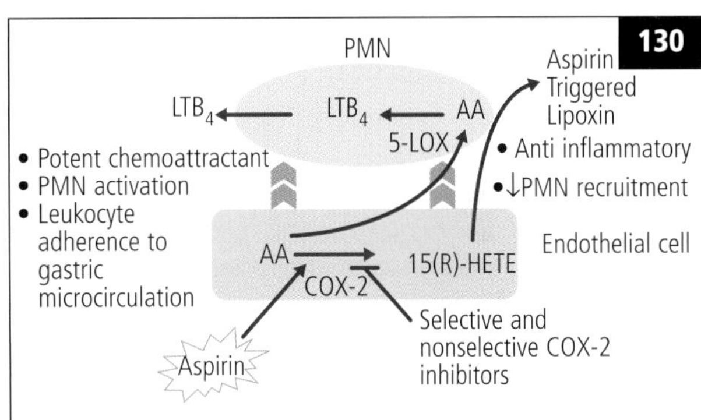

130 Potential for increased GI damage from the concurrent use of aspirin with another NSAID resides with the aspirin triggered lipoxin (ATL) pathway. ATL is a protective mechanism with aspirin consumption, which is blocked with the concurrent administration of another NSAID, giving rise to an alternative pathway for arachidonic acid that actually enhances the potential for aspirin toxicity.[55]

Table 42 Pharmacologial agents for NSAID gastrointestinal prophylaxis and treatment.

Group	Generic name	Brand name	Dose
Proton pump inhibitors (PPI)	Omeprazole	Prilosec	Canine: 0.7 mg/kg, PO
	Lansoprazole	PrevAcid	
	Rabeprazole	AcipHex	
	Pantoprazole	Protonix	
	Esomeprazole	Nexium	
PG analog	Misoprostol	Cytotec	Canine: 2–5 μg/kg, tid, PO
H_2 blockers	Cimetidine	Tagament	Canine/feline: 10 mg/kg, tid, PO, IV, IM; Feline: 3.5 mg/kg, bid, PO or 2.5 mg/kg, bid, IV
	Ranitidine	Zantac	Canine: 2 mg/kg, tid, PO, IV
	Famotidine	Pepcid	Canine/feline: 0.5 mg/kg, sid, PO, IV, IM, SQ or 0.25 mg/kg, bid, PO, IV, IM, SQ
	Nizatidine	Axid	Canine: 2.5–5 mg/kg, sid, PO
Mucosal sealant	Sucralfate	Carafate	Canine: 0.5–1 g, tid–bid, PO; feline: 0.25 g, tid–bid, PO

WASHOUT

Washout between NSAIDs is poorly researched, however one survey report[3] suggests that failure to implement a washout between different NSAIDs may put the patient at risk for gastrointestinal pathology. One must consider the reason for changing NSAIDs when considering a washout period. If the reason for change is efficacy in the healthy dog, 'washout' is a lesser issue than if the reason for change is intolerance. With intolerance, a minimal washout time should be no less than the time required to recover from adverse clinical signs. Most agree that washout following aspirin is a unique scenario, due in part to the phenomenon of aspirin triggered lipoxin (ATL).[55] Five to seven days' washout following aspirin is probably adequate. One study has been conducted where injectable carprofen was followed at the next once a day dosing with deracoxib.[56] In this study of a limited number of healthy dogs, no difference was noted in following injectable carprofen with either oral carprofen or oral deracoxib. Pain relief during a washout period can be obtained by the use of other class drugs, e.g. acetaminophen, tramadol, amantadine, gabapentin or opioids.

ENHANCING RESPONSIBLE NSAID USE

Every pet owner who is discharged with medication, including NSAIDs, should have the following questions addressed:

- What is the medication supposed to do?
- What is the proper dose and dosing interval?
- What potential adverse response(s) are possible?
- What should I do if I observe an adverse response?

Both verbal and written instructions should be given. Preadministrative urinalysis and blood chemistries are well advised prior to dispensing NSAIDs for two primary reasons. Firstly, the pet may be a poor candidate for any NSAID, i.e. it may be azotemic or have decreased liver function. (These physiological compromises may not preclude the use of NSAIDs, but such a decision must be justified.) Secondly, a baseline status should be established for subsequent comparison, should the patient show clinical signs suggestive of drug intolerance. For the patient on a long-term NSAID protocol, the frequency of laboratory profiling should be determined by clinical signs and age. Minimal effective dose should always be the therapeutic objective, and routine examination of the animal constitutes the practice of good medicine. Since alanine aminotransferase (ALT) is more specific than serum alkaline phosphatase (SAP) as a blood chemistry for liver status, an elevation three to four times laboratory normal should prompt a subsequent liver function test. Because the kidney expresses both COX isozymes constitutively, no one NSAID can be presumed safer than another for renal function, and any patient that is hypotensive or insufficiently hydrated is at risk during NSAID administration.

NSAIDs play a major role in a perioperative protocol for healthy animals, due to their features as anti-inflammatories, analgesics, and antipyretics. NSAID inclusion helps prevent CNS windup and provides synergism with opioids.[56] Surgery cannot be performed without resultant iatrogenic inflammation, and the best time to administer the anti-inflammatory drug is pre-emptively–before the surgery. It is imperative that surgical patients be sufficiently hydrated if NSAIDs are used perioperatively. Under the influence of gaseous anesthesia, renal tissue may suffer from underperfusion, at which point PGs are recruited to assist with this perfusion, and if the patient is under the influence of an antiprostaglandin (NSAID), renal function may be at risk. In human medicine, some suggest that NSAIDs should not be withheld from adults with normal preoperative renal function because of concerns about postoperative renal impairment.[58]

NSAIDs AND BONE HEALING

Among their many uses, COX inhibitors (NSAIDs) are widely administered for musculoskeletal conditions, including postsurgical orthopedic analgesia. It has been hypothesized that these agents may modulate bone, ligament, or tendon healing by inhibiting PG production. Results from animal models do suggest that NSAIDs and COX-2 inhibition may have a minimal effect on bone, tendon, and ligament healing, especially at earlier stages, but bear no significant impact on the ultimate long-term outcome. In a review on the subject,[58] the authors proposed that despite the contribution of PGs in the dynamic process of normal bone healing and pathophysiology, alternative mechanisms may maintain normal bone function in the absence of COX-2 activity. Direct comparison studies suggest that adverse effects of selective COX-2 inhibitors on bone healing are lesser in magnitude than those of non-selective NSAIDs.[58]

EFFICACY

It is difficult to differentiate NSAID efficacy in the perioperative setting, because most clinicians administer NSAIDs as part of a multimodal (balanced) analgesic protocol. Perioperative analgesia from an NSAID alone is rarely sufficient. Injectable carprofen was designed for perioperative use, yet for labeled intramuscular administration; the injectable product has a different pharmacokinetic profile than the oral product, due to its mixed-micelle formulation. Given intramuscularly, the maximum concentration (Cmax) of the injectable (Cmax: 8.0 µg/ml at 1.5–8 hr) is half that of the oral formulation (Cmax: 16.9 µg/ml at 0.5–3 hr), and is reached later,[60] suggesting that it be given several hours prior to surgery for maximal pre-emptive effect. There are few objective pain assessment models for soft tissue, from which to compare NSAID efficacy.

In contrast, force plate gait analysis in an orthopedic model has become the standard for ranking NSAID efficacy in canids on an objective basis.[60] Although several NSAID manufacturers have made public their studies comparing one or two products, none have compared the large group of NSAIDs most commonly used in clinical practice. Dr. Darryl Millis and colleagues at the University of Tennessee reported such a study,[61] conducted independent of commercial support, using the force plate gait analysis model, which is considered to be the gold standard for objective assessment (**131**).

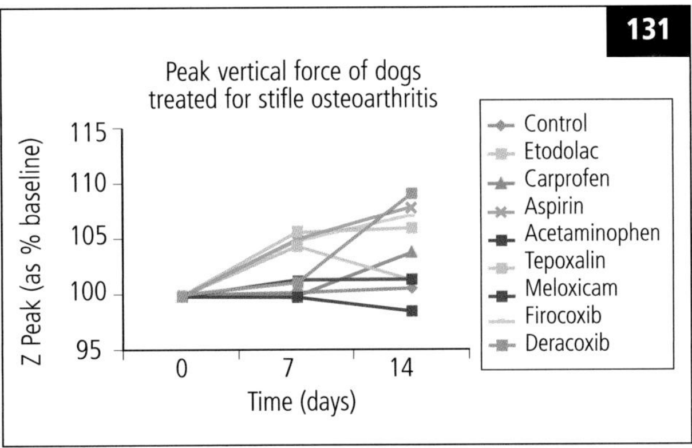

131 Comparative efficacy of contemporary NSAIDs used in veterinary medicine.[61]

Measuring ground reaction forces is the most common way to objectively assess weightbearing in dogs. Using a force plate platform, investigators can compare, with certainty, the degree of lameness over a period of time. In its simplest terms, force plate gait analysis measures ground reaction forces that result when a dog places its limb during a specific gait. The three orthogonal ground reaction forces generated – vertical, craniocaudal, and mediolateral – represent the total forces transmitted through one limb to the ground (**132**). Typically, peak force in the vertical axis is used to objectively measure limb function. When comparing NSAID efficacy, lame dogs (often with long-standing anterior cruciate ligament compromise) are walked over a force plate during a given treatment regimen. Comparing the relative amount of weight

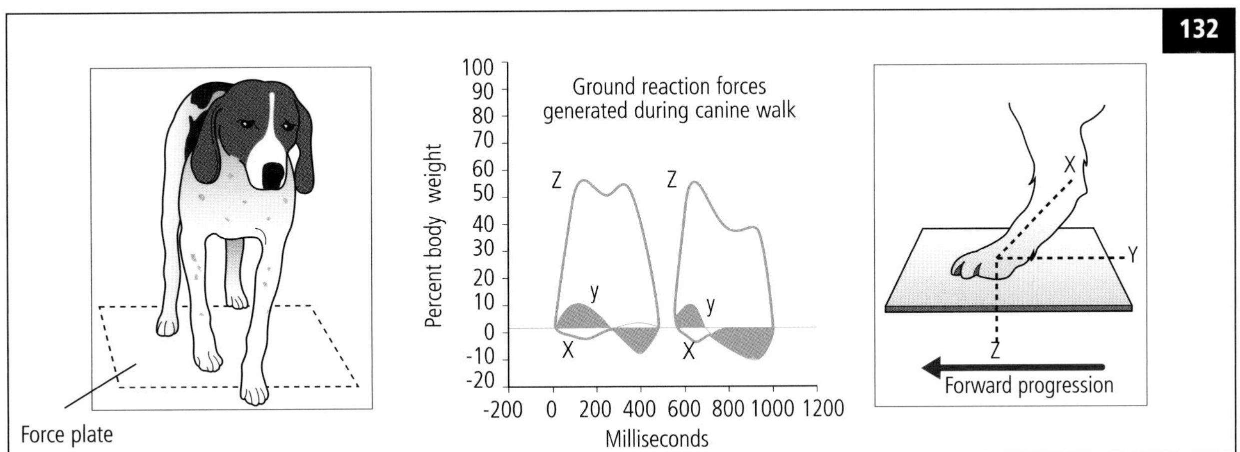

132 Each gait generates a specific pattern of ground reaction forces. The first peak in vertical forces (Z) of the m-shaped pattern of the walk represents the peak vertical forces associated with initial paw strike. Y and X represent the craniocaudal and mediolateral forces, respectively. Breaking and propulsion impulses are indicated by the shaded areas of the craniocaudal graphs.

placed by the compromised limb on the force plate under different NSAID regimens, generates a relative rank of NSAID efficacy, or pain relief. See *Table 43*.

Kinematic gait analysis, or motion analysis, is used less frequently than force platform analysis, but its use is increasing, mostly in research laboratories. Kinematic evaluation measures changes in joint angles with gait, the velocity and acceleration of changes in joint angles, and stride length, as well as gait swing and stance times. Kinematic evaluation is often combined with force platform gait analysis, providing a powerful method of detecting abnormalities and response to therapy.

Objective measurement of lameness severity in cats is quite difficult, as cats do not comply with force plate protocols. However, pressure mats have been used to reveal the distribution of pressures associated with paw contact,[63] so that pressures on each digital pad and on the metacarpal pad could be measured quantitatively following onychectomies. Use of the pressure mat to evaluate lameness in cats will likely see further development. The use of acceleration-based activity monitors may also allow for future objective measurement of improved mobility following treatment for osteoarthritic conditions in the cat.[64]

Table 43 Comparison of NSAID efficacy studies used for US FDA approval.

Drug	Primary assessment method	Ground reaction force assessment
Carprofen	Subjective owner and veterinary assessment indicated improvement more likely in treated dogs	No significant difference between placebo dogs and treated dogs
Etodolac	Ground reaction forces	Peak vertical force improved 0.4%, 2.3%, and 1.6% with placebo, low-dose, and high-dose treatments, respectively. Vertical impulse improved 0.4%, 0.13%, and 0.22%, respectively
Deracoxib	Ground reaction forces	Peak vertical force improved 7.4% with treatment vs. placebo. Vertical impulse improved 4.9% with treatment compared with placebo
Tepoxalin	Subjective changes compared with carprofen, no placebo comparison. Subjective improvement similar to carprofen	Not measured
Meloxicam	Subjective assessment of lameness, weightbearing, pain on palpation, and overall improvement compared with placebo. Significant improvement noted on day 14 of one 14-day study. Significant improvement noted in the parameter of overall assessment on day 7 by veterinary assessors and on day 14 by owners in a second study	Not measured
Firocoxib	Subjective comparison to etodolac. No comparison to placebo. Subjective efficacy comparable to etodolac	Ground reaction forces were determined in a subset of patients. Results were comparable between firocoxib and etodolac

ADMINISTRATION

TIME OF ADMINISTRATION

Time of administration is a common question arising from NSAIDs labeled for dosing once daily: i.e. should the drug be administered in the morning or in the evening? Some argue that morning administration is most logical, taking advantage of Cmax during that time of the day when the dog might be most active. Others suggest the NSAID should be dosed so that Cmax is reached to ensure maximal rest for the animal, proposing that the animal performs best following a good night's rest. There is no consensus.

WITH OR WITHOUT FOOD

Many of the contemporary NSAIDs are labeled for use either with or without food. Administration with food takes advantage of the increased production of gastric bicarbonate and associated buffering. Feeding an NSAID together with food may enhance acceptability in some dogs.

NSAID COMPATIBILITY WITH OTHER AGENTS

NSAIDs are highly protein bound and may compete with binding of other highly protein bound drugs, particularly in the hypoproteinemic animal, resulting in altered drug concentrations. Fortunately, the number of other highly protein bound drugs is minimal. *Table 44* lists drugs and agents that may be

Table 44 **NSAIDs: potential drug interactions.**[64]

Drug	May increase the toxicity of	May decrease the efficacy of	Toxicity may be increased by
Classical NSAIDs (clinically significant COX-1 inhibition)	Warfarin, methotrexate, valproic acid, midazolam, furosemide, spironolactone, sulfonylureas, heparin	Furosemide, thiazide, ACE inhibitors, β blockers	Aminoglycosides, furosemide, cyclosporine (renal), glucocorticoids (gastrointestinal), heparin, gingko, garlic, ginger, ginseng (hemorrhage)
Coxibs and relatively COX-2 selective agents	Warfarin, methotrexate, valproic acid, midazolam, furosemide, spironolactone, sulfonylureas	Furosemide, thiazides, ACE inhibitors, β blockers	Aminoglycosides, furosemide, cyclosporine (renal), Glucocorticoids (gastrointestinal)
Phenylbutazone, acetaminophen	Warfarin, sulfonylureas		Phenobartital, alcohol, rifampin, metoclopramide

influenced by the concurrent administration of NSAIDs. Because pet owners tend to be using more and more 'natural' products, some of which can potentially influence the concurrent use of an NSAID (*Table 45*), it is advisable to ask owners for a complete listing of everything they are giving their pet by mouth.

NSAIDs AND CANCER

Human studies have shown that patients receiving long-term NSAID therapy have a reduced risk of colorectal cancer.[66] Such observations have led to research into the role of NSAIDs as a preventative measure against cancer development and as adjunctive antineoplastic therapy. Published data also suggest that control of oncological pain can impact on the course of cancer progression.[67]

PGs play a major role in cancer development including inhibition of immune surveillance, promotion of angiogenesis, and inhibition of apoptosis.[68,69] High levels of PGs are found in tumors of many types that may exert effects in an autocrine or paracrine fashion, and upregulation of COX-2 has been directly associated with tumor aggression.[70]

In addition to decreasing PG production via inhibition of COX-2, NSAIDs also have COX-independent anticancer mechanisms including activation or inhibition of cellular signaling pathways via upregulation or inhibition of oncogenes. Preliminary results of a study involving deracoxib, a COX-2 selective inhibitor, as therapy for transitional cell carcinoma have demonstrated stable disease in nine of nine dogs.[71] Many oncologists are now prescribing COX-2 inhibitors in conjunction with traditional modalities of surgery, radiation therapy, and chemotherapy for a variety of tumors.

CATS AND NSAIDs

There are approximately 69 million cats in the US[72] and approximately 10 million in the UK.[73] Radiographically detectable DJD is apparently detectable in as high as 90% of cats over 12 years of age.[74] Efficacy of NSAIDs for relief of chronic pain in the cat is difficult to demonstrate, but empirically embraced. Probable reasons for the relative void of evidence base for NSAIDs in cats include:

- Assumption by pharmaceutical manufacturers that the market for cat analgesics is not financially rewarding.
- Difficulty of identifying pain in cats, and therefore indications for administration.
- Scarcity of information about NSAIDs in cats.
- Potential risk of NSAID toxicity in cats.

Salicylate toxicity in cats is well established.

Table 45 Potential herb–drug interactions.[65]

Herb	Interacting drugs	Results
St. John's wort	Cyclosporine, fexofenadine, midazolam, digoxin, tacrolimus, amitriptyline, warfarin, theophylline	Decreased plasma drug concentrations
Gingko	Warfarin, heparin, **NSAIDs** Omeprazole	Bleeding Decreased plasma concentrations
Ginseng	Warfarin, heparin, **NSAIDs**, opioids	Bleeding Falsely elevated serum digoxin levels (laboratory test interaction with ginseng) Decreased analgesic effect (laboratory test interaction with ginseng)
Garlic, chamomile, ginger	Warfarin, Heparin, **NSAIDs**	Bleeding

Cats present a unique susceptibility to NSAID toxicity because of slow clearance and dose-dependent elimination. Cats have a low capacity for hepatic glucuronidation of NSAIDs,[75] which is the major mechanism of metabolism and excretion for this class of drug.

Acetaminophen toxicity in cats results in methemoglobinemia, liver failure, and death. *Cats are particularly susceptible to acetaminophen toxicity* due, in part, to defective conjugation of the drug and conversion to a reactive electrolytic metabolite.

Because of its delivery form as an elixir, meloxicam is sometimes used preferentially in small dogs and cats. Only carprofen,meloxicam and robenacoxib are approved for cats (country dependent). The manufacturer of meloxicam has recommended reducing the original approval dose from 0.2 to 0.1 mg/kg because of some initial gastrointestimal problems. This suggests particular attention be given to accurate dosing of small dogs and cats. As with all NSAIDs in dogs or cats, gastric ulcerations have been observed.

LOOKING TO THE FUTURE

NSAIDs are the fastest growing class of drugs in both human and veterinary medicine because of their relatively safe resolution of a wide range of pathological conditions. Based upon current understanding of their mode of action, future NSAIDs will likely *not* be developed to be 'stronger longer', i.e. supremely COX-2 selective, with a very long half-life. Instead, NSAID development may well offer species- and/or disease-specific molecules, increased safety profiles, and augmenting benefits such as NO inhibition. At present this class of drug offers immense benefits, constrained most often only by issues of safe, responsible use.

IMPROVING SAFETY

The following guidelines can be used to minimize risk factors for NSAID ADEs:

- Proper dosing.
- Administer minimal effective dose.
- Dispense in approved packaging together with owner information sheets.
- Avoid concurrent use of multiple NSAIDs and NSAIDs with corticosteroids.
- Refrain from use of aspirin.
- Provide pet owners with both oral and written instructions for responsible NSAID use.
- Conduct appropriate patient chemistry/urine profiling. Do not use in patients with reduced cardiac output or in patients with overt renal disease.
- Conduct routine check-ups and chemistry profiles for patients on chronic NSAID regimens. Do not fill NSAID prescriptions without conducting patient examinations.
- Caution pet owners regarding supplementation with over-the-counter NSAIDs.
- Administer gastrointestinal protectants for at-risk patients on NSAIDs.
- Avoid NSAID administration in puppies and pregnant animals.
- NSAIDs may decrease the action of angiotensin converting enzyme (ACE) inhibitors and furosemide, a consideration for patients being treated for cardiovascular disease.
- Geriatric animals are more likely to be treated with NSAIDs on a chronic schedule, therefore their 'polypharmacy' protocols and potentially compromised drug clearance should be considered.
- Provide sufficient hydration to surgery patients administered NSAIDs.
- Report ADEs to the product manufacturers.

SUMMARY

NSAIDs are a magnificent class of agents that have changed the practice of both human and veterinary medicine. Their utilization will likely continue for decades to come as we learn more specific applications and features of these molecules. Additionally, NSAIDs are market leaders for pharmaceutical companies, and public awareness is a tenet in the overall marketing strategy for these agents. Consequently, this class of drug is not only a fundamental cornerstone of medical practice, but also an area of public scrutiny. As with all medications, adverse reactions from NSAIDs are possible, however the benefits far outweigh problems associated with their use. With responsible use of NSAIDs, we must always strive for the minimal effective dose, within established dosing ranges, and assess the benefit:risk ratio for each individual patient.

See *Table 46, Table 47*. (*overleaf*)

Table 46 US FDA approved NSAIDs with product details.

	Deramaxx®	**Rimadyl®**	**Previcox®**	**Metacam®**	**EtoGesic®**	**Zubrin®**
Company	Novartis	Pfizer	Merial	Boehringer-Ingelheim	Fort Dodge	Schering-Plough
Active ingredient	Deracoxib	Carprofen	Firocoxib	Meloxicam	Etodolac	Tepoxalin
Formulation	25 mg, 75 mg, 100 mg scored chewable tablets	Caplets/ chewable tablets: 25, 75, 100 mg scored caplets or scored chewable tablets; SC injectable: 50 mg carprofen/ml	Chewable tablets containing 57 or 227 mg, palatability 68%	Liquid suspension: to be squirted on food. Injectable: 5 mg/ml, SC or IV	150 mg, 300 mg scored tablets	Rapidly disintegrating tablets of 30, 50, 100, or 200 mg
Dosage	For the control of pain and inflammation associated with orthopedic surgery in dogs: 3–4 mg/kg. Give prior to surgery for postoperative pain. For the control of pain and inflammation associated with OA in dogs: 1–2 mg/kg daily	Oral and injectable: 4.4 mg/kg once daily or 2.2 mg/kg twice daily. For postoperative pain, administer 2 hr before the procedure	5 mg/kg oral once daily; tablets are scored and dosage should be calculated in ½ tablet increments	0.2 mg/kg injectable once or oral once: followed by 0.1 mg/kg oral suspension daily; cats: 0.3 mg/kg presurgical one-time dose (contraindicated to follow in cats with another NSAID or meloxicam)	10–15 mg/kg once daily. Adjust dose until a satisfactory clinical response is obtained reduced to minimum effective dose	10 mg/kg orally or 20 mg/kg on the initial day of treatment, followed by a daily maintenance dose of 10 mg/kg

– Continued on facing page

Table 46 US FDA approved NSAIDs with product details – ***Continued.***

	Deramaxx®	**Rimadyl®**	**Previcox®**	**Metacam®**	**EtoGesic®**	**Zubrin®**
Indications	For the control of pain and inflammation associated with orthopedic surgery in dogs weighing ≤1.8 kg. For the control of pain and inflammation associated with OA	For the relief of pain and inflammation associated with OA in dogs and the control of postoperative pain in soft tissue and orthopedic surgeries in dogs	For the control of pain and inflammation associated with OA in dogs	Control of pain and inflammation associated with OA in dogs; postoperative pain and inflammation associated with orthopedic surgery, ovariohysterectomy and castration in cats when administered prior to surgery	For the management of pain and inflammation associated with osteoarthritis in dogs	Control of pain and inflammation associated with osteoarthritis in dogs
Mechanism of action	A coxib class drug that uniquely targets COX-2 while sparing COX-1	Inhibition of COX enzyme; *in vitro* selective against COX-2	Inhibition of COX activity; *in vitro* studies show it to be highly selective for COX-2 in canine blood	MOA not on label; oxicam class NSAID	Inhibition of COX activity; inhibits macrophage chemotaxis	COX and LOX inhibitor: 'dual pathway inhibitor of AA metabolism'
Maximum concentration (Tmax)	2 hours	Oral: Cmax of 16.9 µg/ml at 0.5–3 hr. Injectable: Cmax of 8.0 µg/ml at 1.5–8 hr		Dogs: 2.5 hr (inj) and 7.5 hr (oral). Cats: 1.5 hr postinjection	1.08–1.6 hr	2.3±1.4 hr
Half-life	3 hr	8 hr in dog	7.8 hr	Dogs: 24 hr. Cats: 15 hr after injection	7.6–12 hr	2.0±1.2 hr converts to the active metabolite which has a long half-life

– Continued overleaf

Table 46 US FDA approved NSAIDs with product details – *Continued.*

	Deramaxx®	Rimadyl®	Previcox®	Metacam®	EtoGesic®	Zubrin®
Metabolism and excretion	Metabolism primarily liver; excretion to feces is 75%, urine excretion is 20%	Liver bio-transformation: 70–80% in feces and 10–20% in urine. Some enterohepatic circulation	Primarily hepatic metabolism and fecal excretion	Not on label	Primarily hepatic metabolism and fecal excretion; enterohepatic recirculation	Primarily hepatic with excretion through feces 99%, minor urine
Side-effects within licensing studies. Serious adverse reactions associated with this drug class can occur without warning and in rare situations result in death	Vomiting, incisional lesions	Black or tarry stools, hypo-albuminemia, dermatological changes, increased liver enzyme levels, idiosyncratic hepato-toxicosis	Vomiting, diarrhea, decreased appetite. (Use of this product at doses above the recommended 5 mg/kg in puppies less than 7 months of age has been associated with serious ADEs, including death)	Vomiting, soft stools, diarrhea, inappetance, epiphora, autoimmune hemolytic anemia, thrombo-cytopenia, polyarthritis, pyoderma	Weight loss, fecal abnormalities, hypoproteinemia, small intestine erosions	Vomiting, diarrhea, gastric lesions, decrease in total protein, albumin and calcium, death
Packaging	30 count, 90 count	14, 60, 150 count. 20 ml bottle of injectable	10 and 30 count blister packs, 60 count bottles	Oral: 1.5 mg/ml: 10, 32 and 100 ml dropper bottles. Inj: 5 mg/ml in a 10 ml vial	7, 30, and 90 count	Boxes containing 10 foil blisters each

– *Continued on facing page*

Table 46 US FDA approved NSAIDs with product details – *Continued.*

	Deramaxx®	**Rimadyl®**	**Previcox®**	**Metacam®**	**EtoGesic®**	**Zubrin®**
Marketing status	By prescription only	By prescription only	By prescription only	By prescription only	By prescription only	By prescription only
Protein binding	>90%	>99%	>96%	>99%	>99%	>98%
Bio-availability	>90%	>90%	38%	Nearly 100%	Nearly 100%	
Concurrent use statement	Concomitant use with any other anti-inflammatory drugs, such as other NSAIDs and corticosteroids, should be avoided or closely monitored	Concomitant use with any other anti-inflammatory drugs, such as other NSAIDs and corticosteroids, should be avoided or closely monitored	Concomitant use with any other anti-inflammatory drugs, such as other NSAIDs and corticosteroids, should be avoided or closely monitored	Concurrent use with potentially nephrotoxic drugs should be carefully approached. Concomitant use with other anti-inflammatory drugs, such as NSAIDs and corticosteroids, should be avoided or closely monitored	Concomitant use with other anti-inflammatory drugs, such as other NSAIDs and corticosteroids, should be avoided or closely monitored	Concomitant use with any other anti-inflammatory drugs, such as other NSAIDs and corticosteroids, should be avoided or closely monitored
Pre-prescribing advice	Thorough history and physical exam; appropriate laboratory tests	Thorough history and physical exam; appropriate laboratory tests	Thorough history and physical exam; appropriate laboratory tests	Thorough history and physical exam; appropriate laboratory tests	Thorough history and physical exam; appropriate laboratory tests	Geriatric examination; appropriate laboratory tests
Miscella-neous			*In vitro:* showed more COX-2 inhibition than COX-1	Not evaluated for intramuscular injection	*In vitro:* showed more COX-2 inhibition than COX-1	Give with a meal to enhance absorption

Table 47 NSAID pharmacokinetic parameters and dose recommendations for dog and cat. Comparison of nonsteroidal anti-inflammatory drug elimination half-lives in cats and dogs and relationship with clearance mechanism.[73] Correlation to base dosing intervals is undetermined.

NSAID	Dog Half-life (hours)	Dose/route	Ref.	Cat Half-life (hours)	Dose/route	Ref.	Species difference?	Clearance mechanism/s
Aceta-minophen	1.2	100 mg /kg PO	76	0.6	20 mg /kg PO	76	Cat > dog	Glucuronidation and sulfation
	1.2	200 mg /kg PO	76	2.4	60 mg /kg PO	76		
				4.8	120 mg /kg PO	76		
Aspirin	7.5–12	25 mg /kg PO	77	22	20 mg /kg IV	78	Cat > dog	Glucuronidation and glycination
				37.6	IV?	79		
Carprofen	5	25 mg PO	80	20	4 mg /kg IV	78	Cat > dog	Glucuronidation and oxidation
	8.6	25 mg bid PO	80	19	4 mg/kg SC, IV 7 days	81		
	7	25 mg SC	80					
	8.3	25 mg bid SC 7 days	80					
Flunixin	3.7	1.1 mg/ kg IV	82	1–1.5	1 mg/kg PO, IV	83	Cat > dog	Glucuronidation and active transport
				6.6	2 mg/ kg PO	84		

– Continued on facing page

Table 47 NSAID pharmacokinetic parameters and dose recommendations for dog and cat – *Continued.*

NSAID	Dog half-life (hours)	Dose/route	Ref.	Cat half-life (hours)	Dose/route	Ref.	Species difference?	Clearance mechanism/s
Ketoprofen	1.6 for S-ketoprofen	1 mg/kg PO racemic	85	1.5 for S-ketoprofen	2 mg/kg IV racemic	86	Cat = dog	Glucuronidation and thioesterification
				0.6 for R-ketoprofen	2 mg/kg IV racemic	86		
				0.9 for S-ketoprofen	1 mg/kg PO racemic	86		
				0.6 for R-ketoprofen	1 mg/kg PO racemic	86		
				0.5 for S-ketoprofen	1 mg/kg IV S-ketoprofen	87		
				0.5 for R-ketoprofen	1 mg/kg IV R-ketoprofen	87		
Meloxicam	12	0.2 mg/kg PO	85	15	0.3 mg/kg SC	Label	Cat < dog	Oxidation
	24	0.2 mg/kg PO, SC, IV	88					
Piroxicam	40	0.3 mg/kg PO, IV	89	12	0.3 mg/kg PO, IV	90	Cat < dog	Oxidation

6 NUTRACEUTICALS

INTRODUCTION

The world market for pet nutraceuticals was worth \$960 million in 2004. About 60% of this was to dogs, a quarter to cats and 10% to horses.[1] Joint health products for pets accounted for nearly half of the market, followed by vitamins, minerals, amino acids, and antioxidants collectively constituting 20%. The widespread interest in nutraceuticals began in 1997 with publication of the book entitled 'The Arthritis Cure', by Dr. Jason Theodosakis. Three years later US sales of nutraceuticals topped \$640 million.[2]

BACKGROUND

Nutraceuticals are natural, bioactive chemical compounds that have health-promoting, disease-preventing or medicinal properties. They are prescribed drugs in some limited number of countries, but are primarily provided as dietary supplements delivered over the counter. *A supplement that can be administered orally to promote good health and is not a drug is considered a nutraceutical.* As functional foods, nutraceuticals are part of the daily diet as food and drink. Functional food is characterized (from traditional food) 'if it is satisfactorily demonstrated to affect beneficially one or more target functions in the body, beyond adequate nutritional effects in a way which is relevant to either the state of well-being and health or the reduction of the risk of a disease'.[3]

Dietary supplements are regulated by the FDA in a different manner from either over-the-counter or prescription drugs. As laid out in the Dietary Supplement Health and Education Act of 1994 (US), the manufacturer is responsible for determining that the supplement is safe and that any representations or claims made about it are adequately substantiated. Dietary supplements do not need to be approved by the FDA before they are marketed, and subsequently do not carry consumer confidence of FDA endorsement.

DJD, or OA, poses major therapeutic problems in pets as well as humans. Treatment with NSAIDs is designed to reduce pain and inflammation, hallmarks of the disease. Yet long-term use of NSAIDs, notably with complications of inappropriate use,[4] has been associated with adverse effects including gastrointestinal ulceration, hepatic toxicity, renal failure, and, in some cases, negative effects on chondrocytes and cartilage matrix formation.[5] Such issues have led researchers to seek alternatives/adjuncts to NSAIDs for managing OA. Originally these compounds were considered to serve as building blocks for cartilage and exogenous sources of cartilage matrix components. The long-standing rationale for using nutraceuticals is that provision of precursors of cartilage matrix in excess quantities may favor matrix synthesis and repair of articular cartilage.

According to the North American Veterinary Nutraceutical Association (NAVNA), a nutraceutical is 'a nondrug substance that is produced in a purified form and administered orally to provide compounds required for normal body structure and function with the intent of improving health and well-being'. Further, the NAVNA defined a *chondroprotective* as an agent that intends to: 'stimulate cartilage matrix production by chondrocytes, inhibit matrix degradation, and potentially inhibit periarticular microvascular thrombosis'. The two most popular nutraceuticals are glucosamine and chondroitin sulfate. See *Table 48*.

UNDERSTANDING THE CONCEPTS

OA involves cartilage loss from enzymatic degradation of the extracellular matrix (**133**). This results in loss of proteoglycans and the cleavage of type II collagen.[6] (See Chapter 2 for further explanation.) MMPs and aggrecanases play a major role among the degradative enzymes. MMPs are similar in structure but differ somewhat in their preferred substrates. Collagenases (MMP-1, -8, and -13) cleave the intact triple helix of collagen.[7] Thereafter, the collagen fragments are susceptible to further proteolysis by gelatinases (MMP-2 and -9), enzymes that can also cleave aggrecan.[8] Stromelysins (MMP-3, -10, and -11) are capable of degrading aggrecan, denatured type II collagen, and small proteoglycans of the extracellular matrix.[9] Aggrecanases are principal mediators of aggrecan degradation, releasing core protein and GAG constituents of aggrecan into the synovial fluid.[10] A number of cytokines, most importantly IL-1, are considered central to the induction of degradative enzyme and inflammatory mediator synthesis. Cytokines appear to be first produced by cells of the synovial membrane[11] and later by activated chondrocytes.[12] Generally, IL-1 is presumed to enhance cartilage degeneration and inhibit efforts at repair.

To understand the supposition behind the use of nutraceuticals, and particularly chondroprotectives, several tenets must be understood.

GAGs are long-chain polymers of disaccharides. There are three major types in cartilage: chondroitin sulfate-4 and -6; keratan sulfate; and dermatin sulfate. Chondroitin is the prevalent form in cartilage. GAGs are vital in the hydration of cartilage, as they are the primary water-binding constituents within the matrix.

Table 48 Nutraceuticals used for OA.

Ascorbic acid	Hyaluronic acid
Avocado/soybean unsaponifiables	Hydrolysate collagen
Boswellia serrata	Methylsulfonylmethane
Bromelain	Milk and hyperimmune milk
Cat's claw	Omega-3-PUFAs
Chondroitin sulfate	Phycocyanin
Cetyl myristoleate oil	*Ribes nigrum*
	Rosa canina
Curcumin	S-adenosylmethionine (SAMe)
Chitosan	Selenium
Devil's claw	Strontium
Flavonoids	Silicium
Glucosamine SO_4/ Acetyl/HCl	Turmeric
Green lip mussel	Vitamin D
Ginger	Vitamin E
	Willow

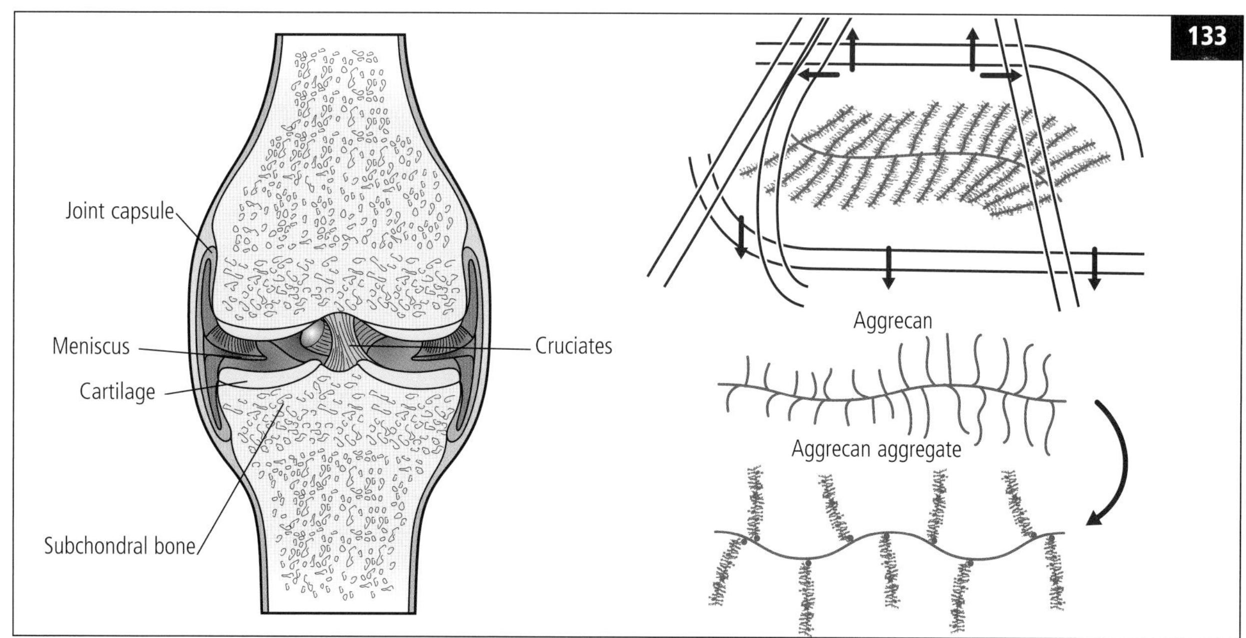

133 Although a disease of the total joint, OA characteristically involves the loss of cartilage. This results from the degradation of aggrecan aggregates and cleavage of type II collagen. (see also 72–76 chapter 2)

CHONDROITIN SULFATE

Chondroitin sulfate is one of two primary GAGs responsible for binding of water in cartilage. The other primary GAG is keratan sulfate. Loss of GAGs, particularly chondroitin sulfate, occurs early in OA. This loss contributes to alterations in water binding in cartilage and subsequently to impaired cartilage mechanics and accelerated cartilage breakdown. Chondroitin sulfate appears to inhibit degradative enzymes, such as metalloproteinase, associated with OA. These degradative enzymes break down the cartilage and hyaluronan in synovial fluid.

Chondroitin-4 has been derived primarily from mammalian tissues, whereas chondroitin-6 is derived primarily from aquatic species including shark cartilage.

The proposed mechanisms of action for chondroitin sulfate are somewhat similar to those of glucosamine: stimulation of GAG synthesis, and inhibition of degradative enzyme synthesis, including MMPs.[13] In contrast to glucosamine, chondroitin sulfate is shown to inhibit IL-1-induced type II collagen degeneration,[14] and improves synovial fluid viscosity by increasing hyaluronic acid concentration.[15]

The molecular weight of chondroitin sulfate directly influences its absorption after oral administration, where higher gastrointestinal permeability is achieved for low-molecular-weight chondroitin sulfate.[16] The form and source of chondroitin sulfate also, apparently, influence its pharmacokinetic profile; in humans, chondroitin sulfate of bovine origin is superior to chondroitin sulfate obtained from shark cartilage due to differences in molecular mass, degree of sulfation, and relative amounts of iduronate and glucuronate.[17,18] Due to size (range from 6–50 kDa), the form of chondroitin sulfate that is ultimately available after oral administration may be affected by intestinal degradation and metabolism within the liver.[19] The gastric mucosa contains several GAG-degrading enzymes, such as exoglycosidases, sulfatases, and hyaluronidase-like enzymes, capable of digesting chondroitin sulfate. This and the fact that charged molecules with a molecular mass exceeding about 180 kDa are unlikely to be absorbed without an active carrier system, suggest the parent chondroitin sulfate is unlikely to be absorbed intact. The monosaccharide building blocks of chondroitin sulfate (glucuronic acid and N-acetylglucosamine) created by its digestive hydrolysis might be absorbed, yet these hydrosylates likely show different biological and biochemical properties to those of the parent structure, for which beneficial attributes have been proposed.

Clearly, all chondroitin sulfate is not the same. Chondroitin sulfate is expensive, and it is possible that some suppliers may dilute chondroitin sulfate with compounds that include sugars like maltose, or other GAGs, such as dermatan sulfate, keratan sulfate, heparin or hyaluronic acid, that can cause analytical methods to overestimate contents. Therefore, despite language like ‘quality tested’ appearing on labels, there is no basis to compare one product against another or to judge the quality of different products. ConsumerLab.com reported in 2007 that 73% of ‘joint formulas’ tested, failed to meet their own label claim for chondroitin content.[20] It is incumbent on the consumer to be knowledgeable about the product and the manufacturer. Consumers should buy from manufacturers that use United States Pharmacopeia (USP) grade materials. They should stay away from products that are backed only by testimonials and not supported by scientific research. ‘We believe what’s happening with chondroitin is economic adulteration. Some manufacturers substitute with cheaper materials that look like the more expensive, real ingredients,’ says Dr. Tod Cooperman, MD, president of ConsumerLab.com, an independent testing group that tests and publishes data on human and veterinary supplements for labeling accuracy and product purity.[20]

In a placebo-controlled double-blind study in dogs with OA, owners and veterinarians were unable to distinguish between dogs supplemented with chondroitin sulphate or placebo after 12 weeks of follow-up.[21]

GLUCOSAMINE

Glucosamine action *in vitro* includes a reduction in proteoglycan degradation and inhibition of the synthesis and activity of degradative enzymes and inflammatory mediators, such as aggrecanases, MMPs, NO, and PGE_2, with anabolic effects of GAG stimulation and proteoglycan production, including aggrecan; but no effect on type II collagen.[13] Glucosamine also appears to inhibit NF-κB activity.[22]

Glucosamine is a hexosamine sugar proposed to act as a precursor for the disaccharide units of GAG. Nutritional glucosamine is suggested to provide the body with extra ‘building blocks’ for the creation of the cartilage matrix. Most glucosamine in the body is in the form of glucosamine-6-phosphate,[23] while glucosamine is commercially available in three forms: glucosamine hydrochloride, glucosamine sulfate, and N-acetyl-D-glucosamine. Apparently, the form of glucosamine influences its activity. Glucosamine hydrochloride and glucosamine sulfate appear to inhibit equine cartilage degeneration more consistently than N-acetyl-D-glucosamine *in vitro*.[24] In addition, there is a suggestion that GAG synthesis may be through promotion of incorporation of sulfur into cartilage.[25]

Investigators have reported that in human patients, glucosamine sulfate increases the expression of cartilage aggrecan core protein and downregulates, in a dose-dependent manner, MMP-1 and -3 expression.[26] Such transcriptional effects are supported by reports that glucosamine sulfate increases proteoglycan synthesis with no effect on their physicochemical form, on type II collagen production or on cell proliferation, in a model of human osteoarthritic chondrocytes.[27]

Osteoarthritic cartilage is characterized by articular surface fibrillation, which has been associated with a significant decrease in chondrocyte adhesion to extracellular matrix proteins and, more specifically, to fibronectin (**134**).[28]

Investigators of this observation suggest that activation of protein kinase C, considered to be involved in the physiological phosphorylation of the integrin subunit, could be one of the possible mechanisms through which glucosamine sulfate restores fibrillated cartilage chondrocytes adhesion to fibronectin, thus improving the repair process in osteoarthritic cartilage.[29] In trials assessing improvement in long-term symptomatic evaluation of human knee OA, it was observed that glucosamine hydrochloride does not induce symptomatic relief in knee OA to the same extent as glucosamine sulfate.[30,31] This raises the question of the importance of sulfate and its contribution to the overall effects of glucosamine. Glucosamine sulfate is very hygroscopic and unstable. Consequently, during manufacturing, varying amounts of potassium or sodium chloride are added to improve stability. Due to concerns over valid labeling, commercially available capsules or tablets of glucosamine sulfate were analysed. The amount of free base varied from 41–108% of the mg content stated on the label; the amount of glucosamine varied from 59–138% even when expressed as sulfate.[32] Therefore, the results obtained with one single preparation of glucosamine sulfate, even when registered as a drug in Europe, cannot be extrapolated to the vast majority of over-the-counter preparations sold without the appropriate quality controls.

Persiani *et al.*[33] reported that glucosamine is bioavailable both systemically and in the joint after oral administration of crystalline glucosamine sulphate in human osteoarthritic patients. 'The formulation used is the original crystalline glucosamine sulphate 1500 mg once-a-day soluble powder preparation which is a prescription drug in most European and extra-European countries and differs from glucosamine formulations available in the US and other countries. In fact, the US Dietary Supplements Health and Education Act of 1994 documented the appearance of several poorly characterized dietary supplements containing either inadequate active ingredient quantity, or other glucosamine salts (e.g. hydrochloride), derivatives (e.g. N-acetyl-glucosamine), or dosage forms and regimens. This might also provide an explanation for the finding that when other salts, formulations, and/or daily regimens have been used in clinical trials, the results have not been favorable. In particular, the recently completed National Institutes of Health (NIH)-sponsored Glucosamine/Chondroitin Arthritis Intervention Trial (GAIT) trial in knee OA, indicated that the symptomatic effect of glucosamine hydrochloride at the dose of 500 mg tid did not differ significantly from placebo. This confirmed the skepticism concerning the several confounders and problematic study design of some trials, and the possible suboptimal exposure of the patients to the active molecule that might also come from the adopted dose and dosing interval.'

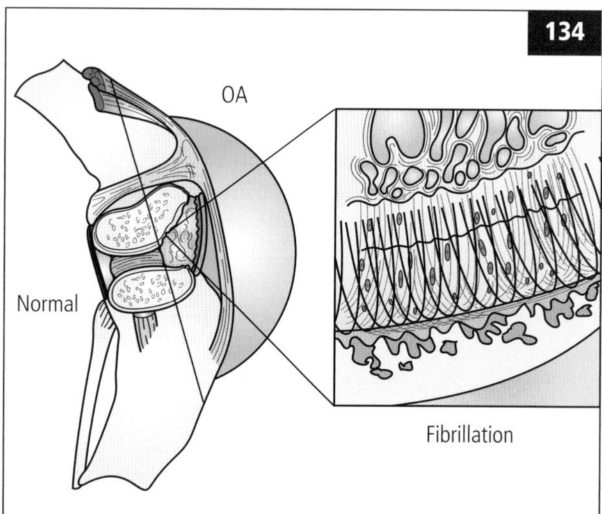

134 Articular cartilage fibrillation has been associated with loss of chondrocyte adhesion to fibronectin in the extracellular matrix.

It is interesting to note that the only clinically relevant results in the GAIT study were observed in the subgroup of more severe patients when glucosamine hydrochloride was combined with chondroitin sulfate, supporting the hypothesis that increasing the sulfate concentration may have therapeutic effects.[34]

Some[33] suggest it is unlikely that the clinical effects of glucosamine (sulfate) are linked to a mere stimulation of GAG synthesis, but support the theory that glucosamine sulfate inhibits IL-1-induced gene expression, possibly via the suppression of the cytokine intracellular signaling pathway and NF-κB activation, thus reversing the proinflammatory and joint degenerating effects of IL-1. Crystalline glucosamine sulfate reportedly inhibits IL-1-stimulated gene expression of COX-2, iNOS, TNF-α, IL-6, IL-1, MMP-3, and aggrecanase 2.[35] Largo *et al.*[36] found that glucosamine sulfate inhibits NF-κB activation and PGE_2 synthesis induced by IL-1β in human chondrocytes, where NF-κB is considered a key regulator of tissue inflammation, since it controls the transcription of a number of proinflammatory genes that regulate the synthesis of cytokines, chemokines, and adhesion molecules. NF-κB activity has been shown to be essential for MMP-1 and MMP-3 upregulation.[37] Glucosamine sulfate also inhibited the gene expression and the protein synthesis of COX-2 induced by IL-1β, while no effect on COX-1 synthesis was seen.

Kuroki *et al.*[38] have shown that within a canine articular cartilage and synovium explant co-culture system, glucosamine or chondroitin sulfate alone retards increased expression of proteinases and inflammatory mediators associated with IL-1, while the combination of glucosamine plus chondroitin sulfate primarily retarded detrimental effects on matrix molecules.

Some[39] have questioned the potential for biological activity of glucosamine, pointing out that the bioavailability from a single or multiple dose of glucosamine hydochloride is only 10–12% in dogs.[40] It is questionable whether substantial amounts of glucosamine reach circulation following oral ingestion,[41] and it is proposed that glucosamine is not essential for the biosynthesis of cartilage; glucosamine is only one of many substrates from which other metabolites are derived for the synthesis of cartilage matrix.[41]

GLUCOSAMINE AND CHONDROITIN SULFATE IN COMBINATION

Orally administered glucosamine hydrochloride and chondroitin sulfate in combination has become a popular nutraceutical offering. In a multicenter, double-blind, placebo- and celecoxib controlled study (GAIT study) of 1583 human patients with stifle joint OA receiving 1500 mg glucosamine, 1200 mg chondroitin sulfate, or both revealed that the supplementations did not reduce stifle joint pain better than placebo.[42] In a subgroup of that same study, patients with moderate-to-severe pain, the response of the combination glucosamine plus chondroitin sulfate was significantly better. In this same subgroup, the positive control, celecoxib, showed no response. Worthy of note is that the study was conducted under pharmaceutical rather than dietary supplement regulations, therefore agents identical to the ones used may not be commercially available. Nevertheless, 'analysis of the primary outcome measure did not show that either supplement, alone or in combination, was efficacious.'[42] In contrast, some nutraceutical manufacturers cite the GAIT study results as testimonial that where an evidence-based efficacious drug (celecoxib) does not work, the glucosamine and chondroitin sulfate combination does (**135**)!

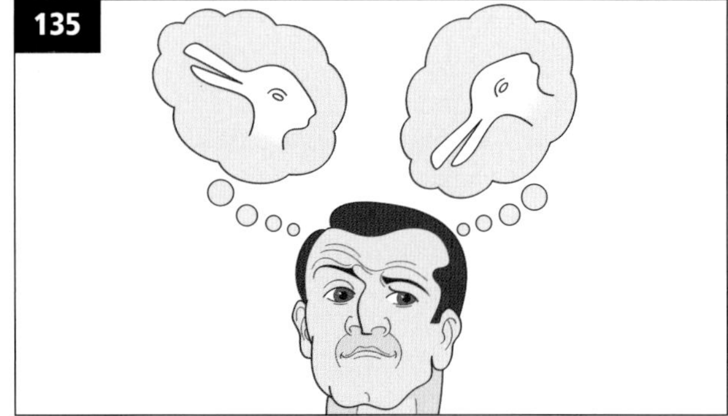

135 Results from the GAIT study are not conclusive; some suggest it shows glucosamine and chondroitin sulfate combination is not effective, while others interpret the data to suggest it is (rabbit or duck?).

Subsequent to the GAIT study, in an editorial appearing in the *New England Journal of Medicine*, Dr. Marc Hochberg, MD, states, 'If patients choose to take dietary supplements to control their symptoms, they should be advised to take glucosamine sulfate rather than glucosamine hydrochloride and, for those with severe pain, that taking chondroitin sulfate with glucosamine sulfate may have an additive effect.'[43]

Studies of *in vivo* or *in vitro* efficacy of veterinary products are limited, and efficacy claims are frequently made from subjective assessments which include owner testimonials or clinical trials lacking peer review. A literature review suggests the bioavailability of these products in dogs after oral intake is limited and is insufficient to prevent or treat OA, whereas parenteral application (either intramuscular or intra-articular) seems to approach the *in vitro* effect. Further, efficacy data are confused by reference to data gained by *in vitro* research, studies in other than target species, or not gained with objective, placebo-controlled, double-blinded studies or any studies at all.[44,45] The Arthritis Foundation recommends that when a supplement has been studied with good results, find out which brand was used in the study, and buy that product.[46]

AVOCADO/SOYBEAN UNSAPONIFIABLES

Avocado/soybean unsaponifiables (ASU) has become a nutraceutical compound of recent investigative interest. The unsaponifiable portions of avocado and soybean oils are extracted via hydrolysis, and the extracts have been shown to effectively treat several connective tissue diseases.[47] Synergism between the avocado and soya components, and their relative ratios, appear to be important.[48] *In vitro* studies show that ASU extracts reduce proinflammatory mediators, including IL-6, IL-8, macrophage inflammatory protein-1β, NO, and PGE_2 by human articular chondrocytes exposed to IL-1β.[49]

It has been observed that osteoblasts isolated from subchondral OA bone demonstrate an altered phenotype from normal.[50] They produce increased amounts of alkaline phosphatase, osteocalcin, TGF-β_1, insulin-like growth factor-1, and urokinase plasminogen activator. OA osteoblasts are also resistant to parathyroid hormone stimulation, possibly contributing to abnormal bone remodeling and bone sclerosis in OA.[51]

OA is a total joint disease, which includes the involvement of subchondral bone. Abnormal remodeling of the subchondral bone plate exposed to excessive nonphysiological mechanical loads makes it stiffer, and no longer effective as a shock absorber, thus increasing mechanical strain on overlying cartilage. It is proposed that intervention that reduces bone sclerosis might slow progressive cartilage degradation. In addition, because microcracks, vascular channels, and neovascularization provide a link between subchondral bone and cartilage, IL-6, TGF-β and perhaps other factors produced by osteoblasts may contribute to the abnormal remodeling of OA cartilage.[52]

Since tidemark microcracks appear early in OA cartilage, it is speculated that soluble mediators produced by sclerotic subchondral osteoblasts may modulate chondrocyte metabolism and contribute to cartilage degradation. Aligning this theory together with ASU prevention of inhibitory effects of osteoarthritic subchondral osteoblasts on aggrecan and type II collagen synthesis by chondrocytes, investigators propose that ASU may act via a new mechanism of action at the subchondral bone level in protecting cartilage.[53] Among study horses, ASU failed to ameliorate increasing lameness, response to joint flexion, or synovial effusion; however, GAG synthesis in the articular cartilage was increased compared with placebo-treated, osteoarthritis-affected joints.[54] Investigators concluded that ASU extracts may have an anabolic effect directly on chondrocytes to increase GAG synthesis and, hence, help prevent articular cartilage damage by enhancing the articular cartilage matrix structure. In a canine study,[55] ASU (4 mg/kg every three days or daily) increased both TGF-β_1 and TGF-β_2 levels in the stifle synovial fluid. TGF-β_1 levels reached maximum values at the end of the second month and then decreased after the third month, while TGF-β_2 levels marginally increased during the first two months, followed by a marked increase at the end of the third month. TGF-β is a stimulator of extracellular matrix production, like collagen type II and proteoglycan, in chondrocytes.[56]

PHYCOCYANIN

Phycocyanin, composed of two protein subunits with covalently bond phycobilins that are the light-capturing part of the blue pigment in blue–green algae, is considered the active agent in PhyCox®, commercialized as PhyCox-JS®, (Teva Animal Health, St. Joseph MO, USA). However, there are some data suggesting that C-phycocyanin is a selective COX-2 inhibitor.[57] Phycocyanin has been shown to have antioxidant and anti-inflammatory properties *in vitro* and *in vivo* (rodents).[58,59] Other ingredients in PhyCox-JS, which may contribute to product efficacy, include glucosamine, flaxseed oil, turmeric, eicosapentaenoic acid (EPA), and docosahexaenoic acid (DHA). PhyCox-JS is not a drug, but positioned as an animal nutraceutical of natural botanical origin (PhyCox). There are no pharmacokinetic studies for phycocyanin in the dog. The observational study done by the manufacturer was based on owner observations of dogs on the ingredient PhyCox and not the commercial product PhyCox-JS, and study design was weak. Further, PhyCox-JS has not been thoroughly studied in use together with an NSAID.

EICOSAPENTAENOIC ACID

Both AA and EPA act as precursors for the synthesis of eicosanoids, important molecules functioning as hormones and mediators of inflammation (**136**). The amounts and types of eicosanoids synthesized are determined by the availability of the polysulfated fatty acid precursor and by the activities of the enzyme system. The eicosanoids produced from AA, the principal precursor under most conditions, appear to be more proinflammatory than those formed from EPA (**137**).

Ingestion of oils containing omega-3 fatty acids results in a decrease in membrane levels of AA because the omega-3 fatty acids replace AA in the substrate pool and reduce the capacity to synthesize inflammatory eicosanoids. Inflammatory eicosanoids produced from AA are, therefore, depressed when dogs consume foods with high levels of omega-3 fatty

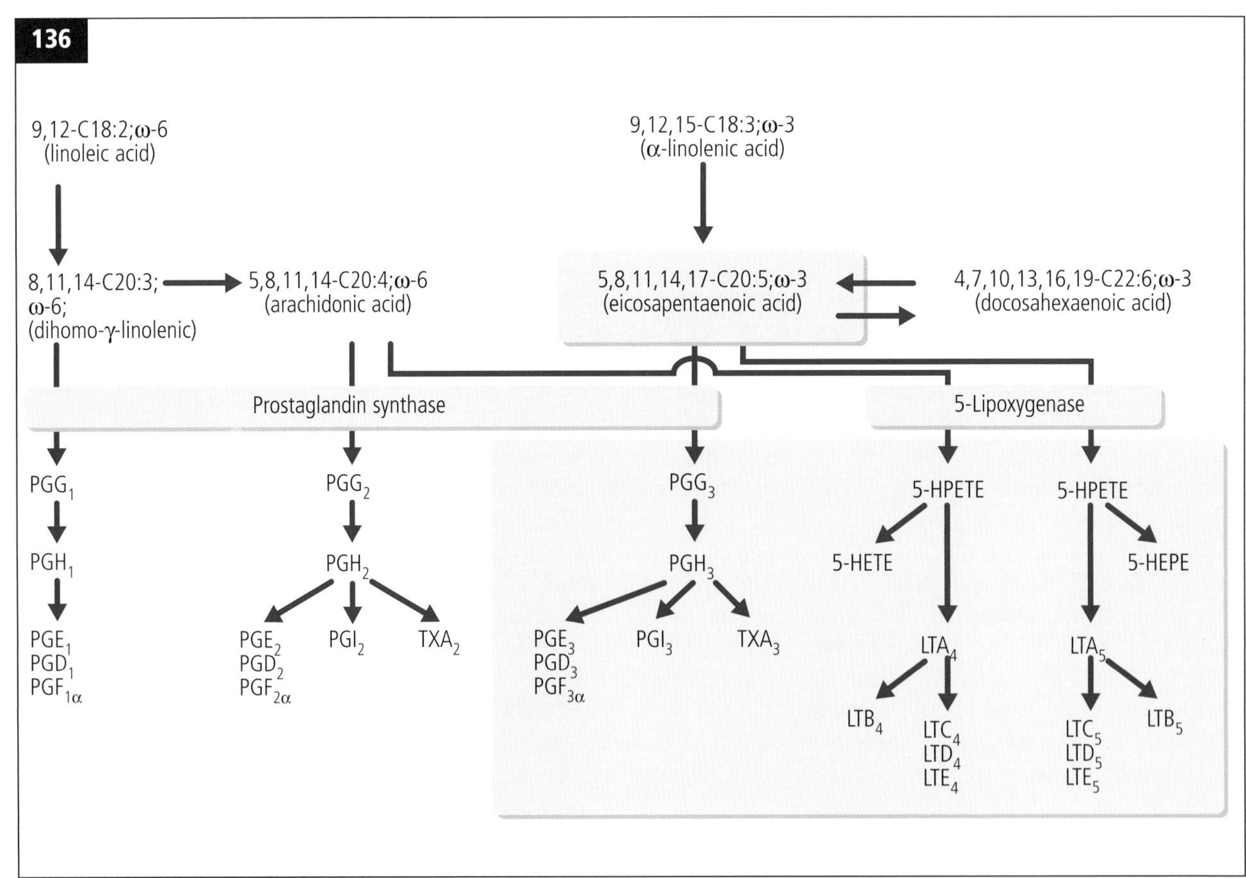

136 EPA is the substrate for synthesis of many eicosanoids which act as mediators of inflammation. (HEPE = hydroxyeicosapentaenoic acid; HETE = hydroxyeicosatetraenoic acid; HPETE = hydroperoxyeicosatetraenoic acid)

acids. In addition, EPA is thought to exert its therapeutic effect on OA by reducing expression of genes encoding for cartilage-degrading enzymes (aggrecanases) within the chondrocytes.[60] *In vitro* studies revealed that by exposing normal canine cartilage to EPA before addition of the catabolic agent, oncostatin M, to initiate processes that mimic the cartilage damage that occurs during the pathogenesis of OA, cartilage degeneration was abrogated.[61] Food containing high concentrations of total omega-3 fatty acids and EPA as well as a low omega-6:omega-3 ratio appears to decrease the severity of OA clinical signs as early as 21 days after initiation of implementation.

Flaxseed oil and fish oil are both rich in omega-3 fatty acids. Fish oil is rich in EPA and DHA, while flaxseed oil contains alpha-linolenic acid (ALA). For ALA in flaxseed oil to have an anti-inflammatory effect, it must be converted to EPA. Efficiency of ALA conversion to EPA is very low (<10%), with most ALA being used for energy. Accordingly, a small amount of fish oil is more effective at providing EPA and DHA than a large quantity of flaxseed oil containing ALA.

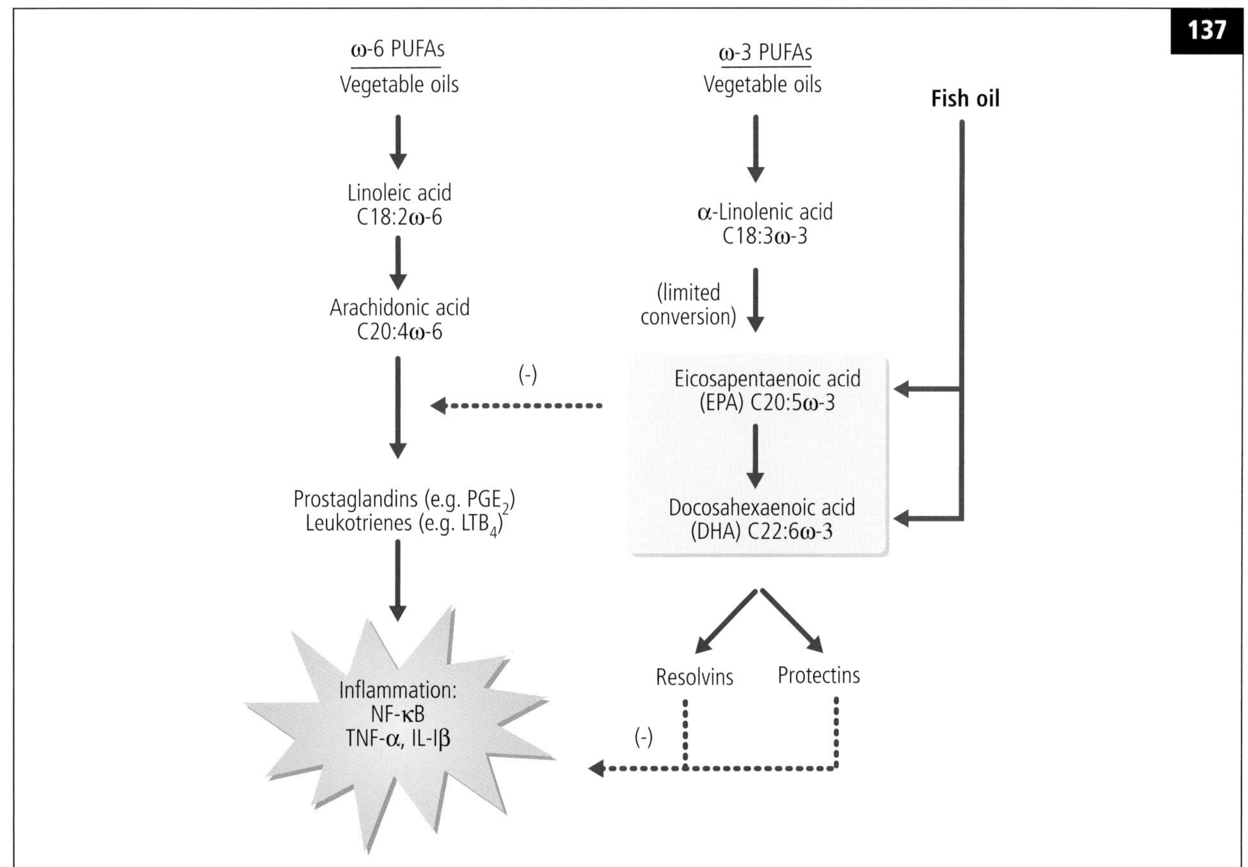

137 Whereas AA-derived eicosanoids tend to be proinflammatory, EPA-derived eicosanoids tend to be less inflammatory/suppress the inflammatory process. (PUFA = polyunsaturated fatty acids)

HYALURONIC ACID

The proteoglycan aggrecan molecule of articular cartilage is attached via a link protein to HA. The entire complex is referred to as a proteoglycan or aggrecan aggregate (**138**). HA acts as an aggregating factor between the collagen, proteoglycan aggregate, and cartilage structural network as a whole. Synovial fluid contains high concentrations of HA, derived from type B synoviocytes embedded within the intimal lining of the joint capsule. The viscoelastic properties of synovial fluid are determined by HA, and with the progression of OA, HA concentrations decrease with a resultant decrease in the viscoelastic properties of the synovial fluid. Intra-articular injection of HA, called viscosupplementation, has demonstrated significant improvement of symptoms in patients with OA.[62]

By definition, injectable HA (e.g. Legend®) is not a nutraceutical. However, it can be considered a chondroprotective agent and there are several commercially available forms of HA, differing by treatment regimens, total dosing, and average molecular weights. Support for use of HA resides in the improvement of OA symptoms with few side-effects. It is unlikely that sustained beneficial effects of HA therapy result from temporary restoration of the synovial fluid lubrication and viscoelasticity.[63] Perhaps HA therapy has disease-modifying biological activity and an impact on OA progression. Four potential mechanisms have been proposed for the beneficial clinical effects noted from HA therapy:

- Restoration of elastic and viscous properties of the synovial fluid.
- Biosynthetic–chondroprotective effect of exogenous hyaluronans on cells (hyaluronans can induce endogenous synthesis of HA by synovial cells, stimulate chondrocyte proliferation, and inhibit cartilage degradation).[60,64–66]
- Anti-inflammatory effects.[67,68]
- Analgesic effect.[69,70]

Pozo *et al.* reported that intra-articular HA reduced nerve impulse activity in nociceptive afferent fibers in a cat model of acute arthritis.[71]

S-ADENOSYLMETHIONINE

SAMe is a nucleotide-like molecule synthesized from methionine and ATP by all living cells. SAMe is particularly important to hepatocytes and plays a pivotal role in the biochemical pathways of transmethylation, transulfuration, and amino-propylation. A therapeutic application of SAMe in joint disorders is derived from pain reduction and improved joint function,[72,73] based on potential antioxidant and anti-inflammatory activity.[74] There are very few studies reporting the effect of SAMe on articular chondrocytes or matrix. One study in dogs

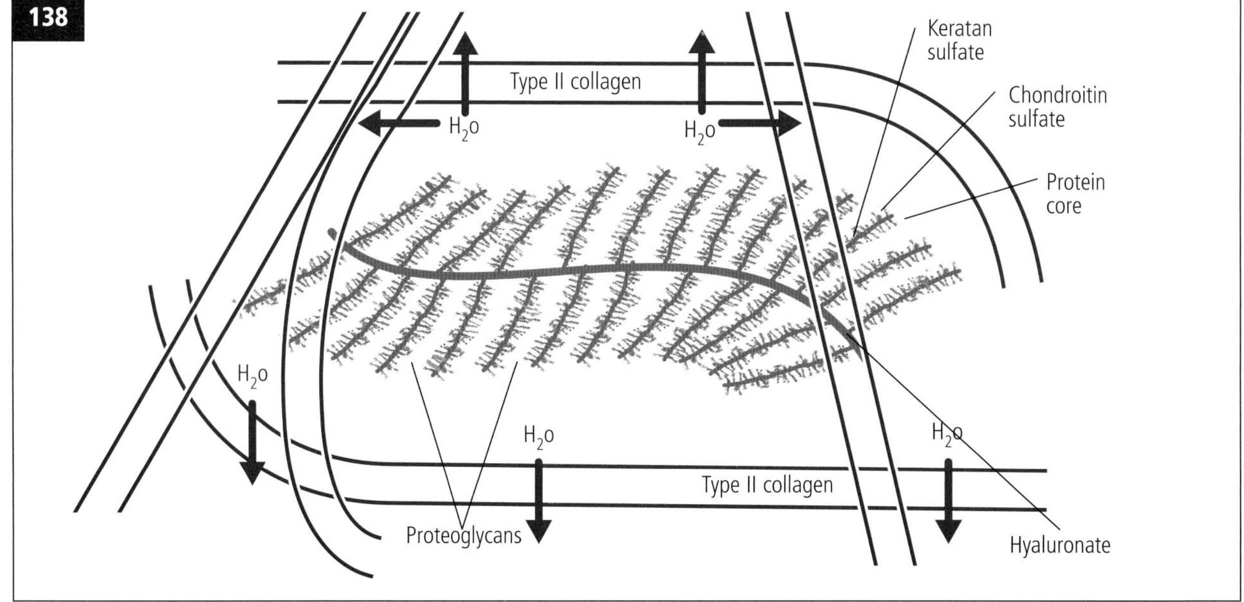

138 Hyaluronic acid is an integral part of the aggrecan aggregate, as well as synovial fluid.

reported an *in vitro* detrimental effect,[75] while one study in humans showed an *in vitro* positive effect.[76] Lippiello *et al.* have reported that the enzymatic inhibition of proteoglycan synthesis by MMP-3 *in vitro* is reversed by the combination of glucosamine and SAMe, but not with either agent alone.[77]

CURCUMINOIDS

Studies to support existing *in vitro* evidence for nutraceutical alleviation of clinical signs for OA are lacking. To date, green tea extract and other Asian herbal remedies have not been evaluated in companion animal models or in animals with spontaneous disease. Curcuminoids, types of phytonutrients extracted from turmeric, have been found to exert some anti-inflammatory effects in certain animal models and *in vitro* assays. A curcuminoid extract in dogs with OA was found to yield no treatment effect using the objective assessment of force-plate analysis, although subjective assessment by the observer was positive.

SUMMARY

Clearly, credible evidence-based support for most nutraceuticals is meager. Arguably, the success of nutraceuticals is being driven by consumers' desire to 'do no harm'. And the role of nutraceuticals is shrouded with vagaries, innuendo, and misinformation. Preliminary information guiding nutraceutical use should be considered with care. Results should be gathered in the target species (i.e. the dog) and not in small laboratory animals, in man, bovine or from *in vitro* studies. Dosage, duration, and route of the agent should be taken into account. Since most of these products are not pharmaceuticals, neither purity nor content is under control, although the package or informational materials may suggest otherwise.

Hyaline articular cartilage harvested from joints of different animal species respond very differently to a variety of catabolic stimulants that are commonly used by researchers to establish *in vitro* models of cartilage degradation that are believed to mimic mechanisms of cartilage degradation in the pathogenesis of DJDs. Innes *et al.*[78] have pointed out that exposure to IL-1α or β, TNF-α, oncostatin M, and retinoic acid can all cause significant increases in cartilage proteoglycan degradation when bovine articular cartilage explant culture systems are used, but similar results are not seen with the canine. Species differences may be due to species variability of catabolic stimulants themselves, which may have different affinities for receptors and other downstream regulators that manifest their metabolic effects on cartilage metabolism. Differences in catabolic responses to cytokines in dogs highlight the difficulty in extrapolating results between species.

Perhaps the best advice for pet owners is to spend their money where the science is strong. Adding a nutraceutical will, likely, do no harm, but evidence-based endorsement is weak. Perhaps variability in testimonials for various nutraceutical efficacies resides in genetic predisposition of yet unidentified subpopulations for their activity.

139 shows the molecular structure of some nutraceuticals and a chondroprotectant.

Polysulfated glycosaminoglycoside (chondroprotectant)

Chondroitin sulfate (nutraceutical)

Glucosamine (nutraceutical)

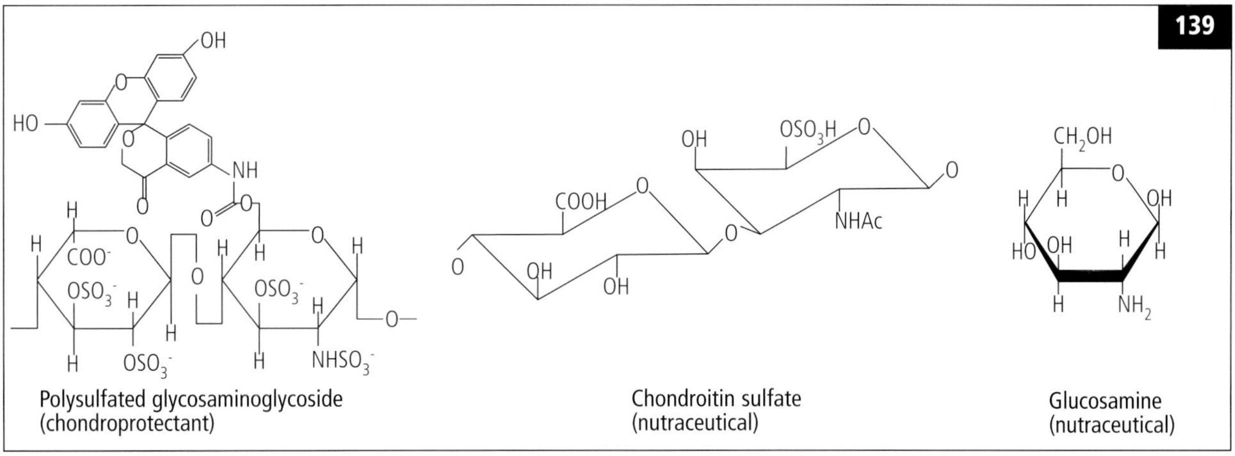

139 Molecular structure of different nutraceuticals and chondroprotectant.

7 MULTIMODAL MANAGEMENT OF PAIN

INTRODUCTION

In addition to pre-emptive analgesia, *multimodal* (or balanced) analgesia has changed the way we treat pain.[1] Multimodal analgesia denotes simultaneous administration of two or more analgesic drugs belonging to different classes (**140**). (Multimodal can also denote different delivery methods and therapies.)

Dosages of each drug can typically be reduced because various classes of drugs have additive or synergistic analgesic effects when given together[2] (e.g., opioid, α_2 agonist,[3] NSAID). As a result, adverse side-effects from each of the drugs in the combination can be anticipated to be less due to the lower dosing of each respective drug. For nearly 2 decades the concept of 'multimodal analgesia' has

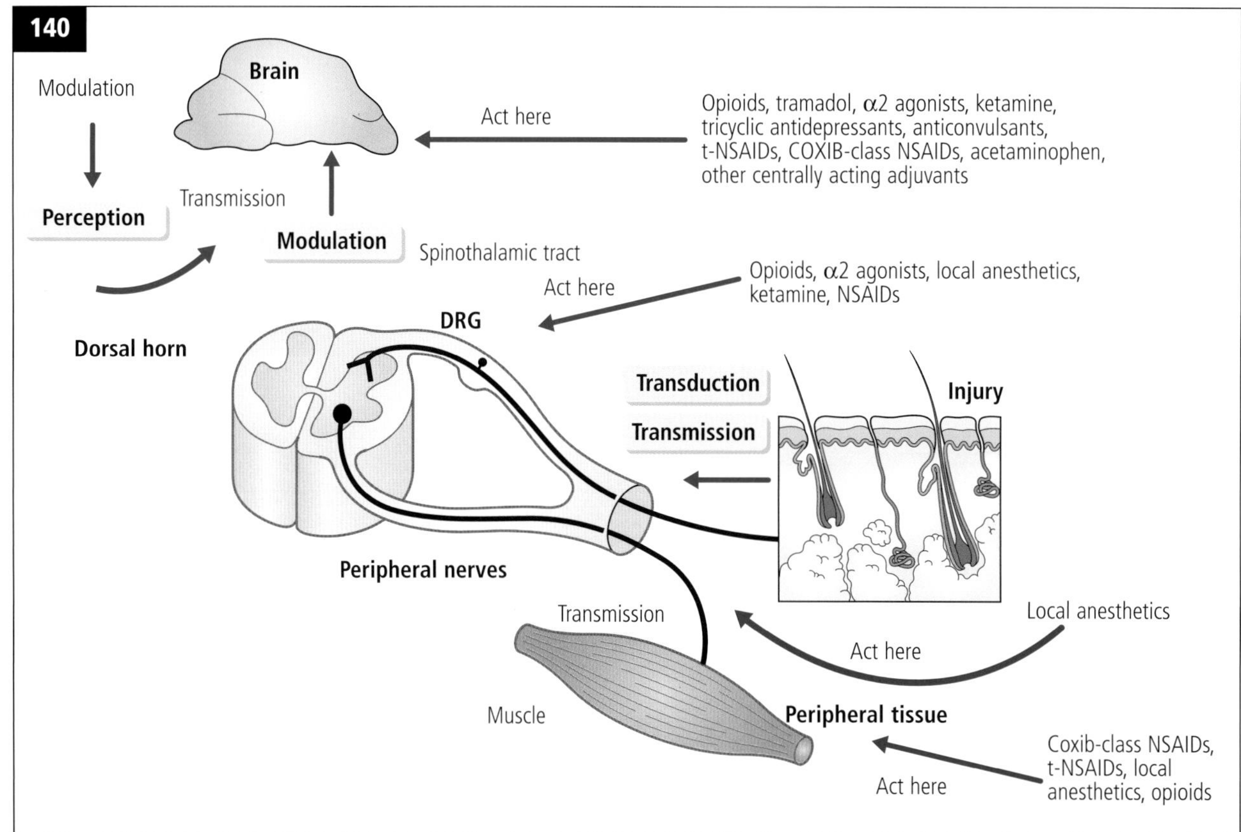

140 Multimodal analgesia denotes the simultaneous administration of different classes of drugs, attempting to block the four physiological processes of transduction, transmission, modulation, and perception.

created important advances in the approach to providing analgesia in both acute[4,5] and chronic pain in humans.[6] Nociception results in pain via multiple pathways, mechanisms and transmitter systems,[7] and it is naïve to consider that a single therapy would be as effective as several different drugs acting on multiple components of the nociceptive system (**141**).

Although there is no published evidence base that multimodal drug therapy is of benefit over monomodal therapy in veterinary patients suffering from chronic painful conditions such as OA, implementation seems implicit.[8]

Herein arises the question: 'What drugs should go into the cocktail?' Drugs comprising the cocktail

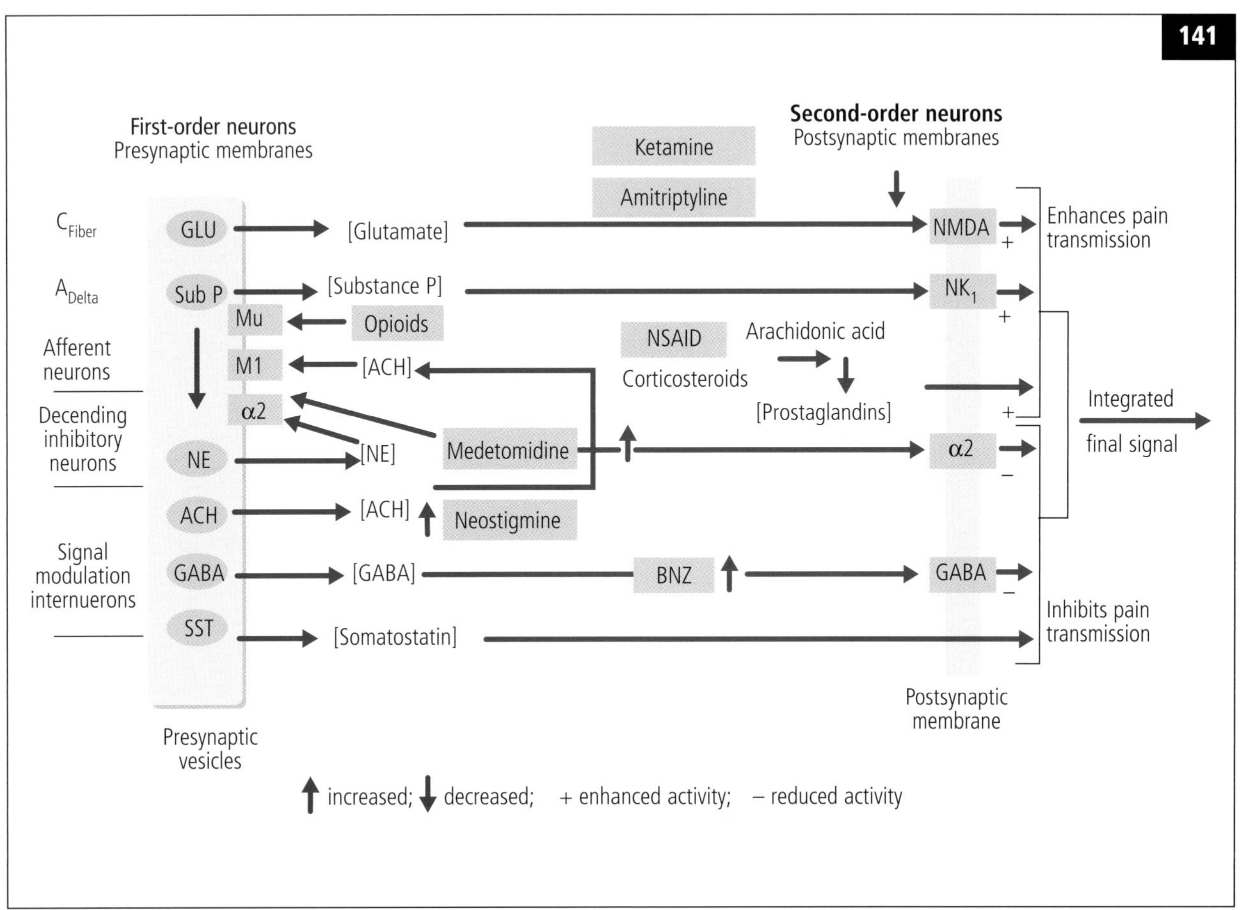

141 Simplistic drawing of nociceptor transmission from the first- to second-order neuron. Most analgesic drugs express their mode of action via a single pathway, transmitter or receptor, and pain is the result of a complex nociceptive network. Therefore, it is naïve to expect a single drug to block the entire 'network'.
(ACH = acetylcholine; BNZ = benzodiazepines)
(Adapted from Tranquilli WJ, *et al.* Pain Management For The Small Animal Practitioner. Teton New Media 2004, 2nd edition (with permission))

should be from different classes (so they can work by different modes of action and not compete for the same substrates or receptor sites) that block as many of the four physiological processes underlying pain: transduction, transmission, modulation, and perception (*Table 49*, **142**).

Table 49 Pain-recognition processes.

Physiological process	Definition
Transduction	Conversion of energy from a noxious stimulus (mechanical, thermal, or chemical) into nerve impulses by sensory receptors (nociceptors)
Transmission	Transference of neural signals from the site of transduction (periphery) to the CNS (spinal cord and brain)
Modulation	Alterations of ascending signals initially in the dorsal horn and continues throughout the CNS. This includes descending inhibitory and facilitatory input from the brain that influences (modulates) nociceptive transmission at the level of the spinal cord
Perception	Receipt and cognitive appreciation of signals arriving at higher CNS structures as pain

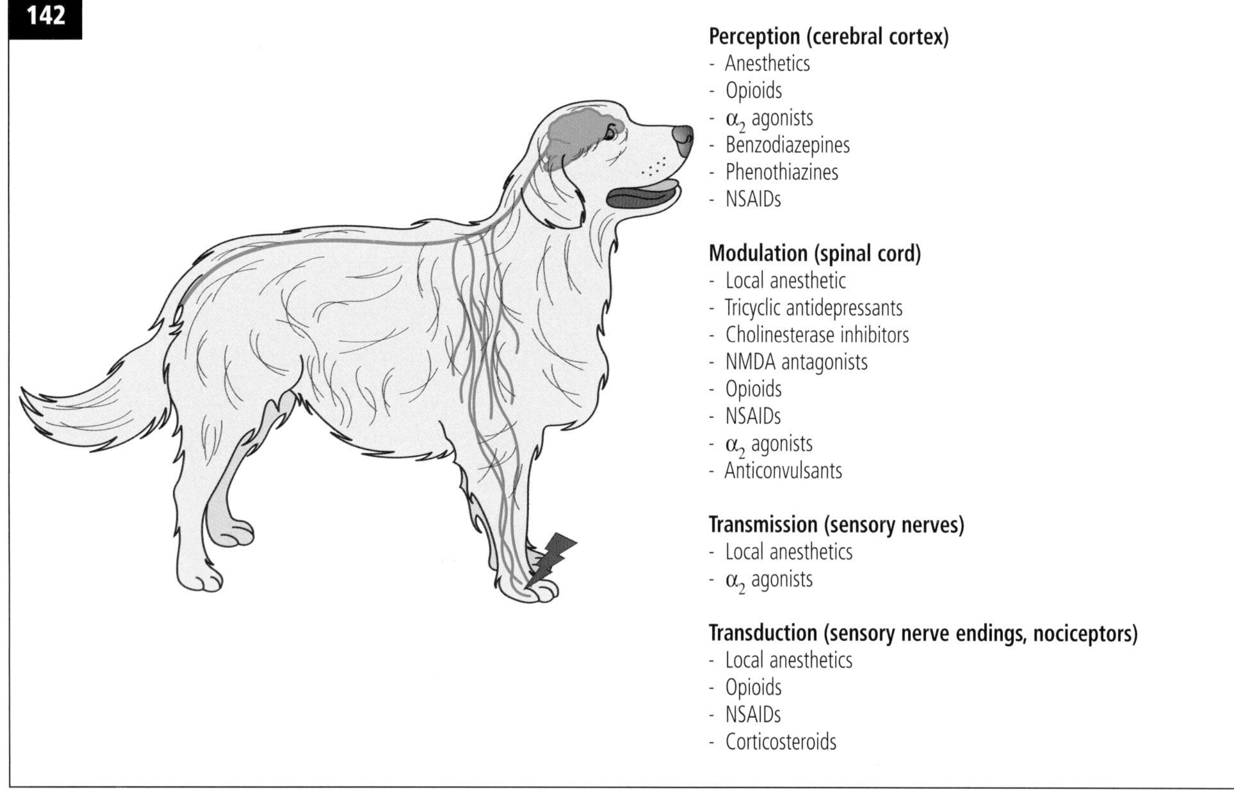

142 Drug classes listed are more effective than others in blocking each of the physiological processes of transduction, transmission, modulation, and perception.

DRUG CLASSES FOR MULTIMODAL USE

A popular combination for multimodal use consists of drugs from the opioid and NSAID classes (*Table 50*). This combination is commonly used postoperatively and for addressing the World Health Organization's cancer pain ladder recommendation for mild-to-moderate and moderate-to-severe pain. There are several opioid/NSAID combination drugs

Table 50 Comparison of opioid and NSAID pharmacology.

	Opioids	**NSAIDs**
Mechanism	Predominantly central	Predominantly peripheral
Availability	Controlled substances	Noncontrolled/some available over the counter
Therapeutic ceiling	No	Yes
Tolerance	Yes	
Addiction	Possible	Not possible
Gastrointestinal side-effects		
Nausea and vomiting	More frequent	Less frequent
Constipation	Frequent	No
Gastric ulceration	No	Possible
Gastrointestinal bleeding	No	Possible
Respiratory side-effects	Depression	Infrequent
Effects on pupil	Yes	No
Cognitive impairment	Yes	No

Table 51 **Some NSAID–opioid commercial drug combinations available for human use. Acetaminophen is not included in this table because acetaminophen is not technically a NSAID: it has analgesic properties, but *not* anti-inflammatory properties.**

Combination	Trade name	Strength (mg)
Aspirin + caffeine + dihydrocodeine	Synalgos	356.4 + 30 + 16
Aspirin + caffeine + propoxyphene	Darvon Compound-65	389 + 32.4 + 65
Aspirin + carisoprodol + codeine	Soma compound w/codeine	325 + 200 +16
Aspirin + codeine	Empirin w/codeine #3 Empirin w/codeine #4	325 + 30 325 + 60
Aspirin + hydrocodone	LortabASA	500 + 5
Aspirin + oxycodone	Persodan-Demi Percodan	325 + 2.25 325 + 4.5
Ibuprofen + oxycodone	Combunox	400 + 5
Ketoprofen + hydrocodone	Vicoprofen	200 + 7.5

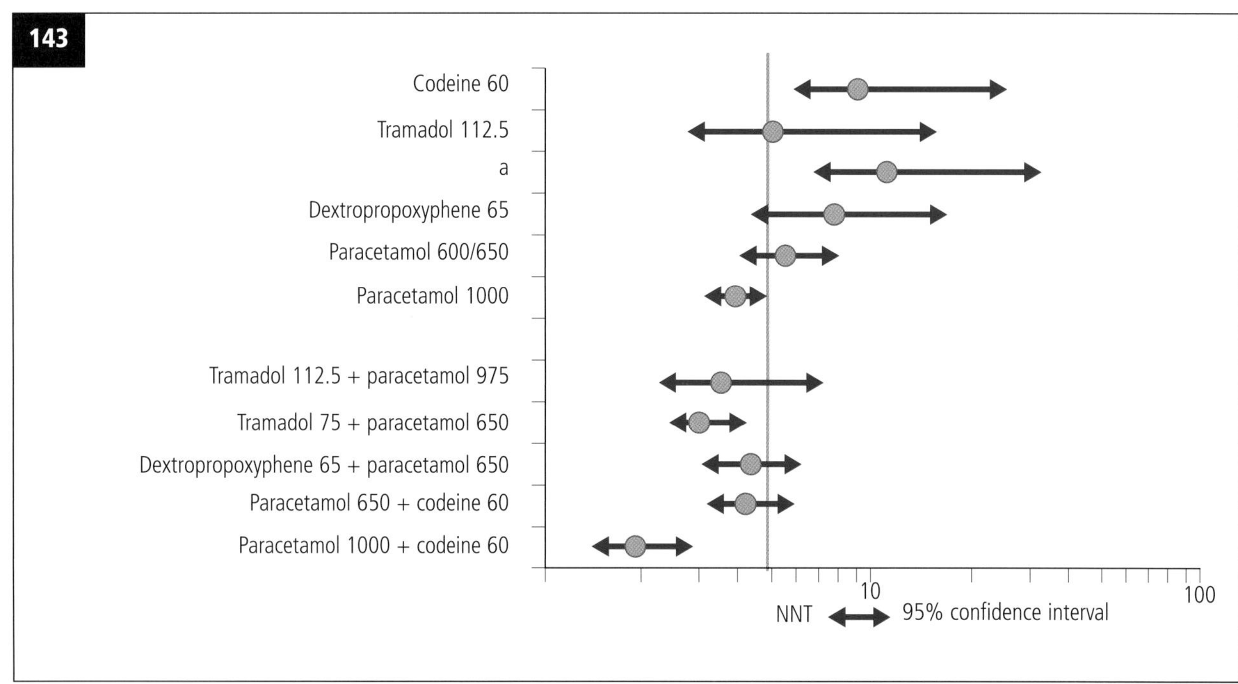

143 Numbers needed to treat demonstrates the increased efficacy when paracetamol is administered together with a different class of drug. (paracetamol = acetaminophen)

commercially available for human use (*Table 51*). **143** shows a comparison of numbers needed to treat human patients, comparing single drug administrations to combinations.[9] Increased efficacy is obvious when paracetamol is combined with various opioids. *Table 52* lists commonly used veterinary protocols.

Table 52 Various drugs commonly used in multimodal protocols.

Drug	Dose	Species	Route	Duration	Comments
Morphine	0.5–1.0 mg/kg	Canine	IM, SC, IV	3–4 hr	Caution with IV administration: histamine release–give slowly
	0.05–0.1 mg/kg	Feline	IM, SC	3–4 hr	
	0.2 mg/kg: loading, IM	Canine: 0.1–0.5 mg/kg/hr. Feline: 0.05–0.1 mg/kg/hr	IM then continuous rate infusion (CRI) (IV)		
	0.1 mg/kg preservative-free	Canine/feline	Epidural	12–24 hr	
	1–5 mg in 5–10 ml saline	Canine	Intra-articular		
Meperidine	3–5 mg/kg	Canine/feline	IM, SC	1–2 hr	Do *not* give IV (histamine release)
Methadone	0.1–0.5 mg/kg	Canine/feline	IM, SC, IV	2–4 hr	NMDA antagonist activity
Oxymorphone	0.05–0.1 mg/kg	Canine	IM, IV, SC	3–4 hr	Minimal histamine release
	0.03–0.05 mg/kg	Feline	IM, SC	3–4 hr	
Hydromorphone	0.1–0.2 mg/kg	Canine/feline	IM, IV, SC	2–4 hr	Minimal histamine release. Hyperthermia may be seen in cats
Fentanyl	5 μg/kg + 3–6 μg/kg/hr	Canine	IV	Infusion	
	2–3 μg/kg + 2–3 μg/kg/hr	Feline	IV	Infusion	
Fentanyl patch	25 μg/hr	Canine: 3–10 kg		1–3 days	24 hr to reach peak concentrations
	50 μg/hr	Canine: 10–20 kg		1–3 days	
	75 μg/hr	Canine: 20–30 kg		1–3 days	
	100 μg/hr	Canine: >30 kg		1–3 days	
	25–50 μg/hr	Feline		≤6 days	6 hr to reach peak concentrations
Butorphanol	0.1–0.2 mg/kg	Canine/feline	IM, IV, SC	dog: 1hr; cat: 2–4 hr	Low oral bioavailability
(10 mg/ml)	0.2–0.4 mg/kg IV; then 0.1–0.2 mg/kg/hr	Canine/feline	CRI		
Pentazocine	1–3 mg/kg	Canine/feline	IM, IV, SC	2–4 hr	
Nalbuphine	0.03–0.1 mg/kg	Canine/feline	IM, IV, SC	2–4 hr	

– *Continued overleaf*

Table 52 Various drugs commonly used in multimodal protocols – *Continued.*

Drug	Dose	Species	Route	Duration	Comments
Buprenorphine	10–30 µg/kg	Canine/feline	IM, IV, SC	4–10 hr	15–30 minute onset. Excellent buccal mucosa absorption in cats and dogs
Tramadol	2–10 mg/kg	Canine	PO	12–24 hr	Nonscheduled. µ agonist activity. Serotonin and norepinephrine reuptake inhibitor. NMDA antagonist at lower doses, GABA receptor inhibitor at high concentrations
	5 mg/kg (suggested)	Feline	PO		
Codeine	1–2 mg/kg	Canine	PO		
Alpha$_2$ agonist					
Medetomidine/ dexmedetomidine	2–15 µg/kg	Canine	IM, IV	0.5–1.5 hr	Sedation, bradycardia, vomition
	5–20 µg/kg	Feline	IM, IV	0.5–1.5 hr	
1.0 mg/ml	1 µg/kg IV, then 1–2 µg/kg/hr	Canine/feline	CRI		
	1–5 µg/kg	Canine/feline	Epidural		
	2–5 µg/kg	Canine/feline	Intra-articular		
Xylazine	0.1–0.5 µg/kg	Canine/feline	IM, IV	0.5–1.0 hr	
(Antagonist) yohimbine	0.1 mg/kg IV; 0.3–0.5 mg/kg IM	Canine/feline			
(Antagonist) atipamezol	0.05–0.2 mg/kg IV	Canine/feline			2–4 times the medetomidine dose
NMDA antagonist					
Ketamine	0.5 mg/kg; IV then 0.1–0.5 mg/kg/hr	Canine/feline	CRI		
Amantadine	3–5 mg/kg	Canine/feline	PO	24 hr	Neuropathic pain
Dextromethorphan	0.5–2 mg/kg	Canine	PO, SQ, IV		D-isomer of codeine; weak NMDA antagonist NOT RECOMMENDED due to side-effects[10]
Methadone	0.1–0.5 mg/kg	Canine/feline	IM, SC	2–4 hr	Opioid derivative

– *Continued on facing page*

Table 52 Various drugs commonly used in multimodal protocols – *Continued.*

Drug	Dose	Species	Route	Duration	Comments
Tricyclic antidepressant					
Amitriptyline	1.0 mg/kg	Canine	PO	12–24 hr	Enhanced noradrenergic activity
	0.5–1.0 mg/kg	Feline	PO	12–24 hr	
Calcium channel modulator					
Gabapentin	5–10 mg/kg	Canine/feline	PO	12–24 hr	VDCC inhibitor
Adjunct					
Acepromazine	0.025–0.05 mg/kg	Canine	IM, SC, IV	8–12 hr	3 mg maximum total dose; used to potentiate or prolong analgesic drug effect
	0.05–0.2 mg/kg	Feline	IM, SC	8–12 hr	
Diazepam	0.1–0.2 mg/kg	Canine/feline	IV	2–4 hr	Used to potentiate or prolong analgesic drug effect
	0.25–1.0 mg/kg	Canine/feline	PO	12–24 hr	
Local anesthetics					
Lidocaine (1–2%)	≤6.0 mg/kg	Canine	Perineural	1–2 hr	Onset: 10–15 minutes. Maximum dose: 12 mg/kg (canine); 6 mg/kg (feline)
	≤3.0 mg/kg	Feline	Perineural	1–2 hr	
	2–4 mg/kg IV, then 25–80 µg/kg/min	Canine	IV: CRI		
	0.25–0.75 mg/kg slow IV, then 10–40 µg/kg/min	Feline	IV: CRI		*NOTE: efficacy and safety are not yet proven*
Bupivacaine (0.25–0.5%)	≤2.0 mg/kg	Canine	Perineural	2–6 hr	Onset: 20–30 minutes. Maximum dose: 2 mg/kg (canine or feline)
	≤1.0 mg/kg	Feline	Perineural	2–6 hr	
Mepivacaine (1–2%)	≤6.0 mg/kg	Canine	Perineural	2–2.5 hr	
	≤3.0 mg/kg	Feline	Perineural	2–2.5 hr	

DELIVERY TECHNIQUES

Local and regional administration techniques are re-emerging in popularity. Analgesic infiltration at a nerve trunk or regional administration via spinal injection provides regional analgesia. The principle benefit of regional analgesia is reduced sedation and other side-effects compared with those seen following parenteral administration of some analgesic agents.

Many traditional analgesic drugs, including opioids and α_2 agonists, have a short duration of action and the potential to produce systemic side-effects, including emesis, respiratory depression, drowsiness, and ileus. In contrast local anesthetics are comparatively safe. They are effective and relatively inexpensive. Local anesthetics have the unique ability to produce complete blockade of sensory nerve fibers and suppress the development of secondary sensitization to pain. Therefore, local and regional anesthetic/analgesic techniques are often used with opioids, α_2 agonists, NMDA antagonists, and NSAIDs as part of a multimodal strategy.

LOCAL ANESTHETICS

During the generation of an action potential, VGSCs open and allow sodium ions to flow into the cell, which depolarizes the cell membrane. Local anesthetics bind to a hydrophilic site within the sodium channel on the cell membrane inner surface, and block activation of the channel, thereby preventing depolarization of the cell membrane. Small nerves and myelinated fibers tend to be more responsive to local anesthetics than are large nerves and unmyelinated fibers. Commonly, autonomic fibers (small unmyelinated C fibers and myelinated B fibers) and pain fibers (small unmyelinated C fibers and myelinated Aδ fibers) are blocked before other sensory and motor fibers (differential block). Local anesthetics are also more effective at sensory fibers because they have longer action potentials and discharge at higher frequencies than do other types of fibers (frequency-dependent blockade). In addition, some local anesthetics, such as bupivacaine, can selectively block sensory rather than motor function.[11]

The practice of adding vasoconstrictors, such as epinephrine, to local anesthetics so as to reduce the rate of systemic absorption and prolong the duration of action, has fallen from favor with the availability of longer-acting local anesthetics such as bupivacaine and ropivacaine.

Adverse side-effects of local anesthetics are rare if appropriate dosage recommendations are followed and are most commonly associated with inappropriate intravenous delivery. CNS and cardiovascular disturbances are the most common side-effects. With excessive dosing, the rate of depolarization of individual cardiac cells is reduced, leading to prolonged conduction of the cardiac impulse, arrhythmias, or bradycardia and asystole.[12] Rapid intravenous administration of local anesthetics can decrease vascular tone and myocardial contractility, resulting in the acute onset of hypotension. CNS effects can range from mild to full-blown seizure activity. The toxicity of most local anesthetics reflects potency, and in dogs, the relative CNS toxicity of lidocaine, etidocaine, and bupivacaine is 1:3:5, respectively.[13]

Local anesthetics can be used in a variety of clinical settings to manage or pre-empt pain. Common uses include digital blocks for feline onychectomy, dental blocks for tooth extraction, local infiltration for cutaneous procedures, intra-articular analgesia, body cavity infusion before or after abdominal surgery, soaker catheters for wound analgesia, and epidural deposition for abdominal and/or hindlimb procedures. Most nerves can be blocked with 0.1–0.3 ml of 2% lidocaine or 0.5% bupivacaine solution using a 25-gauge needle. Doses of local anesthetics, especially for cats and small dogs, should always be calculated carefully, and are best administered with the animal under general anesthesia or heavy sedation.

Oncychectomy

Approximately 24% of owned cats in the US are declawed,[14] and postoperative pain is a generally accepted consequence.[15] Effective analgesia can be provided by blocking the radial, ulnar, and median nerves (**144**), although one study[17] refutes this clinical observation. A combination of both lidocaine and bupivacaine (1.5 mg/kg of each) may provide both a quicker onset and longer duration of analgesic effect than when using either drug alone for blockade.

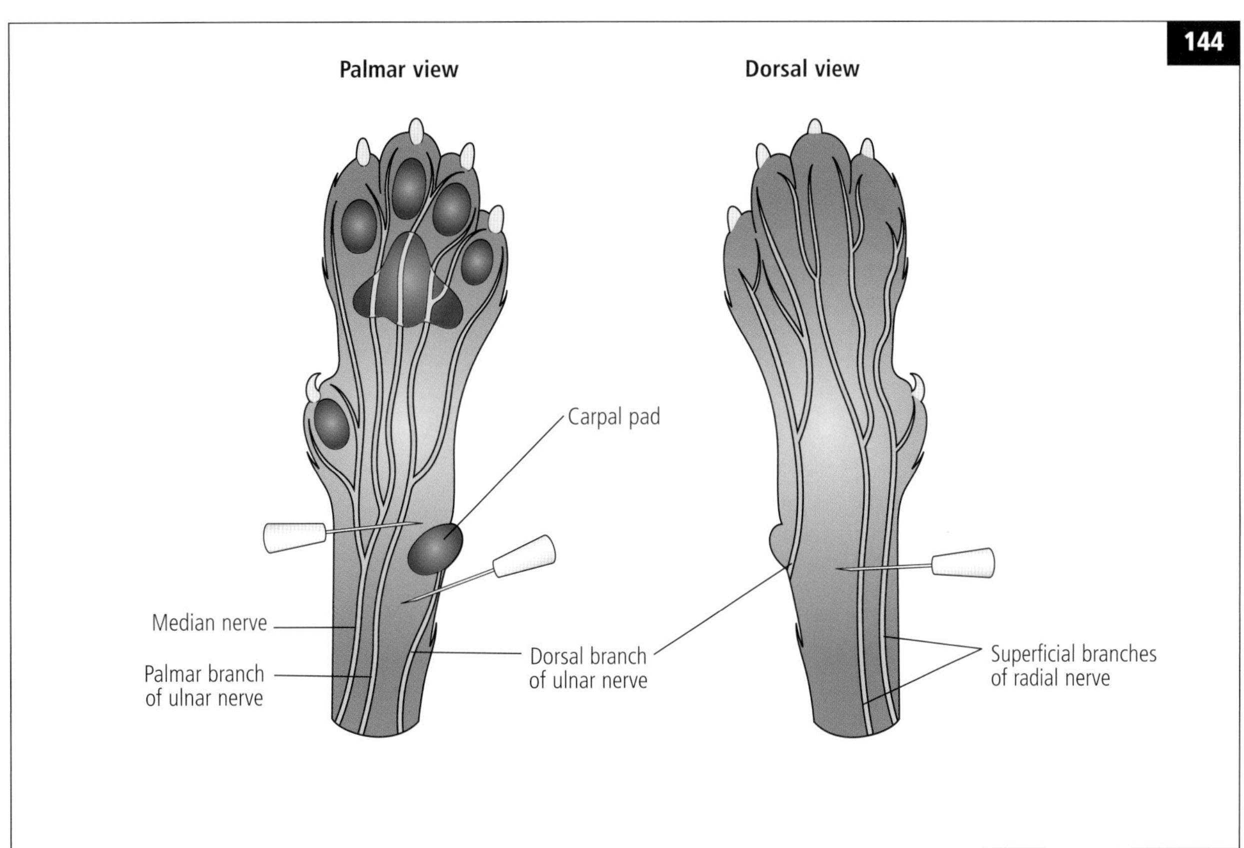

144 Oncychectomy is an excellent example of where analgesia is markedly improved by preemptive local anesthetic blockade. Three sites of local anesthetic deposition effectively blocks the distal extremity. (Adapted from: Tranquilli WJ, *et al*. Pain Management For The Small Animal Practitioner. Teton NewMedia 2004, 2nd edition (with permission))[16]

Table 53 Dental nerve blocks with local anesthetic.

Block	**Mental**	**Mandibular (inferior alveolar)**	**Infraorbital**	**Maxillary**
Effect	Anesthetizes all oral tissues rostral to the second premolar on the ipsilateral side	Affects the bone, teeth, soft tissue and tongue on the ipsilateral side	Anesthetizes the bone, soft tissue, and dentition rostral to, but not including, the upper fourth premolar	Blocks the bone, teeth, soft tissue, and palatal tissue on the ipsilateral side
Location	Mental foramen ventral to the rostral (mesial) root of the second premolar	Lingual side of notch on caudal ventral mandible cranial to the angular process, midpoint between ventral and dorsal borders of the mandible	Infraorbital foramen of the maxilla dorsal to the caudal (distal) root of the upper third premolar	In the open mouth: notch where the zygomatic arch meets the bone surrounding the last maxillary molar

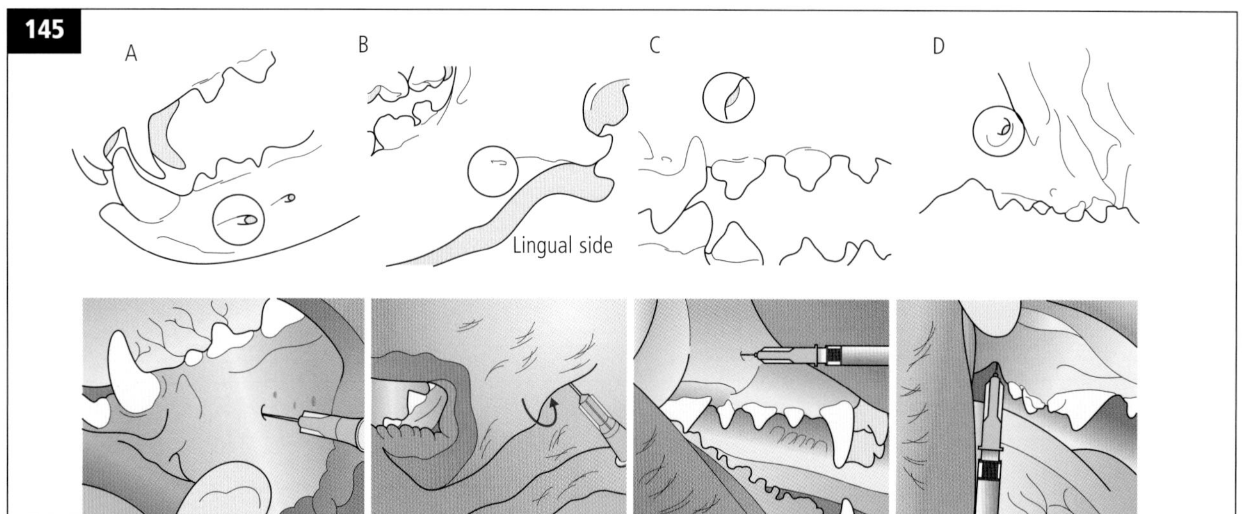

145 Local anesthetic blocks are very effective in providing analgesia for oral cavity procedures. Area blocked is rostral to the injection site. A Mental. B Mandibular. C Infraorbital. D Maxillary.

Dental

Sensory nerve fibers that innervate the bone, teeth, and soft tissues of the oral cavity arborize from the maxillary or mandibular branches of the trigeminal nerve. Four regional nerve blocks can be easily performed to provide analgesia for dental and oral surgical procedures (*Table 53*, **145**).

Dermal

Local anesthetic infiltration is often implemented for removal of tumors or dermal lesions, superficial lacerations, and as preincisional blocks. A small subcutaneous bleb (0.5–2.0 ml) is often sufficient for small lesion removal in the dermis. Infiltrative blocks for removal of subcutaneous masses require a deeper

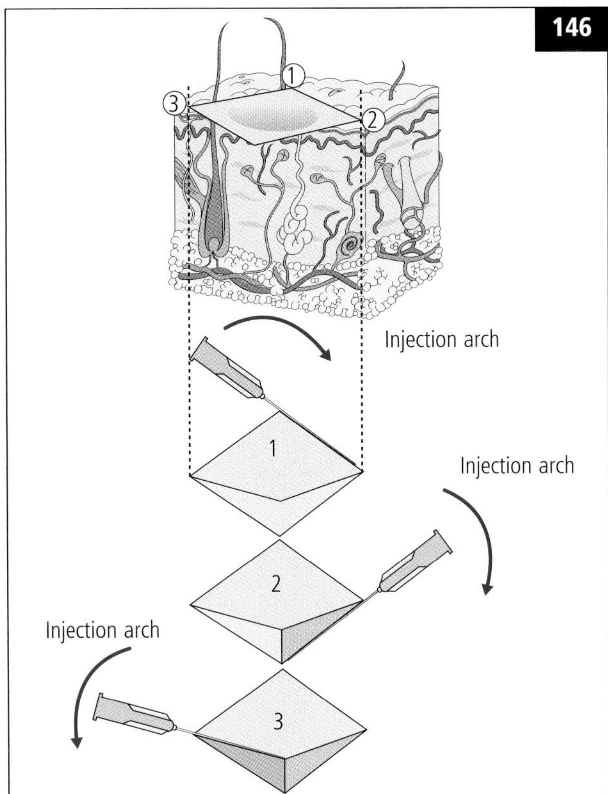

146 Local anesthetic, administered through three injection site archs, will adequately infiltrate an area to be desensitized for procedures such as dermal mass removal. A 1:1 mixture of lidocaine and bupivacaine not to exceed 3.0 mg/kg of lidocaine and 2.0 mg/kg of bupivacaine, takes advantage of the more rapid onset of action of lidocaine together with the longer duration of effect from bupivacaine.

area of desensitization, and an inverted pyramidal area of infiltration works well (**146**).

Body cavities

Intrapleural administration of bupivacaine has been described to manage pain in dogs undergoing intercostal or sternal thoracotomy[18,19] as has peritoneal administration for pancreatitis,[20] and canine ovariohysterectomy.[21] In the awake animal pleural infusion of bupivacaine can be painful, therefore sodium bicarbonate is added. In either case, 0.02 mmol/kg (mEq/kg) of sodium bicarbonate is added to 0.2 ml/kg of 0.5% bupivacaine solution, then saline is added to produce a final volume of 10–20 ml for administration via a thoracostomy tube or abdominocentesis. There is evidence for a reduction of postoperative pain after intra-articular local anesthesia in human patients undergoing arthroscopic knee surgery.[22] In dogs, intra-articular bupivacaine provided pain relief after stifle surgery better than intra-articular morphine.[23]

Other local anesthetic techniques

CRI of lidocaine is also an effective method of delivering local anesthetic (dog: 2–4 mg/kg IV bolus, then 25–80 mg/kg/min; cat: 0.25–0.75 mg/kg slow IV, then 10–40 mg/kg/min; note: efficacy and safety are not yet convincing). Finally, lidocaine is available as a topical patch product (Lidoderm®), 2% jelly, and in a 10% spray formulation.

Specially designed catheters can be utilized for longer-term (days) continuous infiltration of local anesthetic,[24] particularly following procedures such as ear canal ablation (efficacious findings,[25] non-efficacious findings[26]), amputations, and after large soft tissue excision, such as fibrosarcoma removal in cats.[27] Commercial devices are available (Pain Buster®) that include a local anesthetic reservoir connected to a fenestrated catheter or catheters can be constructed from red rubber or polyethylene tubing. Bupivacaine, 0.25%, is diluted to volume and can be given as a bolus: 2 mg/kg (cat: 1 mg/kg) first dose, then 1 mg/kg (cat: 0.5 mg/kg) doses can be given thereafter at intervals >6 hr for 1–2 days.

EPIDURAL ADMINISTRATION

In the 1970s it was discovered that epidural administration of opioids produced profound analgesia in animals with minimal systemic effects.[28] Since that time interest has increased in the epidural route for administration of analgesics, particularly in the delivery of opioids, where the motor paralysis of local anesthesia administration can be avoided. The most frequently administered drugs are the local anesthetics and opioids, but α_2 agonists (xylazine and medetomidine) and combinations of these drugs have also been used (*Table 54*). (*overleaf*)

Epidural drug administration and catheter placement for repeated administration have several advantages:

Table 54 Drug dose and action following epidural administration in dogs.

Drug	Dose (dog)	Approximate onset (minutes)	Approximate duration (hr)
Lidocaine 2%	1 ml/3.4 kg (to T_5) 1 ml/4.5 kg (to T_{13}–L_1)	10	1–1.5
Bupivacaine (0.25% or 0.5%)	1 ml/4.5 kg	20–30	4.5–6
Fentanyl	0.001 mg/kg	4–10	6
Oxymorphone	0.1 mg/kg	15	10
Morphine	0.1 mg/kg	23	20
Buprenorphine	0.003–0.005 mg/kg (in saline solution)	30	12–18

- Requires lower drug doses than systemic injection, and therefore less risk for dose-related side-effects.
- Decreases perioperative injectable and inhalant agent requirement.
- Decreases procedural costs due to the long duration of action and decreased dose of adjunctive drugs.

It has been suggested that epidurals are best utilized together with general anesthesia as part of a balanced (multimodal) analgesia protocol, and this probably plays a noteworthy role in blocking CNS windup. The technique is frequently used for perianal, hindlimb, and abdominal surgery, however analgesia as far rostral as the thoracic limb (using morphine) can be provided in a dose-related manner.[29] Epidural morphine, with or without long-lasting bupivacaine, has been used to relieve pain associated with pancreatitis and peritonitis.[29]

Urine retention and pruritus are reported as possible complications of this technique, although occurrence is rare. The procedure is contraindicated in animals with bleeding disorders because of the potential for hemorrhage into the epidural space with inadvertent puncture of an epidural vessel. Due to the potential for blockade of regional sympathetic nerves, epidurals should not be performed on hypovolemic or hypotensive animals. Injection site skin infection is also a contraindication.

The procedure should be performed in a sterile setting. The site for spinal needle insertion is on the dorsal midline at the lumbosacral space (**147**). In the adult dog the spinal cord ends at approximately the sixth lumbar vertebra, rostral to the injection site. The site for injection is just caudal to the seventh dorsal spinous process, which can be easily identified because it is shorter than the others. Confirmation of correct needle placement can be done by either the 'hanging drop' or 'loss of resistance' technique.[30] Following correct needle placement, the drug(s) is injected slowly to ensure even distribution.

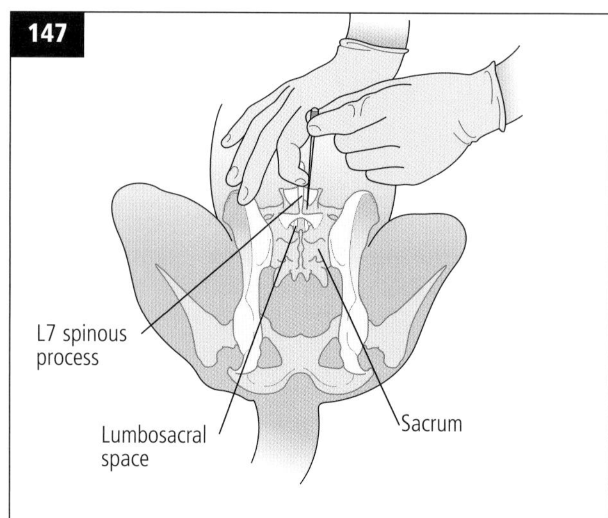

147 Accurate spinal needle insertion comes with practice; however, the skill is not particularly difficult and patient analgesia is noteworthy.[16]

OTHER DELIVERY ROUTES

Oral transmucosal (OTM) drug administration is a relatively new delivery system used in humans, e.g. fentanyl lozenges. This same route has been investigated by Robertson *et al.*[31] as it applies to the efficacy of buprenorphine in cats. Because, in part, the Pk_a of buprenorphine (8.24) is similar to the pH of the cat's mouth (9.0), buprenorphine is readily absorbed across the oral mucous membranes. Absorption by this route, rather than gastrointestinal, avoids hepatic first-pass elimination, because venous drainage is systemic. As a result the onset of analgesic action is as early as 30 minutes and lasts up to 6 hr. This response in the cat is similar to the intravenous administration as assessed by a validated nociception thermal model. OTM administration is easy and avoids multiple injections, making it an excellent delivery form for both in-hospital and take-home use. Apparently, buprenorphine is odorless and tasteless, as cats do not resist OTM administration and do not hypersalivate in response.

ACUPUNCTURE

Acupuncture falls under the categorization of complementary and alternative medicine as part of traditional Chinese medicine, and is utilized in humans in at least 78 countries worldwide.[32] From an historical perspective, little information about acupuncture was available in the US until after President Richard Nixon's visit to China in 1972. However, in 1826 Benjamin Franklin's grandson, a Philadelphia physician, published that acupuncture was an effective treatment for pain associated with rheumatism and neuralgia among prisoners at the Pennsylvania state penitentiary.[33] It is a safe, low-cost modality which is easy to administer and has no side-effects if performed by a trained practitioner; it can be administered stand-alone or as a complement to other medical therapeutics. It is misleading to refer to a single universal form of traditional Chinese acupuncture, as there are more than 80 different acupuncture styles in China alone, in addition to many Japanese, Korean, Vietnamese, European, and American styles.

THEORY OF ACUPUNCTURE

Traditional Chinese medicine places emphasis on function rather than structure. Accordingly, in such practice it is more important to understand the relationships between variables and the functional 'whole' of the patient than to identify the specifics of a single pathology. Basic to the practice of acupuncture is the yin–yang theory, where yin and yang are interdependent but possess similar characteristics (**148**).[34] They can transform into each other, and can consume each other. In this regard, physiology and pathology are variations along a continuum of health and illness.

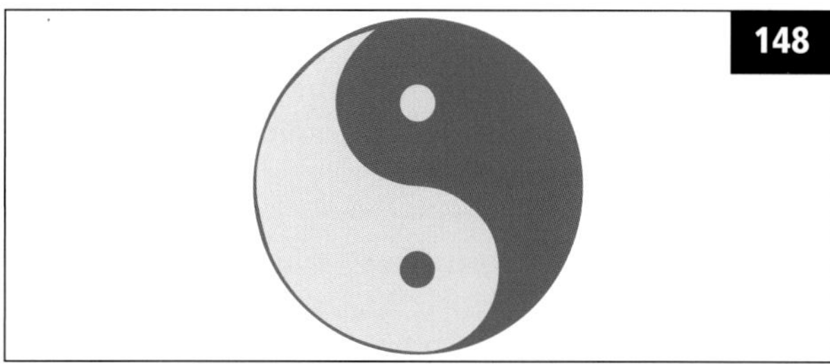

148 The graphic which has come to represent the yin–yang theory.

A common feature shared by all different types of acupuncture is using needles to initiate changes in the soft tissue. Needles and needle-induced changes are believed to activate the built-in survival mechanisms that normalize physiological homeostasis and promote self-healing. Herein, acupuncture can be defined as a physiological therapy coordinated by the brain, which responds to the stimulation of manual or electrical needling of peripheral sensory nerves.[35] Acupuncture can be effective for both peripheral soft tissue pain and internal disorders, but in the case of peripheral soft tissue pain the result appears more predictable because of the local needle reaction.

HYPOTHESIS OF ACUPUNCTURE MECHANISMS

The leading hypotheses include the effects of local stimulation, neuronal gating, the release of endogenous opiates, and the placebo effect. It is further proposed that the CNS is essential for the processing of these effects via its modulation of the autonomic nervous system, the neuroimmune system, and hormonal regulation. Clinical observation suggests that acupuncture needling achieves at least four therapeutic goals:

- Release of physical and emotional stress.
- Activation and control of immune and anti-inflammatory mechanisms.
- Acceleration of tissue healing.
- Pain relief secondary to endorphin and serotonin release.

Keeping in mind that acupuncture therapy is considered to activate built-in survival mechanisms, i.e. self-healing potential, it is effective for those symptoms that can be completely or partially healed by the body. Additionally, each individual has a different self-healing capacity influenced by genetic make-up, medical history, lifestyle, and age, all of which may be dynamically changing.

EASTERN PERSPECTIVES MEET WESTERN PERSPECTIVES

Ancient Chinese thought holds that Qi is a fundamental and vital substance of the universe, with all phenomena being produced by its changes. It is considered a vital substance of the body, flowing along organized pathways known as acupuncture channels, or meridians, helping to maintain normal activities. Traditional Chinese medicine suggests that a balanced flow of Qi throughout the system is required for good health, and acupuncture stimulation can correct imbalances.

Since the mid-1990s, stimulation of acupuncture points has been believed to cause biochemical changes that can affect the body's natural healing. The primary mechanisms involved in these changes include enhanced conduction of bioelectromagnetic signals, activation of opioid systems, and activation of autonomic and central nervous systems causing the release of various neurotransmitters and neurohormones.[36] Approximately 30 years ago it was discovered that acupuncture analgesia could be reversed by naloxone, a pure antagonist to all known opioids.[37] Acupuncture can change concentrations of serotonin and biogenic amines, including opioid peptides, met-enkephalin, leu-enkephalin, β-endorphin, and dynorphin.

Acupuncture can also be explained, in part, by Melzack and Wall's gate theory. When large, unmyelinated Aδ and Aβ fibers are stimulated by acupuncture, impulses from small unmyelinated C fibers, transmitting ascending nociceptive information, are blocked by a gate of inhibitory interneurons.

The strongest evidence for acupuncture efficacy in human cancer has been in the areas of nausea, vomiting, and pain control.[38, 39]

SUMMARY

The term multimodal has come to denote the co-utilization of different delivery modes as well as a variety of different drug-class agents. The objective of this is to provide the patient with a minimal effective dose of each agent and therefore render optimal pain relief with the minimal risk for adverse response.

8 MULTIMODAL MANAGEMENT OF CANINE OSTEOARTHRITIS

INTRODUCTION

For many years, pain was managed by administration of a single pharmacological agent (if it was managed at all), and often only when the animal 'proved' to the clinician that it was suffering. Within the past 10–15 years advancements in the understanding of pain physiology, introduction of more efficacious and safe drugs, and the maturation of ethics toward animals have considerably improved the management of pain that veterinary patients need and deserve.

Following the lead in human medicine, veterinarians have come to appreciate that the network of pain processing involves an incredibly large number of transmitters and receptors, all with different mechanisms, dynamics, and modes of action. From this appreciation comes the conclusion that it is naïve to expect analgesia with a single agent, working by a single mode of action. Multimodal analgesia was initially understood as the administration of a *combination* of different drugs from different pharmacological classes such that they act by different, noncompeting modes of action. However the concept has further expanded to include different methods of delivery, e.g. oral, systemic, transdermal, transbuccal, and epidural as well as nonpharmacological modalities such as acupuncture and physical rehabilitation. Central to the concept is that drug combinations will be synergistic (or at least additive), requiring a reduced amount of each individual drug, and therefore less potential for adverse response to medication. Selection of drugs within the 'cocktail' would be optimal if they collectively blocked all four of the physiological processes associated with pain recognition (i.e. transduction, transmission, modulation, and perception).

SYNERGISM: PERIOPERATIVE BACKGROUND

A study illustrating the concept of synergism was reported by Grimm and others in 2000 (*Table 55*).[1] Whereas the time to positive response in a tail clamping model was 1.5 hr and 2.4 hr for butorphanol (0.2 mg/kg) and medetomidine (5 µg/kg) respectively, the response time for the combination was 5.6 hr rather than 3.9 hr–the sum of each agent taken individually. Synergism is a consistent response when administering an opioid and an α_2 agonist together, making this combination an excellent premedication for surgery.

Table 55 Results of a study by Grimm *et al.*[1] which show that adding an opioid to an α_2 agonist results in a clinical response that is greater than additive; the result is synergistic.

Treatment group	Time until positive response (hr)
Saline control	0.0 ± 0.0
Butorphanol (0.2 mg/kg IM)	1.50 ± 1.50
Medetomidine (5.0 µg/kg IM)	2.36 ± 0.49 (Σ = 3.86) (expectation if effects were additive)
Butorphanol (0.2 mg/kg IM) + medetomidine (5.0 µg/kg IM)	5.58 ± 2.28

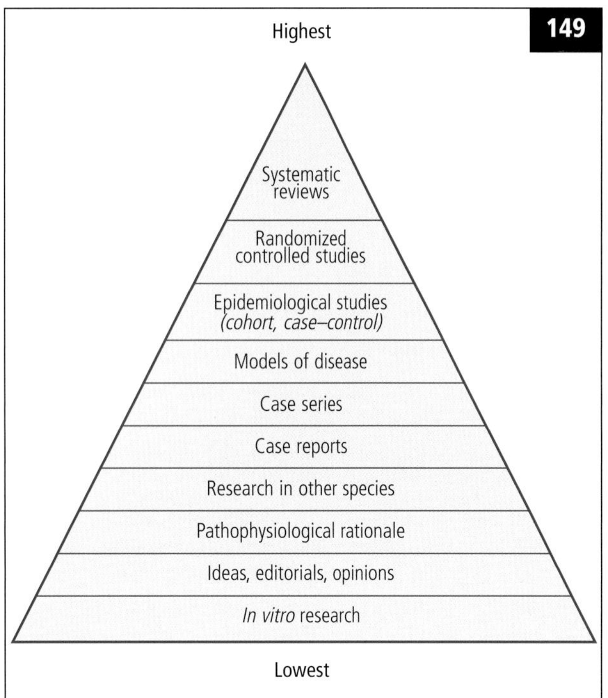

149 The quality of evidence pyramid delineates the origin of confidence a clinician would have in a given treatment protocol.

Further, addition of an NSAID will guard against inflammatory windup and sensitize μ receptors to exogenous opioid effects.[2] From these observations comes recommendation of the optimal surgical premedication protocol to include: an opioid, an α_2 agonist, and a COX-1-sparing NSAID.

Perioperative multimodal analgesia is widely practiced today in veterinary medicine, however monotherapy continues to be common practice for managing the chronic pain of OA. NSAIDs are the foundation for treating OA, and are likely to be the foundation for some years to come. Many clinicians manage the elusive pain of OA simply by sequencing different NSAIDs until satisfactory patient results are found or unacceptable adverse reactions are experienced. However, optimal clinical results are more frequently obtained by implementing a multimodal protocol for OA.

QUALITY OF EVIDENCE

Although contemporary experience precedes published literature, there is a growing evidence base for the multimodal management of OA. This evidence is a collation of clinical expertise, client/patient preferences, available resources, and research evidence, positioned on the evidence pyramid (**149**).

Quality of evidence is an important consideration when making a therapeutic decision, and can be graded from 1 to 4. Grades 1 and 2 compose the highest level of evidence, consisting of systematic reviews (meta-analyses) and well designed, properly randomized, controlled, patient-centered clinical trials. Grade 3 notes a moderate level of evidence, consisting of well designed, non-randomized clinical trials, epidemiological studies (cohort, case–control), models of disease, and dramatic results in uncontrolled studies. Grade 4 is the lower level of evidence encompassing expert opinions, descriptive studies, studies in nontarget species, pathophysiological findings, and *in vitro* studies. Very few reports have been made reviewing the quality of evidence of treatments for OA in dogs.[3]

MULTIMODAL OA TREATMENT PROTOCOL

NONMEDICICAL MANAGEMENT (150)

DIET

Impellizeri *et al.*[4] showed that in overweight dogs with hindlimb lameness secondary to hip OA, weight reduction alone may result in a substantial improvement in clinical lameness. Further, from the Labrador Retriever life-long Nestlé Purina study, Kealy and others[5,6] showed that the prevalence and

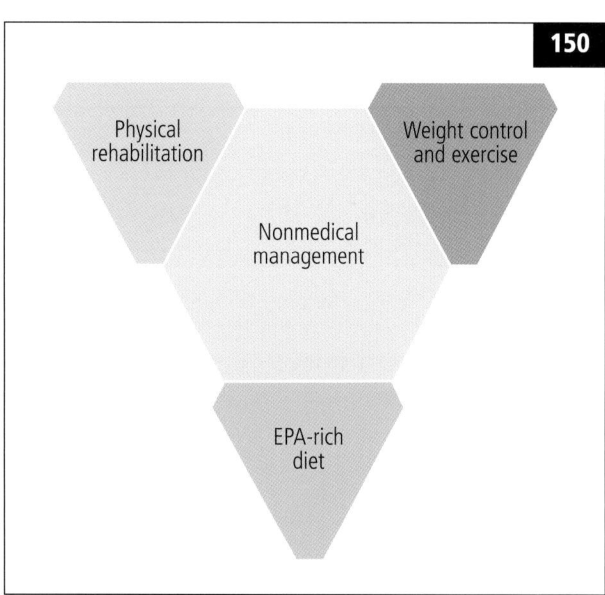

150 The nonmedical management of OA is composed of weight control/exercise, EPA-rich diet, and physical rehabilitation.

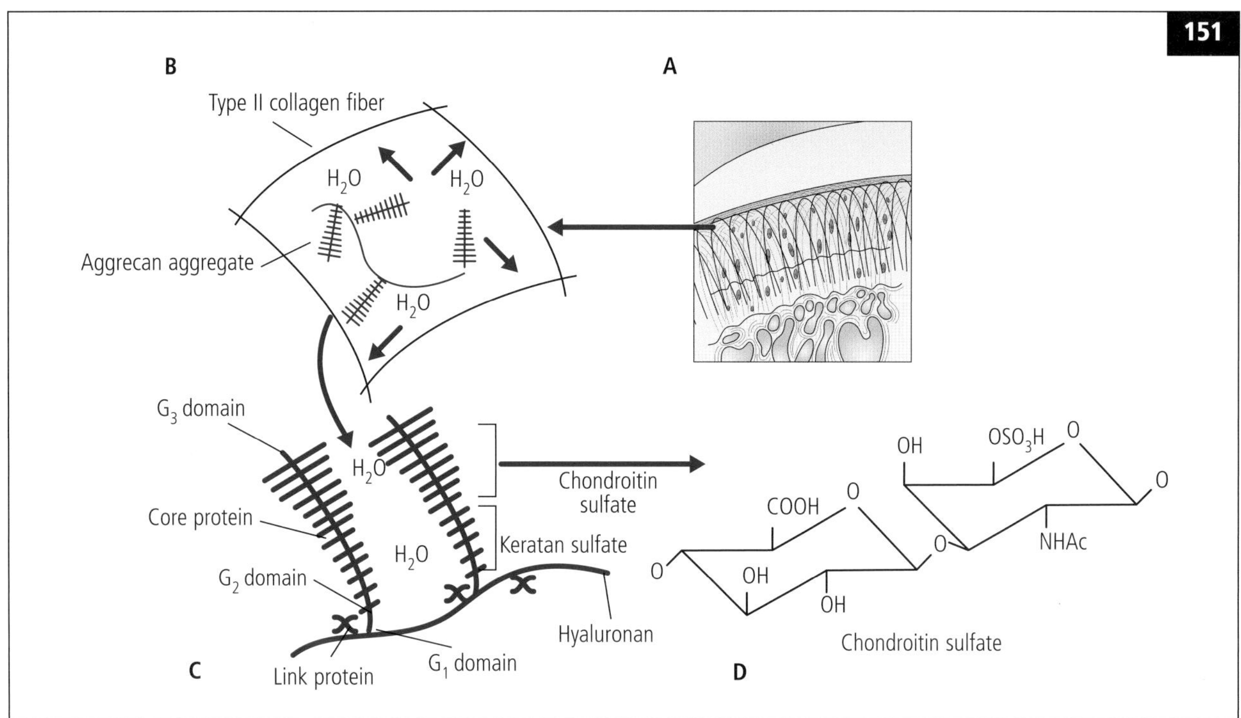

151 The 'functional unit' of articular cartilage is the aggrecan aggregate, wherein a loss of structure results in a loss of function.[7] (A) Cross-section of normal cartilage. (B) Proteoglycans (from chondrocytes), water, and collagen that comprise cartilage. (C) Aggrecan aggregate. (D) Chondrotin sulfate GAG. (Adapted from Johnson SA. *The Veterinary Clinics of North America Small Animal Practice* 1997.)

severity of OA in several joints were less in dogs with long-term reduced food intake, compared with control dogs, and that food intake is an environmental factor that may have a profound effect on development of OA in dogs. Dogs on a restricted diet showed a significant reduction in progression of OA hip scores and lived longer.

Obviously, the content of the diet is critical. The adage, 'you are what you eat' has been given support relative to OA from research conducted on EPA-rich diets by pet food manufacturers.

Aggrecan is the major proteoglycan (by mass) of articular cartilage, consisting of the proteoglycan monomer that aggregates with hyaluronan. Many aggrecan monomers attach to a hyaluronic acid chain to form an aggrecan aggregate. Aggrecan aggregates, type II collagen fibrils, water, and chondrocytes comprise the cartilage matrix wherein structure reflects function (**151**). When structure is altered, so too is function.

A disruption in the normal relationship of collagen and proteoglycans in the articular cartilage matrix is one of the first events in the development of OA. Compared with normal cartilage, OA-affected cartilage behaves like an activated macrophage, with upregulation of IL-1, IL-6, and IL-8 gene expression. Also upregulated in arthritic chondrocytes are PGE_2, TNF-α, NO, and MMP-2, -3, -9, and -13. These enzymes, MMPs, and aggrecanases destroy collagen and proteoglycans faster than new ones can be produced, transitioning the cartilage from an anabolic state to a catabolic state.

Imbalance of TIMPs and MMPs contributes to the pathological breakdown of cartilage (**152**).

Dietary fatty acids can help to correct this imbalance by modulating the production of inflammatory mediators. PGE_2, which increases in inflammatory conditions such as OA, stimulates pain receptors and promotes additional inflammation. On the other hand PGE_3 and LTB_5, the eicosanoid products of EPA, have markedly less biological activity than those derived from AA and are considered anti-inflammatory (**153**). The end result is that when the omega-3 fatty acid EPA replaces AA in cell membranes, the inflammatory cascade is decreased. Further, dog chondrocytes selectively store EPA (and no other omega-3 fatty acid) in the chondrocyte membrane which turns off signal mRNA that prompts production of degradative aggrecanase. See **154**.

Clinical trial results from feeding EPA-rich diets have demonstrated increased serum EPA concentrations, improved clinical performance as assessed by both the veterinarian and the pet owner, improved weightbearing as measured by force plate gait analysis, and have potential for NSAID dose reduction.[9]

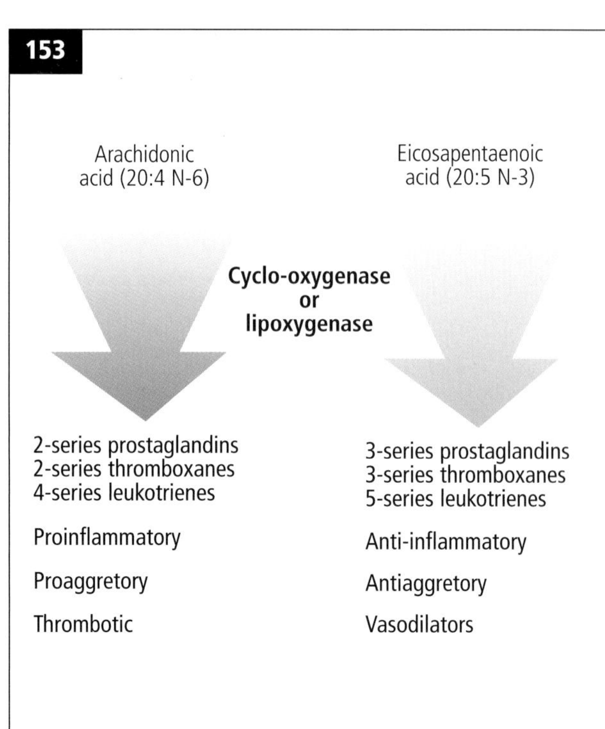

153 Eicosanoid production from AA or EPA.[8]

PHYSICAL REHABILITATION

Physical rehabilitation is a term that defines a broad spectrum of methods from the most advanced techniques used in complex orthopedic surgery recoveries to the simple techniques that can be taught to pet owners for use at home with their pets. The goal is to restore, maintain, and promote optimal function, optimal fitness, wellness, and quality of life as they relate to movement disorders and health.

The chronic OA patient is often reluctant to exercise. This reluctance may be due to the patient's unwillingness or inability. Unwillingness is frequently due to pain which can be managed pharmacologically. However, the inability is often a consequence of decreased muscle mass and decreased joint range of motion, both the sequelae of OA. Physical rehabilitation focuses on the patient's inability to exercise, providing a resultant 'freedom of movement' and serves as a palliation of the disease progression. Frequently, physical rehabilitation together with weight control in earlier stages of OA can be as effective as pharmacological intervention. Techniques of physical rehabilitation easily implemented by pet owners include: leash walking, sit-to-stand exercises, steps, inclines, dancing and wheelbarrowing exercises, treadmill activity, and cavaletti rails.

Weight control/exercise, EPA-rich diet, and physical rehabilitation comprise the nonmedical component of a multimodal OA treatment regimen (**150**).

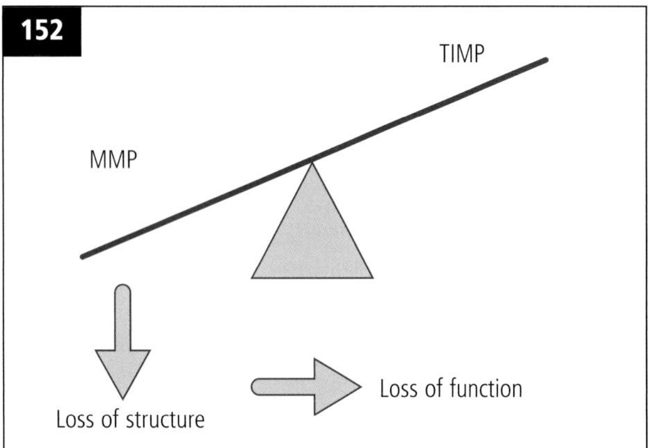

152 Normally, TIMPs counteract the destruction of MMPs, but in the arthritic state TIMPs cannot keep up and catabolism prevails.

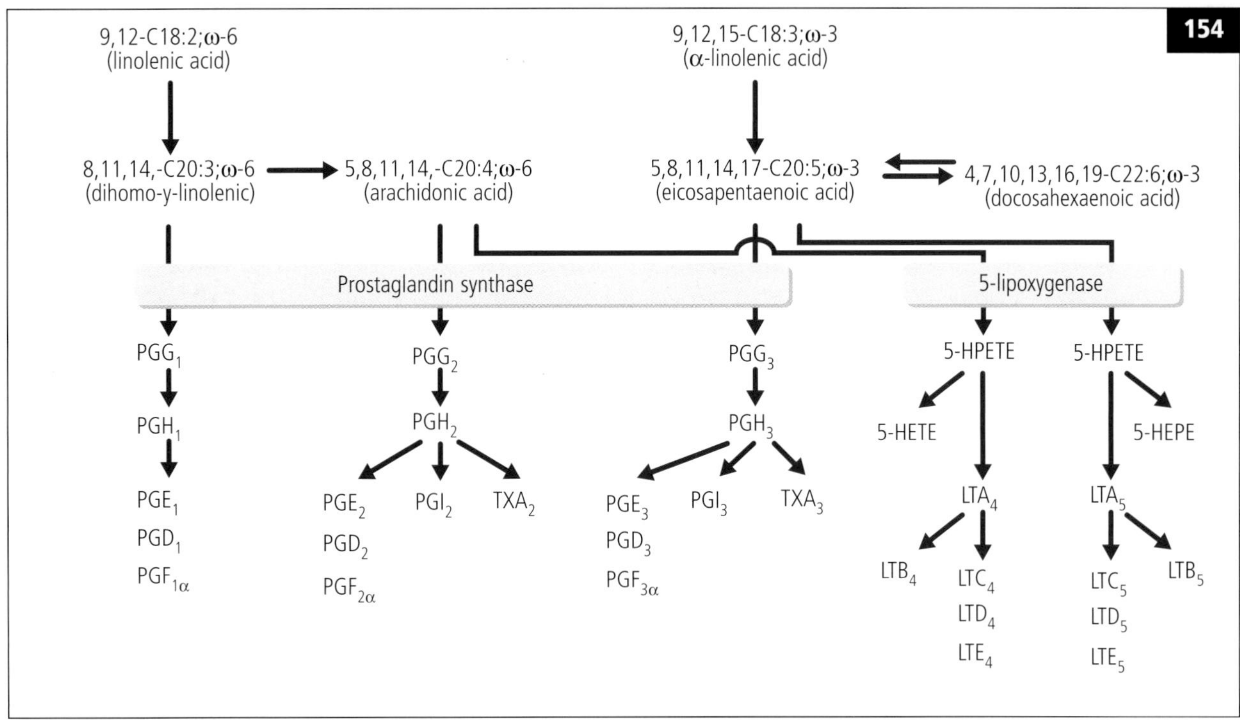

154 Derivation of eicosanoids from omega-6 and omega–3 fatty acids.

MEDICAL MANAGEMENT (155)

NONSTEROIDAL ANTI-INFLAMMATORY DRUGS

OA is one of the most prevalent and debilitating chronic diseases in mammals. Thirty percent of women and 17% of men aged 60 and over have clinical OA, and over 70% of those aged 65 and older show radiographic evidence of the disease.[10] Similarly, it is estimated that one in five adult dogs is arthritic, and pharmaceutical industry marketing surveys suggest the 'average clinic (1½-man practice)' sees approximately 45 new canine OA cases per month.[11]

NSAIDs will likely remain the foundation for treating canine OA based on their anti-inflammatory, analgesic, and antipyretic properties. However, like all drugs, every NSAID has the potential for a patient-dependent intolerance. Further, NSAID adverse responses are over-represented by excessive dosing.[12,13] As OA patients age, and possibly experience renal and/or hepatic compromise, it is imperative that their maintenance NSAID administration be at the minimal effective dose. A multimodal OA treatment protocol is anchored on this tenet of minimal effective dose.

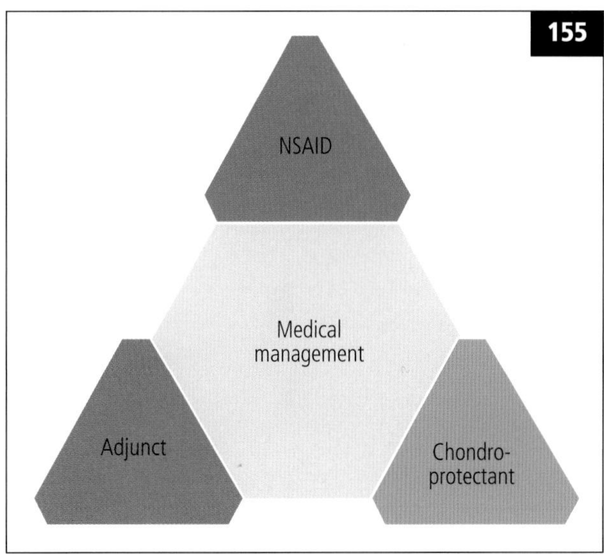

155 The medical management of OA is achieved with NSAIDs, chondroprotectant and analgesic adjunct(s).

NSAIDs relieve the clinical signs of pain. This is achieved by suppression of PGs, primarily PGE_2, produced from the substrate AA within the prostanoid cascade (**156**).

PGE_2 plays a number of roles in osteoarthritis, including (1) lowering the threshold of nociceptor activation, (2) promoting synovitis in the joint lining, (3) enhancing the formation of degradative metalloproteinases, and (4) depressing cartilage matrix synthesis by chondrocytes. In contrast, PGs also play a positive metabolic role such as enhancing platelet aggregation (to prevent excessive bleeding), maintaining integrity of the gastrointestinal tract, and facilitating renal function. Eicosanoid activity is tissue dependent. Therefore, maintaining an optimal balance of PG production in various tissues and organ systems while inhibiting pain is the 'NSAID challenge'.

Coxib-class NSAIDs were developed in an attempt to suppress COX-2-mediated PGs while sparing COX-1-mediated PGs, thereby decreasing the relative risk for gastrointestinal hemorrhage and lesions. Although analogous data in dogs is lacking, nonselective (traditional) NSAIDs increase the relative risk of gastrointestinal bleeding in humans by a factor of 4.7. This might be best illustrated by an observational cohort study[14] in elderly human patients. Relative to intake of no NSAIDs and no coxibs, traditional NSAIDs have an adjusted ratio for increased short-term risk of upper gastrointestinal hemorrhage of 4. This was reduced to 3 by the combination of such nonselective NSAIDs with the PG analog misoprostol. However, the rates were significantly lower for the COX-2 inhibitors, with 1.9 for rofecoxib and 1.0 for celecoxib, the latter being identical to the control group. Overall, dogs may actually be a better (safer usage) target-species for the coxib-class NSAIDs than humans since they tend to have similar (or greater) gastrointestinal issues, but do not have the cardiovascular risk factors, namely atherosclerosis.[15]

The most common complications documented with NSAID use in the dog are associated with overdosing and the concurrent use with other NSAIDs and corticosteroids.[16,17] ADEs are most frequently seen in the gastrointestinal tract followed

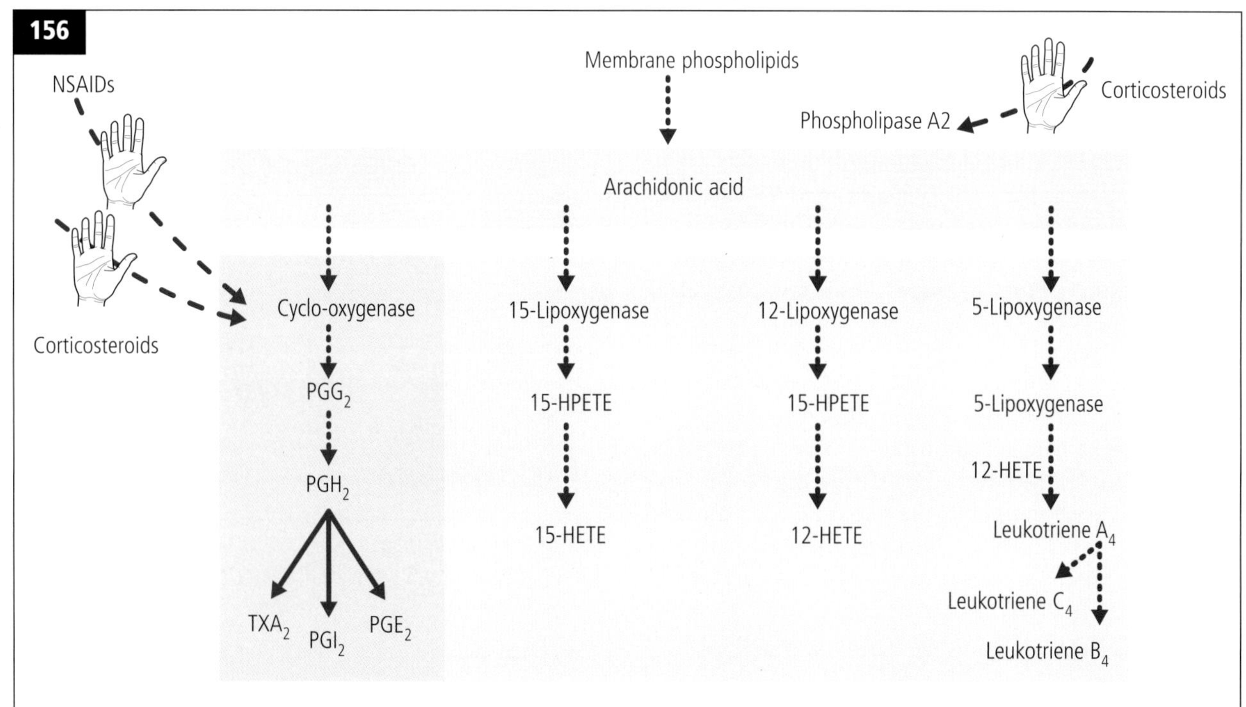

156 Multiple eicosanoids are derived from the AA cascade, which serve various physiological functions. Corticosteroids and NSAIDs block this cascade at points identified in the graphic.

by renal and hepatic systems. US FDA licensing gives the clinician an assurance of safety when individual NSAIDs are administered as labeled, together with consideration of the individual patient. Relative safety of one NSAID to another is an undeterminable prevalence assessment. Prevalence implies a quotient, with the numerator consisting of the number of intolerant dogs over the denominator of how many dogs have been administered the drug. The numerator is impossible to determine because all ADEs are not reported, and all ADEs are not directly causal. The denominator is impossible to determine because there is no means of knowing how many dogs are on a given drug at any point in time. Therefore, accurate quotients cannot be derived or compared in a responsible manner. Nevertheless, the FDA tracks 'global trends' of ADEs in the interests of clinicians and patient wellbeing.

At present, there is no evidence-based guidance to address the contemporary question of 'washout' period when changing from one NSAID to a different NSAID. Empirically, it seems appropriate to follow aspirin with a conservative washout of approximately 7 days. In one study[18] conducted with a limited number of healthy dogs at Colorado State University, there was no significant difference in clinical or clinicopathological data between dogs that were given an injectable NSAID followed by the same molecule in tablet form from those dogs given the injectable NSAID followed by a different coxib-class NSAID.

NUTRACEUTICALS

Next to NSAIDs, nutraceuticals are the fastest growing group of healthcare products in both human and animal health (see Chapter 6). Yet, many do not understand the definition and constraints of a nutraceutical. A nutraceutical is defined as a food additive that is given orally. As such, nutraceuticals are not under regulation by the FDA. In contrast, chondroprotectives are FDA-regulated. Together, chondroprotectants and nutraceuticals are considered disease-modifying osteoarthritic agents (DMOAAs), whereas nutraceuticals are not considered disease modifying osteoarthritic *drugs* (DMOADs). More than 30 nutraceutical products have been listed as potentially active in OA (*Table 56*).[19] ASU is a recent entry to the nutraceutical pool. It is suggested that this compound may promote OA cartilage repair by acting on subchondral bone osteoblasts. ASU has been observed to prevent the inhibitory effect of subchondral osteoblasts on aggrecan synthesis while having no significant effect on MMP, TIMP-1, COX-2, or iNOS expression.[20]

About 21 million Americans have OA.[21] NSAIDs are the foundation for treating OA, however ongoing controversy over conventional medications has created fertile soil for the growth of alternative arthritis remedies, particularly glucosamine and chondroitin. First popularized by the 1997 best-seller *The Arthritis Cure*, by Dr. Jason Theodosakis, these supplements racked up combined sales of $640

Table 56 **More than 30 nutraceuticals are potentially active in OA.**

Ascorbic acid	Avocado/soybean unsaponifiables	*Boswellia serrata*	Bromelain
Cat's claw	Chondroitin sulfate	Cetyl myristoleate oil	Collagen hydrolysate
Curcumin	Chitosan	Devil's claw	Flavonoids
Glucosamine SO_4/acetyl/HCl	Green lipid mussel	Ginger	Hyaluronic acid
Hydolysate collagen	Methylsulfonylmethane	Milk and hyperimmune milk	Omega–3-polyunsaturated fatty acids
Phycocyanin	*Ribes nigrum*	*Rosa canina*	Selenium
Strontium	Silicium	Turmeric	Vitamin D
Vitamin E	Willow		

million in 2000, according to the *Nutrition Business Journal*. Estimated sales of human-use glucosamine and chondroitin sulfate in 2004 approached $730 million. It would appear that popularity of these supplements in the human sector is driving veterinary use. The world market for pet nutraceuticals was worth $960 million in 2004. About 60% of this was given to dogs, a quarter to cats, and 10% to horses.[22]

A meta-analysis of studies evaluating the efficacy of these supplements for OA[23] suggested potential benefit from these agents, but as is often the case with nutraceuticals, questions were raised about the scientific quality of the studies. Therefore, the Glucosamine/chondroitin Arthritis Intervention Trial (GAIT), a 24-week, randomized, double-blind, placebo- and celecoxib-controlled, multicenter, $14 million trial was sponsored by the National Institutes of Health (NIH), to evaluate rigorously the efficacy and safety of glucosamine, chondroitin sulfate, and the two in combination in the treatment of pain due to human OA of the knee. The primary outcome measure of the GAIT study was a 20% decrease in knee pain. Analysis of the primary outcome measure did not show that either supplement, alone or in combination, was efficacious.[24] Prior to the GAIT study, some investigations had suggested efficacy of these supplements. Discrepancies may be explained, in part, by the rigors of the GAIT study imposed by the NIH and the use of only pharmaceutical grade supplements. Many nutraceuticals are least-cost formulations and quality assurance is lacking to nonexistent.[25,26] As a matter of record, in 2005 alone, the FDA rejected 12 research model claims related to products reducing the risk of OA, joint degeneration, cartilage deterioration, and OA-related joint pain, tenderness, and swelling.[27]

The rationale for using nutraceuticals is that provision of precursors of cartilage matrix in excess quantities may favor matrix synthesis and repair of articular cartilage. Glucosamine is an amino monosaccharide (2-amino-2-deoxy-α-D-glucose) that, once modified as N-acetylglucosamine, is proposed to act as a precursor of the disaccharide units of glycosaminoglycans (GAGs) such as hyaluronan and keratan sulfate. Chondroitin sulfate is a GAG consisting of alternating disaccharide subunits of glucuronic acid and sulfated N-acetylgalactosamine. Substitution can occur at the C4 and C6 positions of the N-acetylgalactosaminering to form chondroitin-4-sulfate and chondroitin-6-sulfate. Chondroitin sulfate is a normal constituent of cartilage: the ratio of 4:6 decreasing with age. To date, there is no evidence that nutraceuticals modulate the natural course of OA. Their inclusion in foods is based on theoretical considerations. 'Therefore, although the use of nutraceuticals to treat OA is a reality, the efficiency of these compounds to prevent or slow down OA disease remains a myth.'[19]

The literature contains some support for the use of glucosamine sulfate in humans. It has been observed that glucosamine hydrochloride does not induce symptomatic relief in knee OA to the same extent as glucosamine sulfate.[28] Noteworthy is that glucosamine sulfate is very hygroscopic and unstable, which is why varying amounts of potassium or sodium chloride are added during manufacturing. Dodge *et al.*[29] reported that glucosamine sulfate not only increased the expression of the aggrecan core protein but also downregulated, in a dose-dependent manner, MMP-1 and -3 expression. Some investigators[30] have suggested that the metabolic contribution to OA cartilage from glucosamine sulfate is associated with activation of protein kinase C, considered to be involved in the physiological phosphorylation of the integrin subunit. Herein, the glucosamine sulfate restores fibrillated cartilage chondrocytes' adhesion to fibronectin, thus improving the repair process of OA cartilage by allowing proliferated cells to migrate to damaged areas.

Focusing on the role of IL-1 as an initiating cytokine associated with induction of degradative enzyme and inflammatory mediator synthesis in OA, Neil *et al.*[31] have summarized reports on the impact of glucosamine/chondroitin sulfate on IL-1 (*Table 57*).

Pharmacokinetic studies in dogs reveals that glucosamine hydrochloride is only 10–12% bioavailable from single or multiple doses.[51] At current recommended intake, it is extremely unlikely that relevant concentrations of glucosamine reach the joint,[52] or that substantial amounts of glucosamine get into the circulation following oral ingestion.[53] Glucosamine is expected to be metabolized rapidly by the liver or incorporated into glycoproteins. Glucosamine is not ordinarily available in the circulation as a source of cartilage matrix substrate, cartilage uses glucose for that purpose.

Charged molecules exceeding approximately 180 daltons are likely not to pass the gastrointestinal mucosa and be absorbed unless assisted by a carrier-mediated transport system, therefore it is unlikely that chondroitin sulfate would be absorbed intact via the gastrointestinal tract. The gastric mucosa contains a number of GAG-degrading enzymes, such as exoglycosidases, sulfatases, and hyaluronidase-like

Table 57 Influence of interleukin-1 (IL-1) on articular cartilage matrix components, inflammatory mediators, and degradative enzymes. Columns 3 and 4 note the + or – complementary effect from glucosamine and chondroitin sulfate.

Mediator/matrix molecule	IL-1 effect on chondrocyte biosynthesis	Glucosamine effect	Chondroitin sulfate effect
	References 32–37	(+) inhibits, or (–) fails to inhibit effects induced by IL-1	(+) inhibits, or (–) fails to inhibit effects induced by IL-1
COX-2/PGE_2	Stimulates synthesis	+ References 38, 39	+/– References 44, 47, 48
iNOS/NO	Stimulates synthesis	+ References 38, 40	+/– References 47, 49
MMPs	Induces synthesis, activity, and secretion	+ References 38, 40, 41	+ Reference 48
Aggrecanases/aggrecan	Increased synthesis and activity	References 42, 43	
PGs/GAGs	Decreased synthesis, increased degradation	+ Reference 44	+ References 44, 48, 50
Type II collagen	Inhibits synthesis	– References 44, 45	+ Reference 44
Transcription factors (NF-κB, activator protein 1)	Stimulates increased mRNA expression and activity	+ Reference 39, 46	

enzymes, which should degrade chondroitin sulfate.

Controversy remains over mechanisms by which nutraceuticals may lead to modulation of disease symptoms and cartilage degradation in OA, and which product is preferred for treatment. Perhaps our scientific community lacks the expertise to identify how these products might work. Nevertheless, as a class of agents, nutraceuticals fall short in evidence-based efficacy, lack dose titration studies to validate appropriate doses, and have shown inconsistencies in product quality assurance. Good intentions in the few have been clouded by many! A sound recommendation for consumers is, buyer beware. One might argue that the most responsible advice for recommending a nutraceutical is as an adjunct to a 'science-based' medicinal, in that the nutraceutical may, or may not help. Recommending that the pet owner spend money on a nutraceutical as the first line of treatment lacks convincing scientific underpinning.

CHONDROPROTECTANTS: POLYSULFATED GLYCOSAMINOGLYCAN

Adequan®, a polysulfated glycosaminoglycan (PSGAG), is available as a chondroprotectant as is the hyaluronic acid product Legend™. The products Chondroprotec™ and IChON® are neither a nutraceutical nor a chondroprotectant. Both are licensed as *topical wound devices*, rather than drugs.

Adequan Canine® is a PSGAG characterized as a DMOAD which has met the rigors of FDA registration. Experiments conducted *in vitro* have shown PSGAG to inhibit certain catabolic enzymes which have increased activity in inflamed joints, and to enhance the activity of some anabolic enzymes.[54] PSGAG has been shown to significantly inhibit serine proteinases, which play a role in the IL-1-mediated degradation of cartilage proteoglycans and collagen.[55] PSGAG has further been reported to inhibit some catabolic enzymes such as elastase, stromelysin, metalloproteinases, cathepsin G and B1, and hyaluronidases, which degrade collagen, proteoglycans, and hyaluronic acid.[56,57] It is also reported to inhibit PGE synthesis.[58] PSGAG has shown a specific potentiating effect on hyaluronic acid synthesis by synovial membrane cells *in vitro*.[59]

Within 2 hours of administration, Adequan Canine® enters cartilage, where it reduces proteoglycan degradation, inhibits synthesis and activity of degradative enzymes, stimulates GAG synthesis, and increases hyaluronan concentrations. Clinical data from Millis *et al.* (unpublished, 2005) demonstrated that comfortable angle of extension and lameness scores were both improved following administration of Adequan Canine® at both 4 and 8 weeks following anterior cruciate ligament transection, while the concentration of neutral metalloproteinase was reduced relative to controls. In an era where evidence-based treatment is being emphasized, in this instance, the separation between patient response to FDA-approved drugs and unlicensed agents is, gratifyingly, widening.

Adequan Canine® is most appropriately administered in the early stages of OA (**157**), since once hyaline cartilage is lost, it is lost forever! The strategy in administering this chondroprotective is to delay the time during progression of osteoarthritis that medically aggressive treatment is required (**158, 159**).

Summary of Adequan Canine® activity:

- Reduction in proteoglycan degradation.
- Inhibition of synthesis and activity of:
  - Aggrecanases.
  - MMPs.
  - NO.
  - PGE_2.
- Stimulates GAG synthesis.
- Increases hyaluronan concentrations.

ADJUNCTS

OA is both a chronic disease and an acute disease, with intermittent flare-ups that may render an NSAID ineffective as a sole pharmaceutical analgesic therapy because of 'breakthrough pain' (**160**). Further, chronic pain is not just a prolonged version of acute pain (see Chapter 1). As pain signals are repeatedly generated, neural pathways undergo physiochemical changes that make them hypersensitive to the pain signals and resistant to antinociceptive input. In a very real sense, the signals can become embedded in the spinal cord, like a painful memory.

The main neurotransmitter used by nociceptors synapsing with the dorsal horn of the spinal cord is glutamate, a molecule that can bind to a number of different receptors. Discovering the role of the NMDA receptor in chronic pain has given rise to the efficacious implementation of NMDA antagonists, such as *amantadine*, which is occasionally administered together with voltage-gated calcium channel modulator *gabapentanoids* as adjuncts in a multimodal OA protocol (also finding efficacy in other chronic pain diseases).

The synthetic codeine analog, *tramadol*, is also widely used in veterinary medicine (although not approved in dogs). Approximately 40% of its activity is at the μ receptor. Forty percent of tramadol activity is as an NE reuptake inhibitor and 20% is as a serotonin reuptake inhibitor (see Chapter 4). Since the majority of tramadol activity is other than at the μ receptor, it is a poor substitute for the 'pure' opioids. Further, the efficacy and safety of tramadol alone or in combination with other drugs is unknown in veterinary patients.

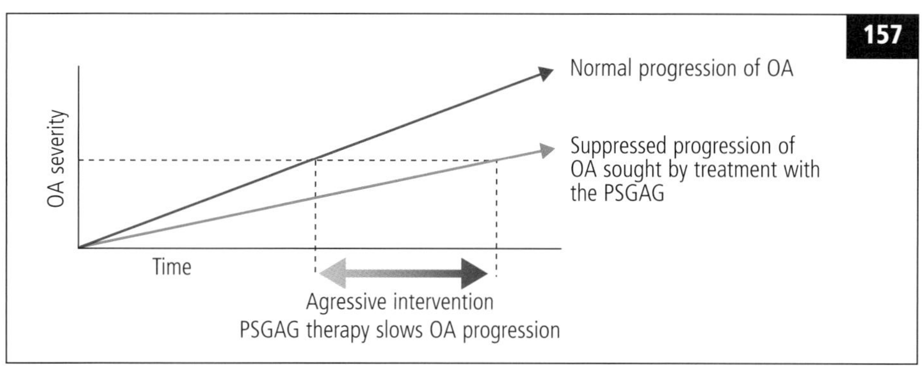

157 The strategy of early PSGAG treatment is to delay the point in time when 'aggressive' treatment is required to keep the patient comfortable.

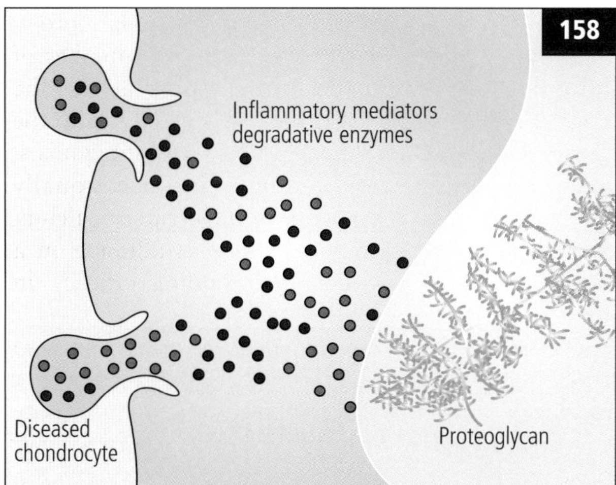

158 Chondrocytes within the cartilage matrix (far left) generate all components of the matrix. In the OA disease state, they also produce enzymes which degrade matrix aggrecan (pink structure). The PSGAG, Adequan Canine®, helps to protect cartilage against the catabolic activity of these degradative enzymes.

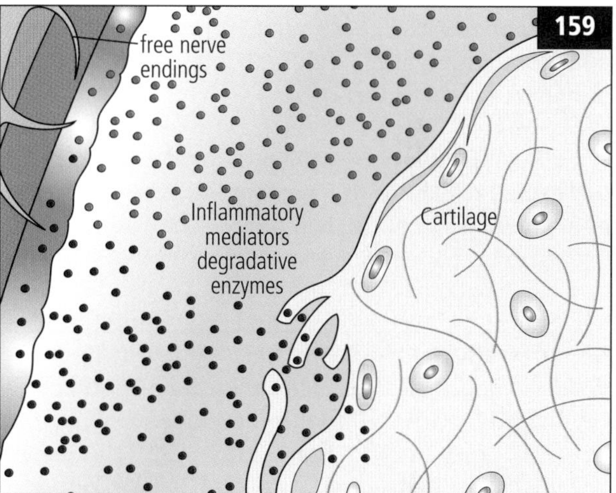

159 As degradative enzymes are released from arthritic cartilage (right), they change the composition of joint fluid. Synoviocytes of the joint lining, sensing these inflammatory mediators act as macrophages, and release even more inflammatory agents into the joint. As weightbearing loads and unloads the cartilage, it acts as a sponge, absorbing and releasing these inflammatory agents within the joint. Hence, the worse it gets, the worse it gets! PSGAG acts to dampen this catabolic activity.

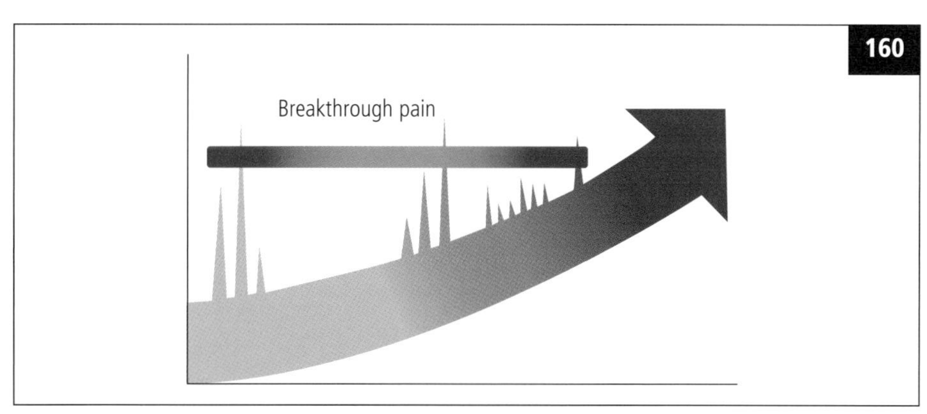

160 OA is both an acute and a chronic disease, with pain that can break through first-to-second (WHO) ladder analgesics.

However, tramadol can be used as an adjunct to opioid or NSAID use. In humans tramadol is able to reduce the amount of sP in synovial fluid as well as IL-6, which seems to correlate with the stage of OA pathology being treated.[60] The American College of Rheumatology and the American Medical Directors Association support the addition of tramadol to an NSAID for the management of chronic pain in humans (**155**).[61,62]

Implementing both the medical (**155**) and non-medical (**150**) management principles to the canine osteoarthritic patient, provides the optimal benefits to the patient (**161**). The evidence base for each component of the multimodal management approach is substantial, (See *Table 58*) and impacts on the tenet of determining the minimal effective dose to maximize safety of therapy.

See **162**.

Following adoption of the multimodal scheme, the question at hand is sequencing the different modalities. Herein, there appears to be two different suggestions. Some suggest starting the patient on non-pharmacologic modalities, such as nutraceuticals, weight loss and diet modifications (dotted line). Thereafter, integrating the pharmacologic agents. However, this approach is challenged by two well founded arguments. Firstly, it is well recognized that most of the non-pharmacologic modalities take 3-4 weeks before a clinical response is observed, and pet owners want to see a response sooner than that Secondly, it is in the patients' best interest to provide analgesia as soon as possible. Anything less could be argued as inhumane—not providing immediate relief to the patient, which it needs and deserves. Accordingly, the solid line path would appear the most ethical.

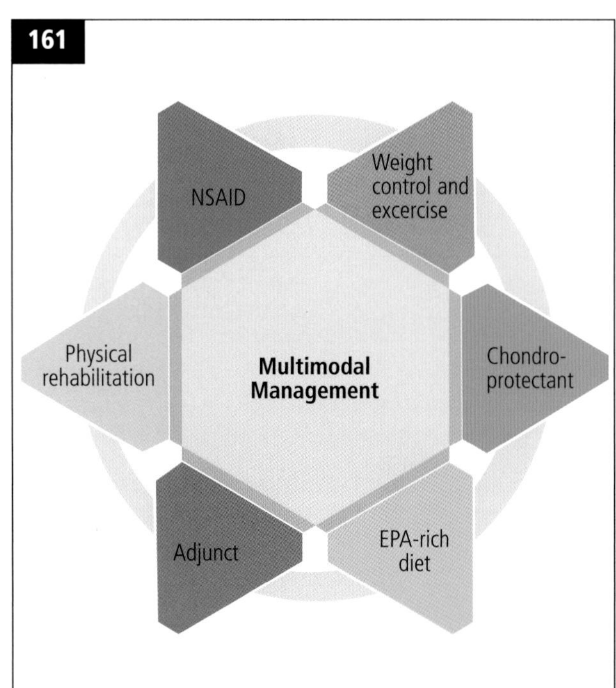

161 Multimodal management of OA.

Table 58 Evidence rank of various therapeutic approaches to OA.

Modality	Selected references establishing evidence base
NSAID	63–66
Chondroprotectant	67–70
Adjuncts	71–74
Weight control/exercise	5, 8, 10, 75–77
EPA-rich diet	78–83
Physical rehabilitation	84–87

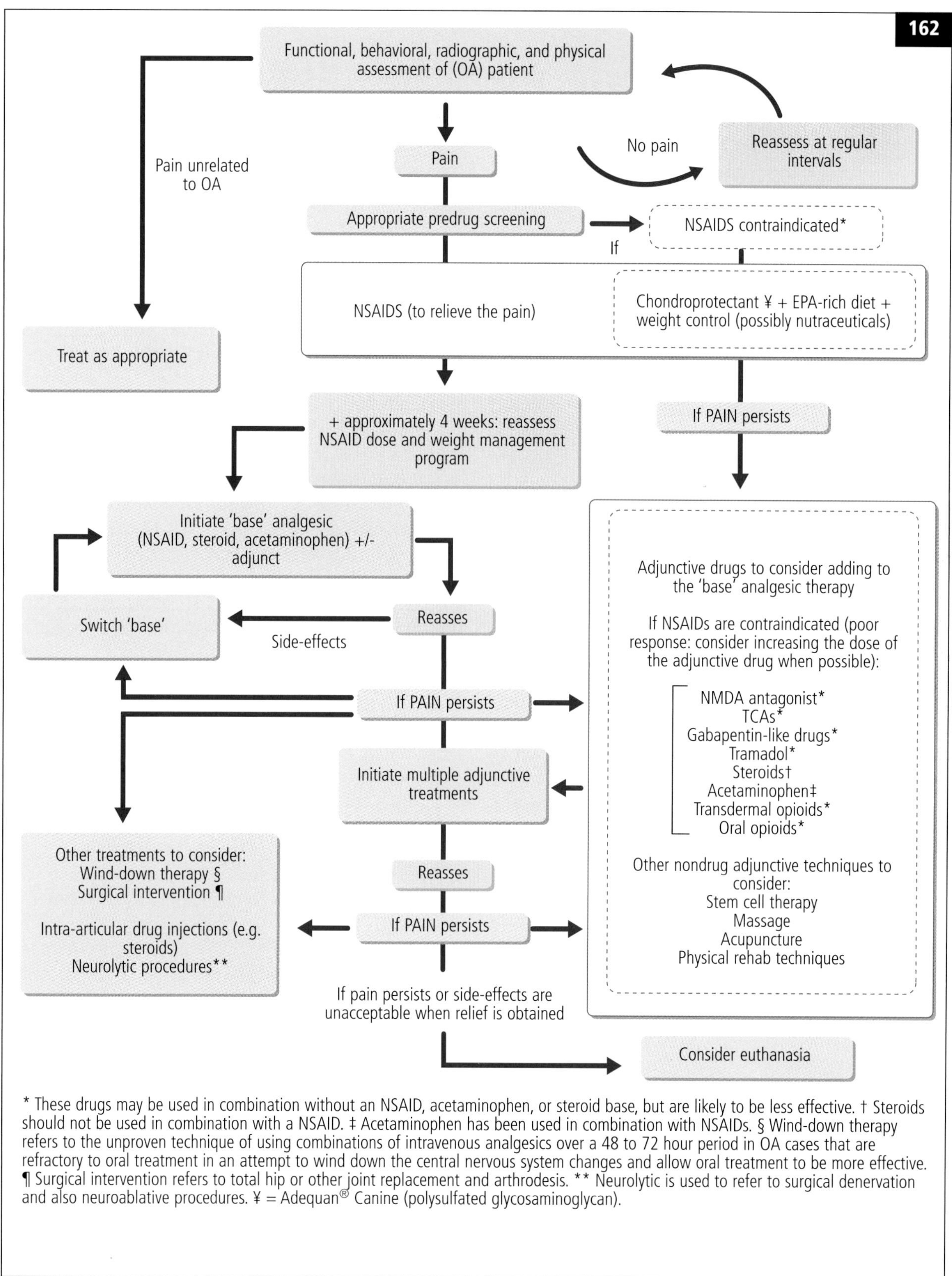

162 Proposed algorithm for implementing a multimodal plan for non-surgical management of the OA patient. Adopted from Lascelles, 2008.

9 CHRONIC PAIN IN SELECTED PHYSIOLOGICAL SYSTEMS: OPHTHALMIC, AURAL, AND DENTAL

OPHTHALMIC PAIN

Ocular pain can be severe, requiring prompt treatment from a welfare perspective as well as to prevent progression of the original disease. Ophthalmic pain in animals is often difficult to identify, but can be inferred from reports of humans with similar anomalies. Keratitis, iritis, and glaucoma result in a dull deep pain that has an inflammatory component. Corneal foreign bodies and erosions produce superficial pain, which is acute and sharp.

The cornea has the highest concentration of free nerve endings in the body and is therefore particularly sensitive to painful stimuli.[1–3] Any ocular surgery, trauma or infection of the corneal epithelium may cause severe and persistent pain that is difficult to manage. Further, human studies have shown that only a limited amount of local anesthetic can be used without causing local toxicity and severe damage to the cornea.[4]

The literature suggests that the ideal topical anesthetic agent for cataract surgery should meet the following criteria: (1) no systemic toxicity and minimal corneal toxicity, (2) no eye irritation, (3) prompt onset, and (4) adequate duration of action.[5] Several topical agents, such as cocaine, tetracaine, and proparacaine have been used in the past for anterior segment surgery; however, cocaine and proparacaine have associated corneal toxicity,[6] and tetracaine does not produce sufficient anesthesia or adequate duration of action.[5] That said, most cataract surgery is done under general anesthesia.

In 1993, Liu *et al.*[7] compared proparacaine and bupivacaine for onset time, corneal epithelial toxicity, and duration of action in rabbit eyes, finding that bupivacaine was less toxic to the corneal epithelium than proparacaine 0.5%, and that increasing the pH of a bupivacaine solution from 5.7 to 6.5 practically doubled the duration of action.

In 1999, Sun *et al.*[8] compared bupivacaine, lidocaine, procaine, and benzocaine. Onset time for all drugs was within 1 minute. Bupivacaine and lidocaine had a longer anesthetic effect than procaine or benzocaine, and the durations of action for lidocaine and bupivacaine in pH-adjusted solutions were significantly longer than those of nonpH-adjusted solutions. These data support results from other studies[7,9,10] documenting that the addition of sodium bicarbonate to solutions of local anesthetic to raise the pH closer to the agent's pKa could reduce the latency, increase the intensity, and prolong the duration of neural blockade without compromising toxicity. For relief of corneal pain, topical local anesthetics can be effective, however they should not be used beyond the perioperative period because they may inhibit corneal re-epithelialization, interfere with lacrimation, and produce corneal swelling and increased corneal epithelial permeability.[11] Regarding pre-emptive analgesia for intraocular surgery in dogs, preliminary studies suggest that systemic lidocaine is effective with few adverse side-effects.[12] Retrobulbar administration of local anesthetics is commonly used for ocular procedures in human medicine.

Because glucocorticoids inhibit the vascular and cellular responses characteristic of early inflammation and also suppress the persistent, nonresolving changes of chronic inflammation, they are commonly used for ophthalmic conditions. In the latter stages of inflammation, glucocorticoids suppress formation of fibroblasts and their collagen-forming activity as well as neovascularization. Accordingly, topical glucocorticoids are effective for treating nonulcerative keratitis by suppressing or preventing neovascular ingrowth and scar tissue formation, and thereby preserve the structure and transparency of the cornea.[13]

Topical glucocorticoid preparations are available as solutions, suspensions, or ointments. Phosphate derivatives provide a clear solution in contrast to acetate and alcohol derivatives, which are less water soluble and are in suspensions. Due to the lipid-rich composition of the corneal epithelium, lipophilic acetate and alcohol corticosteroid preparations penetrate the cornea better than the polar preparations such as sodium salts of the steroid phosphate.[14]

Absorption of glucocorticoid suspensions is slow, and may maintain therapeutic levels for 2–3 weeks in humans, while a substantial amount of active glucocorticoid may remain up to 13 months in subconjunctival depots.[15] Although not assessed in animals, intravitreal administration of triamcinolone acetonide has been suggested for humans as a possible treatment for diabetic macular edema, proliferative diabetic retinopathy, chronic pre-phthisical ocular hypotony, chronic uveitis, and exudative retinal detachment. Vitreous concentrations from clinical injections can be present for up to 1.5 years after the application.[16] Systemic administration of glucocorticoids may either be combined with topical or subconjunctival therapy for treatment of severe or refractory anterior uveitis or used alone for the control of chorioretinitis, optic neuritis, or noninfectious orbital inflammation.[17]

Topical glucocorticoids are considered contraindicated in the presence of corneal ulceration, because of delayed epithelial healing rates, stromal keratocyte proliferation, and collagen deposition. Further, debate over the use of glucocorticoids for the management of ocular infections is unresolved. Steroid-induced cataract has been produced experimentally in cats by topical administration of dexamethasone or prednisolone,[18] and the hypertensive effect of corticosteroids has been documented in Beagles[19] with primary open-angle glaucoma and in normal cats.

All surgical diseases have an inflammatory component. Further, atropine-resistant miosis, rise in intraocular pressure, disruption of the blood–aqueous barrier, vasodilatation associated with vascular permeability in the conjunctiva and iris, and possibly corneal neovascularization are inflammatory effects caused by ocular PGs.[20] Accordingly, NSAIDs can be quite efficacious in minimizing the detrimental effects of the inflammatory response, including pain.

Topical formulations of NSAIDs for ophthalmic use became commercially available worldwide by the early 1990s. They are often considered a safer alternative to topical corticosteroids, avoiding the potential undesirable side-effects associated with topical steroids, such as elevations in intraocular pressure and progression of cataracts (both of which are less common in veterinary medicine than human medicine), increased risk of infection, and worsening of stromal melting by activation of MMPs. Topically applied NSAIDs are commonly used in the management and prevention of noninfectious ocular inflammation following cataract surgery. Additionally, they are used in the management of pain following refractive surgery and in the treatment of allergic conjunctivitis. Topical NSAIDs were first shown to be more effective in intraocular penetration than systemic formulations by Sawa and Masuda[21] and Miyake,[22] who also demonstrated the effects of topical NSAIDs on the prevention of intraoperative miosis and cystoid macular edema. They were first used in cataract surgery for the prevention of intraoperative miosis,[23] and later shown to be effective in controlling the pain following refractive surgery,[24] with potential in the prevention and treatment of cystoid macular edema.[25]

Topical NSAIDs are classified into six groups based on their chemical composition:

- Indoles.
- Phenylacetic acids.
- Phenylalkanoic acids.
- Salicylates.
- Fenamates.
- Pyrazolones.

Salicylates, fenamates and pyrazolones are considered too toxic to be used in the eye.[26] See *Table 59.*(*over page*)

In contrast to postoperative inflammation, many forms of uveitis require prolonged corticosteroid therapy to control the inflammation and discomfort, but with the risk of local toxicity. In some cases NSAIDs are a potential alternative that provide safer treatment.[27]

A comparative study of topical 1.0% suspensions of flurbiprofen, diclofenac, tolmedin, and suprofen showed that diclofenac is more effective than the others in stabilizing the blood–aqueous barrier in canine eyes.[28] In the dog, topical 0.1% indomethacin solution was as effective as topical 1% indomethacin suspension in preventing the increase in permeability of the blood–aqueous barrier and the miotic response induced by aqueous paracentesis.[29] Further, it is reported in dogs that topical indomethacin readily penetrates the cornea and enters the aqueous humor to prevent *in situ* PG synthesis and blood–aqueous breakdown.[30]

In a study comparing effects of orally administered tepoxalin, carprofen, and meloxicam for controlling aqueocentesis-induced anterior uveitis in dogs, as determined by measurement of aqueous prostaglandin E_2

Table 59 Commercially available topical NSAIDs for control of human ophthalmic pain and inflammation.					
Drug name		**Manufacturer**	**Chemical class**	**Formulation**	**Indications**
Generic	**Brand**				
Flurbiprofen	Ocufen®	Allergan	Phenylalkanoic acid	0.03% solution	Inhibition of intraoperative miosis
Suprofen	Profenal®	Alcon	Phenylalkanoic acid	1.0% solution	Inhibition of intraoperative miosis
Ketorolac	Acular®	Allergan	Phenylalkanoic acid	0.5% solution	Seasonal allergic conjunctivitis, postoperative inflammation following cataract surgery
	Acular LS®	Allergan	Phenylalkanoic acid	0.4% solution	Reduction of ocular pain and burning/stinging following corneal refractive surgery
Diclofenac	Voltaren®	Novartis	Phenylacetic acid	0.1% solution	Postoperative inflammation following cataract surgery, reduction of pain and photophobia following refractive surgery
Nepafenac	Nevanac®	Alcon	Phenylacetic acid	0.1% suspension	Pain and inflammation associated with cataract surgery
Bromfenac	Xibrom®	Bausch & Lomb	Phenylacetic acid	0.9% solution	Postoperative inflammation and pain following cataract surgery
Indomethacin	Indocin®	Various	Indole	0.1% solution	Prevention of the inflammation linked with cataract surgery and anterior segment of the eye, inhibition of preoperative miosis and treatment of pain related to refractive surgery
	Indocollyre® Indomelol®			0.5% solution 1% suspension	

(PGE_2) concentrations, Gilmour et al. concluded that tepoxalin was more effective than carprofen or meloxicam for controlling the production of PGE_2 in dogs with experimentally induced uveitis.[31]

Although rare, systemic adverse reactions to topically applied NSAIDs have been reported. The systemic absorption of topically applied ophthalmic preparations is considered minimal, however it is prudent to consider the potential for systemic effects. Severe adverse events associated with topical NSAIDs appear to require potentiation in the form of high total doses, ocular comorbidities or other risk factors such as previous cataract or ocular surgeries, diabetes, or ocular vascular or cardiovascular disease.[32] As with systemic NSAID administration, adverse reactions to topically administered NSAIDs in humans are not infrequently associated with inappropriate use.[33]

Pain associated with corneal ulceration in animals or humans may not always be specifically treated,[34] focusing instead on rapid covering of nerve endings by advancing epithelium, thereby sparing the axons from noxious stimuli. And, although uncomplicated corneal ulcers in dogs may heal in a few days, the dog is likely to experience considerable pain during that time. Dogs being treated for indolent or nonhealing corneal ulcers often require multiple episodes of debridement or surgical intervention[35] and show signs of pain for weeks or months during the slow healing process.

Under such circumstances, topically administered corneal anesthetic agents are inappropriate because of both short duration and toxicosis of the corneal epithelium with associated delay in healing. NSAIDs administered topically have offered some analgesic effects in humans with corneal ulcers[36,37] and may offer benefit in dogs, but can be associated with delayed would healing and corneal melting. Stiles *et al.*[34] have reported that the topical use of 1% morphine sulfate solution in dogs with corneal ulcers provided analgesia for a subjective assessment of at least 4 hours without interference with wound healing. These results are consistent with those observed in the human patient and literature.[38]

Glaucoma is one of the most frequent blinding diseases in dogs, characterized by high intraocular pressure (>25–30 mmHg in dogs; >31 mmHg in cats) that causes characteristic degenerative changes in the optic nerve and retina, with subsequent loss of vision. Glaucoma results from the degeneration of retinal ganglion cells and their axons. Glaucomatous conditions characterized by degenerative retinal ganglion cell death in the absence of elevated intraocular pressure have not been recognized in the dog. The dog has the highest frequency of primary glaucomas of all animals, with the narrow- or closed-angle type being the most common,[39] and the contralateral eye usually develops glaucoma in affected dogs within a few months. **163** illustrates tonometers, used to measure intraocular pressure.

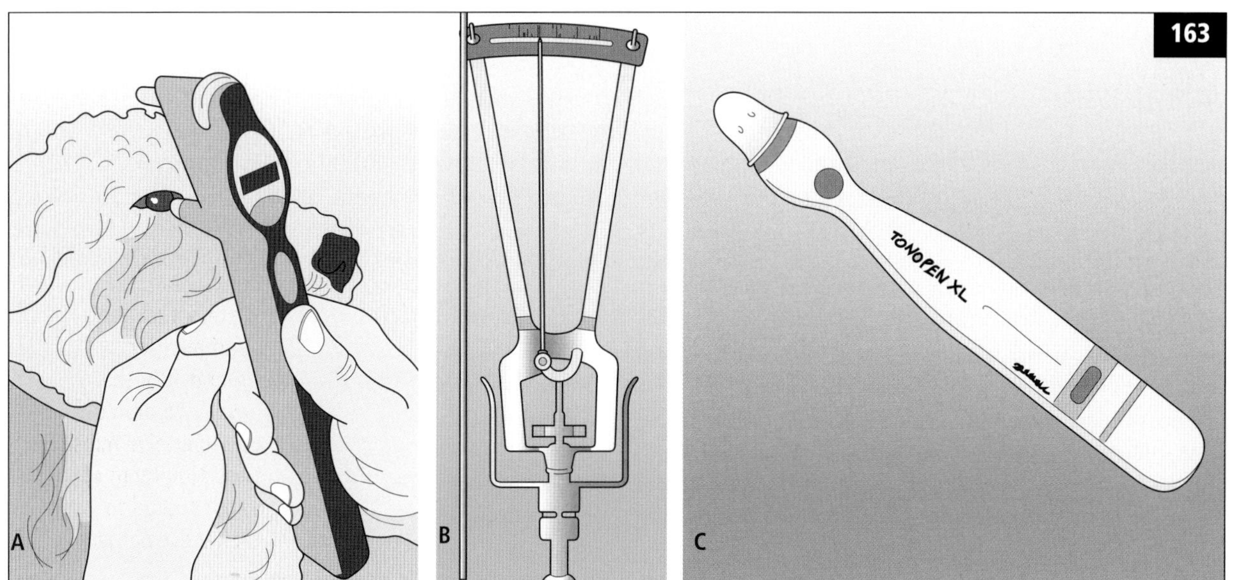

163 (A) Tonovet® a handheld magnetic rebound tonometer for measuring intraocular pressure, (B) the more traditional Schiötz indentation tonometer, and (C) the tonopen applanation tonometer.

While glaucoma in human patients is usually not associated with clinical signs of ocular pain and discomfort, glaucoma in veterinary patients is usually recognized when aggressive clinical signs of the disease are present. Nevertheless, most veterinary textbooks address treatment for controlling intraocular pressures associated with glaucoma, but few address the associated pain. In some cases, enucleation or evisceration may be the only way to relieve the animal's pain. If ocular pain is exacerbated by exposure to bright light, relief may be achieved by reducing ambient illumination.

Glaucoma can be conceptualized as an optic neuropathy associated with characteristic structural damage to the optic nerve and associated visual dysfunction.[40] Hypothesizing that part of the pain in human patients with painful, blind, glaucomatous eyes might be explained by optic neuropathy and optic nerve structural damage causing neuropathic pain, Kavalieratos and Dimou[41] have published a case report of significant pain relief with the administration of gabapentin.

Acupuncture is an area of emerging interest and application in veterinary medicine. There are few prospective controlled studies on the use of acupuncture for ophthalmic pain in people or animals. Nevertheless, there are favorable reports when used in people. Nepp *et al.*[42] reported favorable responses from acupuncture based upon VAS for a variety of painful ophthalmic conditions, including glaucoma, ophthalmic migraine, blepharospasm, and dry eyes. There are also clinical reports of pain relief from KCS in human patients after acupuncture treatment.[43]

AURAL PAIN

Ear disease is a very common ailment of dogs. Approximately 15–20% of all canine patients and approximately 6–7% of all feline patients have some kind of ear disease, from mild erythema to severe otitis media.[44] In dogs, secondary otitis media occurs in approximately 16% of acute otitis externa cases and as many as 50–80% of chronic otitis externa cases.[45] Most patients with chronic otitis externa that has been present for 45–60 days will have a coexisting otitis media, and often an otitis interna. Chronic ear disease is often painful. Manipulation of the pinna or otoscopic examination of the painful ear of a dog or cat can cause discomfort to the patient and may result in aggressive behavior toward the examiner.

The ear canal is an invagination of epidermis forming a hollow skin tube in the inside of the head that begins at the eardrum (**164**). Primary causes of ear disease are skin diseases that also have an effect on the skin lining the ear canal. Cutaneous diseases such as atopy, food hypersensitivity, parasites, foreign bodies, hypothyroidism, and seborrheic disease frequently result in ear disease. Often complicating the condition is longstanding overtreatment of ears with ear cleaners, drugs that irritate the epithelium, and cotton-tipped applicators. It has been theorized that chronic inflammation, more common in the dog than in the cat, may initiate progression of otic lesions from hyperplasia to dysplasia, and perhaps, even to neoplasia.[44]

Perpetuating factors that prevent the ear canal from effectively healing include infections with bacteria and yeasts, improper treatment of the ear, overtreatment of the ear with ear cleaners and medications, and otitis media. The examiner should conduct an otoscopic examination of the ear canals for the following:

- Parasites.
- Patency or stenosis.
- Ulcerations.
- Exudates.
- Foreign bodies.
- Color changes.
- Proliferative changes.
- Tumors.
- Excessive hair or waxy accumulation.

Cytological assessment should accompany every infected ear examination. When signs of vestibular dysfunction are present, peripheral versus central vestibular disease should be identified by performing a cranial nerve examination. In many cases, proper diagnosis and treatment of the underlying pathology resolves the disease. However, in some animals with severe infection and disease, it can be impossible to medicate because of their pain, apprehension, and, often, resulting aggression. In these cases it may be better to recommend surgical intervention to prevent further suffering and to optimize client resources. With the salvage procedure of canine total ear canal ablation, Wolfe *et al.*[46] have reported the favorable use of local lidocaine delivery, as compared to intravenous morphine.

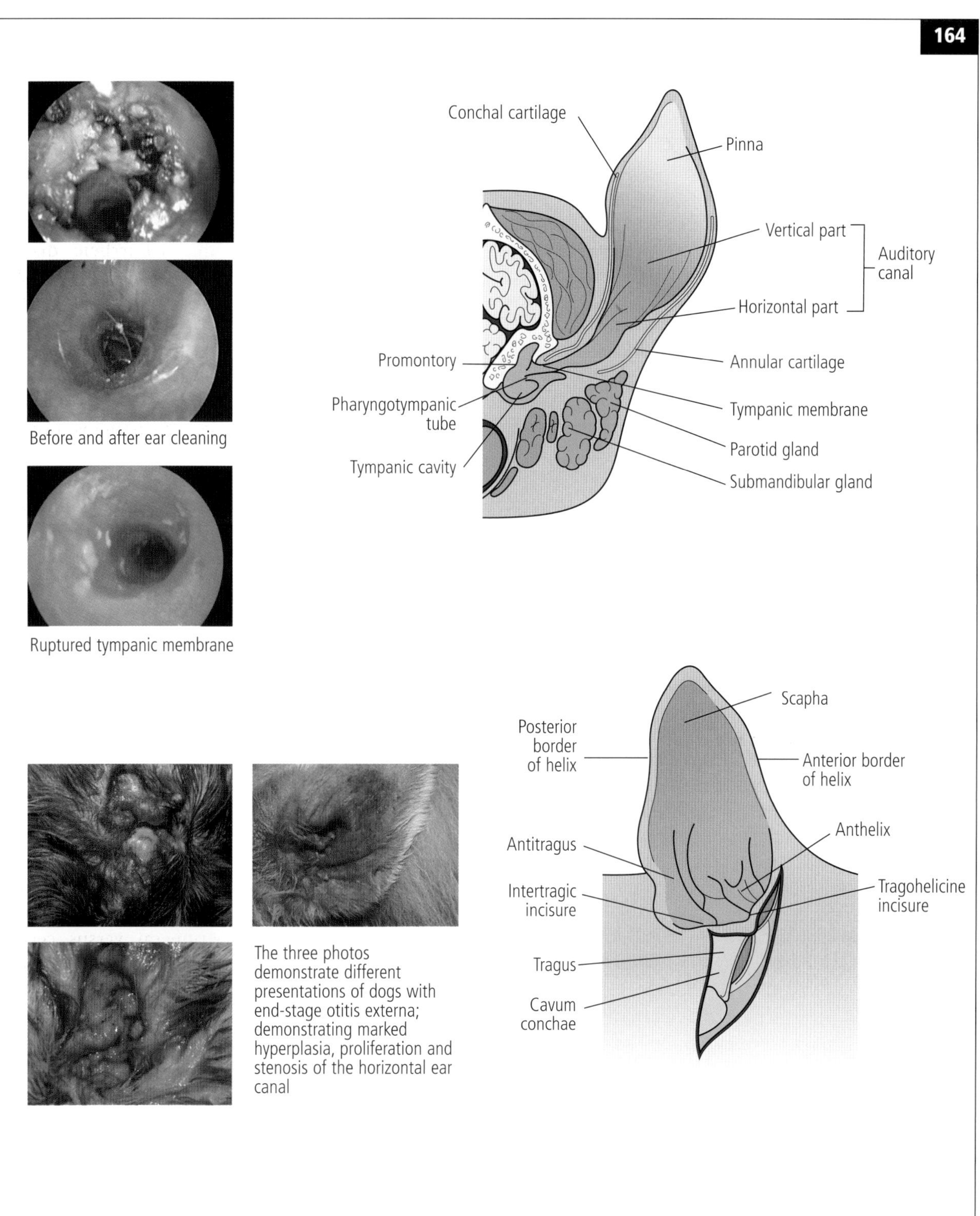

164 Anatomy of the canine ear and related otitis externa clinical observations. Photographs courtesy of Dr Keith Hnilica; otoscopy courtesy of Dr Diane Lewis.

DENTAL PAIN

An estimated 85% of dogs and 75% of cats over 3 years of age display some form of periodontal disease.[47] Gingivitis (inflammation of the gingiva) results from the accumulation of plaque. Bacteria present in plaque induce tissue destruction via production of cytotoxins and degradative enzymes, with the resulting endogenous inflammatory response leading to additional destruction of local tissues. Inflammation along the periodontal space can progress to periodontitis, characterized by active destruction of the periodontal ligament and alveolar bone with pocket formation, recession, or both. Periodontal disease can also progress to endodontic disease if alveolar bone loss advances to the root apex or lateral canal. Untreated, this may result in chronic rhinitis and ophthalmic pathology. Pain associated with periodontal disease is often identified with the patient's reluctance to eat (**165**).

Evidence from animal experiments and clinical trials documents that selective and nonselective NSAIDs are mainly responsible for the stabilization of periodontal conditions by reducing the rate of alveolar bone resorption.[48] It may well be that those 'senior' dogs on long-term NSAID treatment for musculoskeletal disorders are also receiving prophylactic periodontal treatment.

One should remember that analgesics are the second-best means of managing pain; the best means is to diagnose the cause and treat the pathology as quickly as possible.

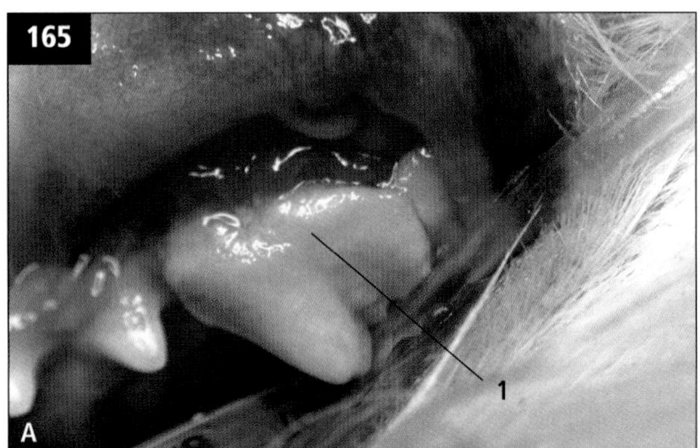

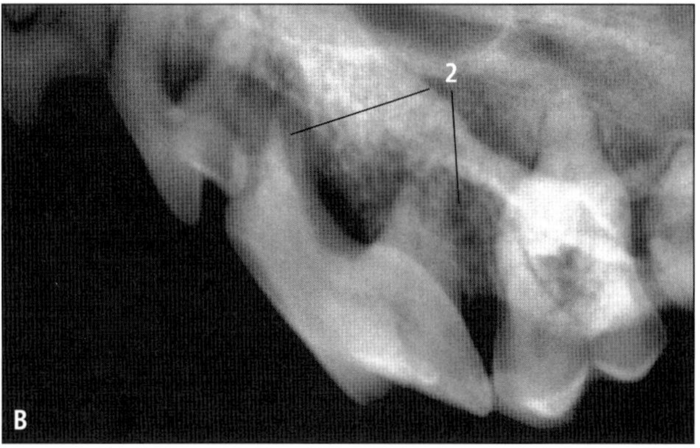

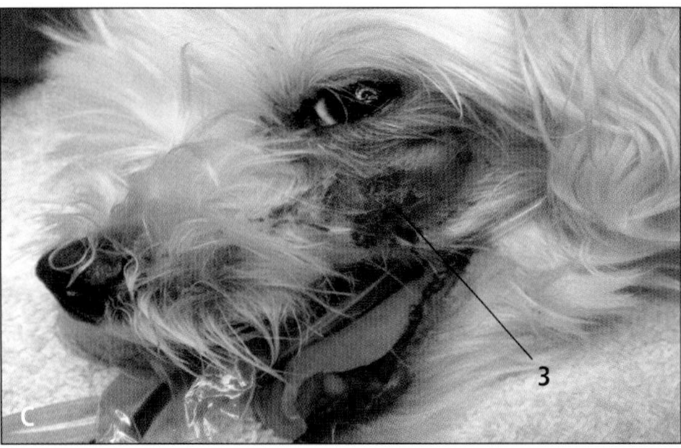

165 Periodontal disease can lead to pain, anorexia, and systemic disease. (A) Bacterial plaque. (B) Alveolar bone erosion. (C) Severe conditions can manifest as fistula with exudative purulent tracts. 1: Bacterial plaque 2: Alveolar bone erosion 3: Suborbital fistula Photographs courtesy of Brett Beckman, DVM, FAVD, DAVDC, DAAPM.

CASE REPORTS

CASE REPORT[1]

Signalment: 16-year-old, controlled diabetic, castrated male cat. The owner reported that the cat was no longer jumping on to the kitchen counter and was eating less.

Physical examination was normal, although an orthopedic examination revealed pain on palpation of either coxofemoral joint and decreased range of motion in both coxofemoral joints.

Radiographs of the hips demonstrated bilateral coxofemoral joint OA with pronounced secondary changes.

Blood/chemistry profiles revealed: packed cell volume (PCV) 39%; total protein (TP) 65 g/l (6.5 g/dl); BUN 13.2 mmol/l (37 mg/dl), creatinine 247.5 μmol/l (2.8 mg/dl); blood glucose 22.03 mmol/l (397 mg/dl).

Previous management included (1) oral ketoprofen, which was discontinued due to vomiting and renal compromise, (2) oral butorphanol, discontinued due to idiosyncratic dermal self-trauma, and (3) transmucosal buprenorphine, which was discontinued after 3 days' dosing because of lethargy and inappetance.

This senior-aged cat could have been given amantadine, tramadol, and/or a chondroprotective. However, the cat responded to acupuncture at 4- to 6-week intervals, with a return of appetite and increased activity. Not all cats respond as well to acupuncture; however, in this case sole management of clinical signs by acupuncture spared any potential organ challenge by therapeutic drugs.

CASE REPORT[2]

Signalment: 5-year-old, female, spayed Siberian husky. Presented for right forelimb lameness.

Physical examination revealed an otherwise healthy patient. Palpation of the right humerus revealed soreness.

Radiographs showed a lesion confirmed by biopsy to be osteosarcoma.

Initial treatment consisted of immediate forelimb amputation. Premedication consisted of a combination of morphine and atropine. Anesthesia was induced with a combination of intravenous midazolam followed by propofol and initially maintained with isoflurane in oxygen. Fentanyl was administered following induction, and intravenous ketamine was administered as an infusion throughout surgery. Postoperatively, the patient was maintained for 24 hr in an intensive care ward and administered continuous infusions of fentanyl and ketamine until discharge on day 2.

Home convalescence included a 3-day treatment of oral morphine and daily NSAID administration.

One month postoperatively, the patient appeared painful, and as the NSAID was continued, oral morphine was again prescribed (twice daily), which the owners increased (to three times daily). Although the owners began dosing the morphine as they felt necessary, the more frequent dosing resulted in unacceptable sedation.

All medications were stopped, and the patient was re-examined. Physical examination at this stage revealed pronounced vocalization when various parts of her body were palpated, especially the area of surgery. Allodynia from neuropathic pain was diagnosed based on the patient's painful response to nonpainful stimulation. Injury of the PNS or CNS, resultant from transection of nerves at the time of amputation, was speculated as etiology of the neuropathic pain.

The patient was administered amantadine for 5 days and morphine for 2 days. Two days following discontinuation of the amantadine, the patient was comfortable. At that time she was administered oral morphine for 5 days, amantadine for 7 days, and gabapentin for 10 days. The patient has maintained a pain-free status since this round of therapy.

Speculation holds that this patient's pain might have been much worse and more difficult to treat had her acute pain not been treated so aggressively.

CASE REPORT[2]

Signalment: 13-year-old, female, Labrador retriever with a 10-year history of hindlimb stiffness, variably medicated with PSGAG (Adequan) injections, glucosamine–chondroitin sulfate-manganese (Cosequin), and aspirin. She was being leash-walked 10 minutes per day, and had free roam in the yard, but was growling at the owner when being helped into the automobile.

Gait analysis revealed 7/10 lameness in both hindlimbs, and 3/10 lameness in both forelimbs. The left-sided limbs appeared worse than the right.

Orthopedic examination showed a decreased range of motion in both elbows and some pain upon manipulation. The left stifle produced crepitus on movement, with considerable pain on manipulation. Painful, aggressive response was elicited with manipulation of both coxofemoral joints, and crepitus was noted in the right coxofemoral joint. Paralumbar muscles were noted to be tense, hard and painful.

There were no neurological abnormalities.

A complete blood cell count was normal.

Alkaline phosphatase was 405 IU/l (normal: 12–150 IU/l), and alanine aminotransferase was 274 IU/l (normal: 5–105 IU/l). Both pre- and postprandial bile acid values were normal.

Initial management: (1) weight loss plan designed to lose 7.2 kg (16 lb) over the following 3 months, (2) physiotherapy of increasing, controlled lead exercise from 10 minutes once daily to 20 minutes 3 times daily over a 6-week period, and (3) discontinue the aspirin, but continue the nutraceutical and begin a different NSAID regimen. A revisit was scheduled for 2 weeks so as to assess clinical progress and liver function.

After 2 weeks, the patient was still lame, but less than previously noted at presentation. The owners reported their dog was 'happier', but had difficulty getting comfortable at night. She was still resistant to joint manipulation. At this point acupuncture therapy was offered, but declined, and amantadine (3 mg/kg orally, once daily) was added to the patient's treatment regimen.

After another 4 weeks, re-examination showed less lameness, but a persistent pain on joint manipulation. Tramadol (4 mg/kg twice daily) was added to the treatment regimen. Two weeks thereafter the owner reported considerable improvement and an orthopedic examination confirmed the owner's impression.

The patient continues the multimodal regimen, showing relapses when components of the regimen are removed, although dosages of each agent are continually being decreased. Painful flare-ups, usually associated with rigorous exercising, are effectively managed with small doses of acetaminophen (5 mg/kg twice daily for 2–4 days). Although a DMOAD and an EPA-rich diet were not integrated into the management regimen of this particular case, they could easily be added in an attempt to further lower current drug dosages.

REFERENCES

CHAPTER 1

1. Lynn B. Capsaicin: actions on nociceptive C-fibres and therapeutic potential. *Pain* 1990;**41**:61–69.
2. Carlton SM, Coggeshall RE. Peripheral capsaicin receptors increase in the inflamed rat handpaw; a possible mechanism for peripheral sensitization. *Neurosci Lett* 2001;**310**:53–56.
3. Sugiura T, Tominaga M, Katsuya H *et al.* Bradykinin lowers the threshold temperature for heat activation of vanilloid receptor 1. *J Neurophysiol* 2002; **88**:544–548.
4. Caterina MJ, Rosen T, Tominaga M, *et al.* A capsaicin-receptor homologue with a high threshold for noxious heat. *Nature* 1999;**398**:436–441.
5. Bernardini N, Neuhuber W, Reeh PW, *et al.* Morphological evidence for functional capsaicin receptor expression and calcitonin gene-related peptide exocytosis in isolated peripheral nerve axons of the mouse. *Neuroscience* 2004; **126**:585–590.
6. La Motte RH, Thalhammer JG, Robinson CJ. Peripheral neural correlates of magnitude of cutaneous pain and hyperalgesia: a comparison of neural events in monkey with sensory judgements in human. *J Neurophysiol* 1983;**50**:1–26.
7. Davis KD, Meyer RA, Campbell JN. Chemosensitivity and sensitization of nociceptive afferents that innervate the hairy skin of monkey. *J Neurophysiol* 1993;**69**:1071–1081.
8. Melzack R, Wall PD. Pain mechanisms: a new theory. *Science* 1965;**150**(699):971–979.
9. Gracely RH, Lynch SA, Bennett GI. Painful neuropathy altered central processing maintained dynamically by peripheral input. *Pain* 1992;**51**:175–194.
10. Choi B, Rowbotham MC. Effect of adrenergic receptor activation on post-herpetic neuralgia pain and sensory disturbance. *Pain* 1997;**69**:55–63.
11. Catterall WA, Goldin AL, Waxman SG. International Union of Pharmacology XXXIX. Compendium of voltage-gated ion channels: sodium channels. *Pharmacol Rev* 2003;**55**:575–578.
12. Tsien RW, Lipscombe D, Madison D, *et al.* Reflections on Ca($^{2+}$)-channel diversity 1988–1994. *Trends Neurosci* 1995;**18**:52–54.
13. Amir R, Argoff CE, Bennett GJ, *et al.* The role of sodium channels in chronic inflammatory and neuropathic pain. *J Pain* 2006;**7**:S1–29.
14. Robinson RB, Siegelbaum SA. Hyperpolarization-activated cation currents: from molecules to physiological function. *Annu Rev Physiol* 2003;**65**:453–480.
15. Costello M, Syring RS. Calcium channel blocker toxicity. *J Vet Emerg Crit Care* 2008;**18**:54–60.
16. Kawabata A, Manabe S, Manabe Y, *et al.* Effect of topical administration of L-arginine on formalin-induced nociception in the mouse: a dual role of peripherally formed NO in pain modulation. *Br J Pharmacol* 1994;**112**:547–550.
17. Wood J, Garthwaite J. Models of the diffusional spread of nitric oxide: implications for neural nitric oxide signalling and its pharmacological properties. *Neuropharmacology* 1994;**33**:1235–1244.
18. Sautebin L, Ialenti A, Ianaro A, *et al.* Modulation by nitric oxide of prostaglandin biosynthesis in the rat. *Br J Pharmacol* 1995;**114**:323–328.
19. Müller CE, Scior T. Adenosine receptors and their modulators. *Pharm Acta Helv* 1993;**68**:77–111.
20. Levine JD, Goetzl EJ, Basbaum AL. Contribution of the nervous system to the pathophysiology of rheumatoid arthritis and other polyarthritides. *Rheum Dis Clin North Am* 1987;**13**:369–383.
21. Sawynok J, Sweeney MI. The role of purines in nociception. Neuroscience 1989;**32**:557–569.
22. Pearson JD, Gordon JL. Vascular endothelial and smooth muscle cells in culture selectively release adenine nucleotides. *Nature* 1979;**281**:384–386.
23. Sosnowski M, Yaksh TL. Role of spinal adenosine receptors in modulating the hyperesthesia produced by spinal glycine receptor antagonism. *Anesth Analg* 1989;**69**:587–592.

24. Djouhri L, Bleazard L, Lawson SN. Association of somatic action potential shape with sensory receptive properties in guinea-pig dorsal root ganglion neurons. *J Physiol* 1998;**513**:857–872.
25. Meyer RA, Ringkamp M, Campbell JN, *et al.* Peripheral mechanisms of cutaneous nociception. In: McMahon SB, Koltzenburg M (eds) *Wall and Melzack's Textbook of Pain.* Elsevier, London, 2006, p22.
26. Pedersen JL, Crawford ME, Dahl JB, *et al.* Effect of preemptive nerve block on inflammation and hyperalgesia after human thermal injury. *Anesthesiology* 1996;**84**;1020–1026.
27. Gu JG, MacDermott AB. Activation of ATP P2X receptors elicits glutamate release from sensory neuron synapses. *Nature* 1997;**389**:749–753.
28. Cao YQ, Mantyh PW, Carlson EJ, *et al.* Primary afferent tachykinins are required to experience moderate to intense pain. *Nature* 1998;**392**:390–394.
29. Dubner R, Ruda MA. Activity-dependent neuronal plasticity following tissue injury and inflammation. *Trends Neurosci* 1992;**15**(3):96–103.
30. Powell JJ, Todd AJ. Light and electron microscope study of GABA-immunoreactive neurons in lamina III of rat spinal cord. *J Comp Neurol* 1992;**315**:125–136.
31. Benn S, Perrelet D, Kato A, *et al.* Hsp27 upregulation and phosphorylation is required for injured sensory and motor neuron survival. *Neuron* 2002;**36**:45–56.
32. Ibuki T, Hama AT, Wang XT, *et al.* Loss of GABA-immunoreactivity in the spinal dorsal horn of rats with peripheral nerve injury and promotion of recovery by adrenal medullary grafts. *Neuroscience* 1997;**76**:845–858.
33. Mendell LM. Modifiability of spinal synapses. *Physiol Rev* 1984;**64**:260–324.
34. Woolf CJ, Salter MW. Neuronal plasticity: increasing the gain in pain. *Science* 2000;**288**:1765–1769.
35. Lei Z, Ruan Y, Yang AN, *et al.* NMDA receptor mediated dendritic plasticity in cortical cultures after oxygen-glucose deprivation. *Neurosci Lett* 2006;**407**:224–229.
36. Zhang X, Verge V, Wiesenfeldhallin Z, *et al.* Nitric oxide synthase-like immunoreactivity in lumbar dorsal root ganglia and spinal cord of rat and monkey and effect of peripheral axotomy. *J Comp Neurol* 1993;**335**:563–575.
37. Pain. Clinical Updates. *IASP* 2005;13(2):1.
38. Fox SM, Mellor DJ, Firth EC, *et al.* Changes in plasma cortisol concentrations before, during and after analgesia, anaesthesia and anaesthesia plus ovariohysterectomy in bitches. *Res Vet Sci* 1994;**57**:110–118.
39. Hansen BD, Hardie EM, Carroll GS. Physiological measurements after ovariohysterectomy in dogs: what's normal? *Appl Anim Behav Sci* 1997;**51**:101–109.
40. Sun WZ, Shyu BC, Shieh JY. Nitrous oxide or halothane, or both, fail to suppress *c-fos* expression in rat spinal cord dorsal horn neurons after subcutaneous formalin. *Br J Anaesth* 1996;**76**:99–105.
41. Wall PD. The prevention of post operative pain. *Pain* 1988;**32**:289–290.
42. Shafford HL, Lascelles BDX, Hellyer PW. Preemptive analgesia: managing pain before it begins. *Vet Med* 2001;**6**:478–491.
43. Tverskoy M, Oz Y, Isakson A, *et al.* Preemptive effect of fentanyl and ketamine on postoperative pain and wound hyperalgesia. *Anesth Analg* 1994;**78**:205–209.
44. Rockemann MG, Seeling W, Bischof C, *et al.* Prophylactic use of epidural mepivacaine/morphine, systemic diclofenac, and metamizol reduces postoperative morphine consumption after major abdominal surgery. *Anesthesiology* 1996;**84**:1027–1034.
45. Lee VC, Rowlingson JC. Pre-emptive analgesia: update on nonsteroidal anti-inflammatory drugs in anesthesia. *Adv Anesth* 1995;V**12**:69–110.
46. Souter AJ, Fredman B, White PF. Controversies in the perioperative use of nonsteroidal anti-inflammatory drugs. *Anesth Analg* 1994;**79**:1178–1190.
47. Malmberg AB, Yaksh TL. Pharmacology of the spinal action of ketorolac, morphine, ST-91, U50488H, and L-PIA on the formalin test and an isobolographic analysis of the NSAID interaction. *Anesthesiology* 1993;**79**:270–281.
48. Vaughn C, Ingram SL, Connor MA, *et al.* How opioids inhibit GABA-mediated neurotransmission. *Nature* 1997;**390**:611–614.
49. Emkey R, Rosenthal N, Wu S-C, *et al.* Efficacy and safety of tramadol/acetaminophen tablets (Ultracet®) as add-on therapy for osteoarthritis pain in subjects receiving a COX-2 nonsteroidal anti-inflammatory drug: a multicenter, randomized, double-blind, placebo-controlled trial. *J Rheumatol* 2004;**31**(1):150–156.
50. Edwards JE, McQuay HJ, Moore RA. Combination analgesic efficacy: individual patient data meta-analysis of single-dose oral tramadol plus acetaminophen in acute postoperative pain. *J Pain Symptom Manage* 2002;**23**(2):121–130.
51. Gillies GWA, Kenny GNC, Bullingham RES, *et al.* The morphine sparing effects of ketorolac tromethamine: a study of a new, parenteral non-steroidal

anti-inflammatory agent after abdominal surgery. *Anaesthesia* 1987;**42**:727–731.
52. Sevarino FB, Sinatra RS, Paige D, *et al.* The efficacy of intramuscular ketorolac in combination with intravenous PCA morphine for postoperative pain relief. *J Clin Anesth* 1992;**4**:285–288.
53. Maier SF, Watkins LR. Cytokines for psychologists: implications of bidirectional immune-to-brain communication for understanding behavior, mood, and cognition. *Psychol Rev* 1998;**105**:83–107.
54. Sjöstrand J. Neuroglial proliferation in the hypoglossal nucleus after nerve injury. *Exp Neurol* 1971;**30**:178–189.
55. Tilders FJ, DeRijk RH, Van Dam AM, *et al.* Activation of the hypothalamus–pituitary–adrenal axis by bacterial endotoxins: routes and intermediate signals. *Psychoneuroendocrinology* 1994;**19**:209–232.
56. Stoll G, Jander S. The role of microglia and macrophages in the pathophysiology of the CNS. *Prog Neurobiol* 1999;**58**:233–247.
57. Coyle DE. Partial peripheral nerve injury leads to activation of astroglia and microglia which parallels the development of allodynic behavior. *Glia* 1998;**23**:75–83.
58. Barres BA, Barde Y. Neuronal and glial cell biology. *Curr Opin Neurobiol* 2000;**10**:642–648.
59. Ridet JL, Malhotra SK, Privat A, *et al.* Reactive astrocytes: cellular and molecular cues to biological function. *Trends Neurosci* 1997;**20**:570–577.
60. Watkins LR, Maier SF. Glia: a novel drug discovery target for clinical pain. *Nat Rev Drug Discov* 2003;**2**:973–985.
61. Cuadros MA, Navascues J. Early origin and colonization of the developing central nervous system by microglial precursors. In: Castellano Lopez B, Nieto-Sampedro M (eds) *Progress in Brain Research*, Vol 132. Elsevier, Amsterdam, 2001, p51–59.
62. Kaur C, Hao AJ, Wu CH, Ling EA. Origin of microglia. *Microsc Res Tech* 2001;**54**:2–9.
63. Lee JC, Mayer-Proschel M, Rao MS. Gliogenesis in the central nervous system. *Glia* 2000;**30**:105–121.
64. Tsacopoulos M. Metabolic signaling between neurons and glial cells: a short review. *J Physiol Paris* 2002;**96**:283–288.
65. Perea G, Araqe A. Communication between astrocytes and neurons: a complex language. *J Physiol Paris* 2002;**96**:199–207.
66. Haydon PG. Glia: listening and talking to the synapse. *Nat Rev Neurosci* 2001;**2**:185–193.
67. Carmignoto G. Reciprocal communication systems between astrocytes and neurons. *Prog Neurobiol* 2000;**62**:561–581.
68. Araque A, Parpura V, Sanzgiri RP, *et al.* Tripartite synapses: glia, the unacknowledged partner. *Trends Neurosci* 1999;**55**:1–26.
69. Chapman GA, Moores K, Harrison D, *et al.* Fractalkine cleavage from neuronal membranes represents an acute event in the inflammatory response to excitotoxic brain damage. *J Neurosci* 2000;**20**:RC87.
70. Milligan E, Zapata V, Schoeniger D, *et al.* An initial investigation of spinal mechanisms underlying pain enhancement induced by fractalkine, a neuronally released chemokine. *Eur J Neurosci* 2005;**22**:2775–2782.
71. Tsuda M, Shigemoto-Mogami Y, Koizume S, *et al.* P2X4 receptors induced in spinal microglia gate tactile allodynia after nerve injury. *Nature* 2003;**424**:778–783.
72. Coull JA, Boudreau D, Bachand K, *et al.* Trans-synaptic shift in anion gradient in spinal lamina I neurons as a mechanism of neuropathic pain. *Nature* 2003;**424**:938–942.
73. Devor M. Response of nerves to injury in relation to neuropathic pain. In: McMahon SB, Koltzenburg M (eds) *Wall and Melzack's Textbook of Pain*. Elsevier, London, 2006, p907.
74. Kirk EJ. Impulses in dorsal spinal nerve rootlets in cats and rabbits arising from dorsal root ganglia isolated from the periphery. *J Comp Neurol* 1974;**155**:165–175.
75. Liu C-N, Wall PD, Ben-Dor E, *et al.* Tactile allodynia in the absence of C-fiber activation: altered firing properties of DRG neurons following spinal nerve injury. *Pain* 2000;**85**:503–521.
76. Wall P, Devor M, Inbal RF, *et al.* Autotomy following peripheral nerve lesions: experimental anaesthesia dolorosa. *Pain* 1979;**7**:103–113.
77. Fried K, Govrin-Lippmann R, Devor M. Close apposition among neighbouring axonal endings in a neuroma. *J Neurocytol* 1993;**22**:663–681.
78. Waxman SG (ed) Sodium channels and neuronal hyperexcitability. Novartis Foundation Symposia 2002, p241.
79. Devor M, Govrin-Lippmann R, Angelides K. Na^+ channel immunolocalization in peripheral mammalian axons and changes following nerve injury and neuroma formation. *J Neurosci* 1993;**13**:1976–1982.
80. Amir R, Liu C-N, Kocsis J D, *et al.* Oscillatory mechanism in primary sensory neurons. *Brain* 2002;**125**:421–435.
81. Vertosick FT. *Why We Hurt. The Natural History of Pain*. Harcourt, Inc., New York, 2000.

82. Pogatzki EM, Raja SN. A mouse model of incisional pain. *Anesthesiology* 2003;**99**(4):1023–1027.
83. Ali Z, Meyer RA, Campbell JN. Secondary hyperalgesia to mechanical but not heat stimuli following a capsaicin injection in hairy skin. *Pain* 1996;**68**:401–411.
84. Tsuda M, Koizumi S, Inoue K. Role of endogenous ATP at the incision area in a rat model of postoperative pain. *Neuroreport* 2001;**12**:1701–1704.
85. Bonica JJ. History of pain concepts and pain theory. *Mt Sinai J Med* 1991;**58**:191–202.
86. Cervero F. Sensory innervation of the viscera: peripheral basis of visceral pain. *Physiol Rev* 1994;**74**:95–138.
87. McMahon SB, Dmitrieva N, Koltzenberg M. Visceral pain. *Br J Anaesth* 1995;**75**:132–144.
88. Strigo IA, Duncan GH, Boivin M, *et al.* Differentiation of visceral and cutaneous pain in the human brain. *J Neurophysiol* 2003;**89**:3294–3303.
89. Unruh AM. Gender variations in clinical pain experience. *Pain* 1996;**65**:123–167.
90. Muir WW 3rd, Wiese AJ, Wittum TE. Prevalence and characteristics of pain in dogs and cats examined as outpatients at a veterinary teaching hospital. *J Am Vet Med Assoc* 2004;**224**:1459–1463.
91. Holdcroft A, Sapsed-Byrne S, Ma D, *et al.* Sex and oestrous cycle differences in visceromotor responses and vasopressin release in response to colonic distension in male and female rats anaesthetized with halothane. *Br J Anaesth* 2000;**85**:907–910.
92. Kamp EH, Jones RC 3rd, Tillman SR, *et al.* Quantitative assessment and characterization of visceral nociception and hyperalgesia in mice. *Am J Physiol Gastrointest Liver Physiol* 2003;**284**:G434–G444.
93. Mogil JS, Chanda ML. The case for the inclusion of female subjects in basic science studies of pain. *Pain* 2005;**117**:1–5.
94. Strigo IA, Bushnell MC, Boivin M, *et al.* Psychophysical analysis of visceral and cutaneous pain in human subjects. *Pain* 2002;**97**:235–246.
95. Häbler HJ, Jänig W, Koltzenburg M. Activation of unmyelinated afferent fibers by mechanical stimuli and inflammation of the urinary bladder in the cat. *J Physiol* 1990;**425**:545–562.
96. Gebhart GF. Pathobiology of visceral pain: molecular mechanisms and therapeutic implications v. central nervous system processing of somatic and visceral sensory signals. *Am J Physiol Gastrointest Liver Physiol* 2000;**278**:G834–G838.
97. Cervero F. Visceral hyperalgesia revisited. *Lancet* 2000;**356**:1127–1128.
98. Petersen P, Gao C, Arendt-Neielsen K, *et al.* Pain intensity and biomechanical responses during ramp-controlled distension of the human rectum. *Dig Dis Sci* 2003;**48**:1310–1316.
99. Bonaz B, Rivière PJ, Siniger V, *et al.* Fedotozine, a kappa-opioid agonist, prevents spinal and supraspinal Fos expression induced by a noxious visceral stimulus in the rat. *Neurogastroenterol Motil* 2000;**12**:135–147.
100. Sengupta JN, Snider A, Su X, Gebhart GF. Effects of kappa opioids in the inflamed rat colon. *Pain* 1999;**79**:171–185.
101. Sarkar S, Hobson AR, Furlong PL, *et al.* Central neural mechanisms mediating human visceral hypersensitivity. *Am J Physiol Gastrointest Liver Physiol* 2001;**281**:G1196–G1202.
102. Sugiura Y, Terui N, Hosoya Y, *et al.* Quantitative analysis of central terminal projections of visceral and somatic unmyelinated (C) primary afferent fibers in the guinea pig. *J Comp Neurol* 1993;**332**:315–325.
103. Ness TJ, Powell-Boone T, Cannon R, *et al.* Psychophysical evidence of hypersensitivity in subjects with interstitial cystitis. *J Urol* 2005;**173**:1983–1987.
104. Alagiri M, Chottiner S, Ratner V, *et al.* Interstitial cystitis: unexplained associations with other chronic disease and pain syndromes. *Urology* 1997;**49**(Suppl):52–57.
105. Whorwell PJ, McCallum M, Creed FH, *et al.* Non-colonic features of irritable bowel syndrome. *Gut* 1986;**27**:37–40.
106. Pezzone MA, Liang R, Fraser MO. A model of neural cross-talk and irritation in the pelvis: Implications for the overlap of chronic pelvic pain disorders. *Gastroenterology* 2005;**128**:1953–1964.
107. Qin C, Foreman RD. Viscerovisceral convergence of urinary bladder and colorectal inputs to lumbosacral spinal neurons in rats. *Neuroreport* 2004;**15**:467–471.
108. McMahon SB, Morrison JFB. Two groups of spinal interneurons that respond to stimulation of the abdominal viscera of the cat. *J Physiol* 1982;**322**:21–34.
109. Mertz H. Review article: visceral hypersensitivity. *Aliment Pharmacol Ther* 2003;**17**:623–633.
110. Cervero F, Laird JMA. Mechanisms of touch-evoked pain (allodynia): a new model. Review article. *Pain* 1996;**68**:13–23.
111. Russo CM, Brose WG. Chronic pain. *Annu Rev Med* 1998;**49**:123–133.
112. Schaible HG, Richter F. Pathophysiology of pain. *Langenbecks Arch Surg* 2004;**389**:237–243.

113. Jacobsen L, Mariano A. General considerations of chronic pain. In: Loeser JD, Butler SH, Chapman SR (eds) *Bonica's Management of Pain*, 3rd ed. Lippincott Williams & Wilkins, Baltimore, MD, 2001, p241–254.
114. Cervero F, Laird JM. From acute to chronic pain: peripheral and central mechanisms. In: Bountra C, Munglani R, Schmidt WK (eds) *Pain: Current Understanding, Emerging Therapies, and Novel Approaches to Drug Discovery*. Marcel Dekker, Inc, New York, 2003, p29–44.
115. Merskey H, Bogduk N. *Classification of Chronic Pain: Descriptions of Chronic Pain Syndromes and Definitions of Pain Terms*, 2nd ed. IASP Press, Seattle, 1994, p222.
116. McMahon SB, Jones NG. Plasticity of pain signaling: role of neurotrophic factors exemplified by acid-induced pain. *J Neurobiol* 2004;**61**:72–87.
117. Villar MJ, Cortés R, Theodorsson E, *et al.* Neuropeptide expression in rat dorsal root ganglion cells and spinal cord after peripheral nerve injury with special reference to galanin. *Neuroscience* 1989;**33**:587–604.
118. Boucher TJ, Okuse K, Bennett DL, *et al.* Potent analgesic effects of GDNF in neuropathic pain states. *Science* 2000;**290**:124–127.
119. Vos BP, Maciewicz RJ. Behavioral evidence of trigeminal neuropathic pain following chronic constriction injury of rats' infraorbital nerve. *J Neurosci* 1994;**14**:2708–2723.
120. Burchiel KJ, Russell LC, Lee RP, *et al.* Spontaneous activity of primary afferent neurons in diabetic BB/Wistar rats. *Diabetes* 1985;**34**:1210–1213.
121. Aley KO, Reichling DB, Levine JD. Vincristine hyperalgesia in the rat: a model of painful vincristine neuropathy in humans. *Neuroscience* 1996;**73**:259–265.
122. Bennett GJ, Xie Y-K. A peripheral mononeuropathy in rat that produces disorders of pain sensation like those seen in man. *Pain* 1988;**33**:87–107.
123. Seltzer Z, Dubner R, Shir Y. A novel behavioral model of neuropathic pain disorders produced in rats by partial sciatic nerve injury. *Pain* 1990;**43**:205–218.
124. Lombard MC, Nashold BS, Albe-Fessard D. Deafferentation hypersensitivity in the rat after dorsal rhizotomy: a possible model of chronic pain. *Pain* 1979;**6**:163–174.
125. Carlton SM, Lekan HA, Kim SH, *et al.* Behavioral manifestations of an experimental model for peripheral neuropathy produced by spinal nerve ligation in the primate. *Pain* 1994;**56**:155–166.
126. Deleo JA, Coombs DW, Willenbring S, *et al.* Characterization of a neuropathic pain model–sciatic cryoneurolysis in the rat. *Pain* 1994;**56**:9–16.
127. Kupers R, Yu W, Persson JKE, *et al.* Photochemically-induced ischemia of the rat sciatic nerve produces a dose-dependent and highly reproducible mechanical, heat and cold allodynia, and signs of spontaneous pain. *Pain* 1998;**76**:45–59.
128. Attal N, Cruccu G, Haanpää M, *et al.* EFNS guidelines on pharmacological treatment of neuropathic pain. *Eur J Neurol* 2006;**13**:1153–1169.
129. Finnerup NB, Otto M, McQuay HJ, *et al.* Algorithm for neuropathic pain treatment: an evidence based proposal. *Pain* 2005;**118**:289–305.
130. Yang L, Zhang F-X, Huang F, *et al.* Peripheral nerve injury induces trans-synaptic modification of channels, receptors and signal pathways in rat dorsal spinal cord. *Eur J Neurosci* 2004;**19**:871–883.
131. Devor M, Govrin-Lippmann R, Angelides K. Na^+ channel immunolocalization in peripheral mammalian axons and changes following nerve injury and neuroma formation. *J Neurosci* 1993;**13**:1976–1992.
132. Catterall WA, Goldin AL, Waxman SG. International Union of Pharmacology. XLVII. Nomenclature and structure–function relationships of voltage-gated sodium channels. *Pharmacol Rev* 2005;**57**:397–409.
133. Masferrer JL, Leahy KM, Koki AT, *et al.* Antiangiogenic and antitumor activities of cyclooxygenase-2 inhibitors. *Cancer Res* 2000;**60**(5):1306–1311.
134. Nelson JB, Carducci MA. The role of endothelin-1 and endothelin receptor antagonists in prostate cancer. *BJU Int* 2000;**85**(Suppl 2):45–48.
135. Dawas K, Loizidou M, Shankar A, *et al.* Angiogenesis in cancer: the role of endothelin-1. *Ann R Coll Surg Engl* 1999;**81**:306–310.
136. Asham EH, Loizidou M, Taylor I. Endothelin-1and tumour development. *Eur J Surg Oncol* 1998;**24**(1):57–60.
137. Honore P, Luger NM, Sabino MA, *et al.* Osteoprotegerin blocks bone cancer-induced skeletal destruction, skeletal pain and pain-related neurochemical reorganization of the spinal cord. *Nat Med* 2000;**6**(5):521–528.
138. Mannix K, Ahmedzai SH, Anderson H, *et al.* Using bisphosphonates to control the pain of bone metastases: evidence-based guidelines for palliative care. *Palliat Med* 2000;**14**:455–461.
139. Mathews KA. Management of Pain. Pain assessment and general approach to management. *Vet Clin North Am Small Anim Pract* 2000;**30**:732–733.

140. Holton L, Reid J, Scott EM, *et al.* Development of a behaviour-based scale to measure acute pain in dogs. *Vet Rec* 2001;**148**:525–531.
141. Wiseman-Orr M, Scott EM, Reid J, *et al.* Validation of a structured questionnaire as an instrument to measure chronic pain in dogs on the basis of effects on health-related quality of life. *Am J Vet Res* 2006;**67**:1826–1836.
142. McMillan FD. Quality of life in animals. *J Am Vet Med Assoc* 2000;**216**:1904–1910.
143. Hielm-Björkman AK, Kuusela E, Markkola A, *et al.* Evaluation of methods for assessment of pain associated with chronic osteoarthritis in dogs. *J Am Vet Med Assoc* 2003;**222**:1552–1558.
144. Gingerich DA, Strobel JD. Use of client-specific outcome measures to assess treatment effects in geriatric, arthritic dogs: controlled clinical evaluation of a nutraceutical. *Vet Ther* 2003;**4**:56–66.
145. Woolf CJ, Borsook D, Koltzenburg M. Mechanism-based classifications of pain and analgesic drug discovery. In: Bountra C, Munglani R, Schmidt WK (eds) *Pain: Current Understanding, Emerging Therapies, and Novel Approaches to Drug Discovery.* Marcel Dekker, Inc, New York, 2003, p1–8.

CHAPTER 2

1. Jehn CT, Perzak DE, Cook JL, *et al.* Usefulness, completeness, and accuracy of Web sites providing information on osteoarthritis in dogs. *J Am Vet Med Assoc* 2003;**223**(9):1272–1275.
2. Wilke VL, Robinson DA, Evans RB, *et al.* Estimate of the annual economic impact of treatment of cranial cruciate ligament injury in dogs in the United States. *J Am Vet Med Assoc* 2005;**227**(10): 1604–1607.
3. Kee CC. Osteoarthritis: manageable scourge of aging. *Nurs Clin North Am* 2000;**35**:199–208.
4. Pfizer Animal Health proprietary market research; survey of 200 veterinarians, 1996.
5. 1999 Rimadyl A&U Study–USA: 039 DRIM 197.
6. Hardie EM, Roe SC, Martin FR. Radiographic evidence of degenerative joint disease in geriatric cats: 100 cases (1994–1997). *J Am Vet Med Assoc* 2002;**220**:628–632.
7. Godfrey DR. Ostoarthritis in cats: a retrospective radiological study. *J Small Anim Pract* 2005;**46**:425–429.
8. Clarke SP, Mellor D, Clements DN, *et al.* Prevalence of radiographic signs of degenerative joint disease in a hospital population of cats. *Vet Rec* 2005;**157**:793–799.
9. Freire M, Simpson W, Thomson A, *et al.* Cross-sectional study evaluating the radiographic prevalence of feline degenerative joint disease. Proceedings of ACVS Annual Meeting, San Diego CA, 2008.
10. Freire M, Hash J, Lascelles BDX. Evaluation of post mortem radiological appearance versus macroscopic appearance of appendicular joints in cats. Proceedings of ACVS Annual Meeting, San Diego CA, 2008.
11. Stamper C. Osteoarthritis in cats: a more common disease than you might expect. *FDA Veterinarian Newsletter* 2008;**23**(2):6–8.
12. Yuan GH, Masukp-Hongo K, Kato T, *et al.* Immunologic intervention in the pathogenesis of osteoarthritis. *Arthritis Rheum* 2003;**48**:602–611.
13. Amin AR. Regulation of tumor necrosis factor-alpha and tumor necrosis factor converting enzyme in human osteoarthritis. *Osteoarthritis Cartilage* 1999;**7**:392–394.
14. Schaible HGT, Ebersberger A, Von Banchet GS. Mechanisms of pain in arthritis. *Ann N Y Acad Sci* 2002;**966**:343–354.
15. Kidd BL, Photiou A, Inglis JJ. The role of inflammatory mediators on nociception and pain in arthritis. *Novartis Found Symp* 2004;**260**:122–133.
16. Kontinnen YT, Kemppinen P, Segerberg M, *et al.* Peripheral and spinal neuronal mechanisms in arthritis with particular reference to treatment of inflammation and pain. *Arthritis Rheum* 1994;**37**:965–982.
17. Koki A, Khan NK, Woerner BM, *et al.* Cyclooxygenase-2 in human pathological disease. *Adv Exp Med Biol* 2002;**507**:177–184.
18. Seki H, Fukuda M, Lino M, *et al.* Immunohistochemical localization of cyclooxygenase-1 and -2 in synovial tissues from patients with internal derangement or osteoarthritis of the temporomandibular joint. *Int J Oral Maxillofac Surg* 2004;**33**:687–692.
19. Knorth H, Dorfmuller P, Lebert R, *et al.* Participation of cyclooxygenase-1 in prostaglandin E2 release from synovitis tissue in primary osteoarthritis in vitro. *Osteoarthritis Cartilage* 2004;**12**:658–666.
20. Lascelles BDX, King S, Marcelin-Little DJ, *et al.* Expression and activity of COX-1 and 2 in joint tissues in dogs with naturally occurring osteoarthritis. (In press.)
21. Muller-Ladner U, Gay RE, Gay S. Structure and function of synoviocytes. In: Koopman WJ (ed) *Arthritis and Allied Conditions*, 13th ed. Williams & Wilkins, Baltimore, 1997, p243.
22. Arnoldi CC, Djurhuus JC, Heerfordt J, *et al.* Intraosseous phlebography, intraosseus pressure measurements and 99mTc polyphosphate scintigraphy

in patients with painful conditions in the hip and knee. *Acta Orthop Scand* 1980;**51**:19–28.

23. Poole AC. The structure and function of articular cartilage matrices. In: Woessner JF, Howell DS (eds) *Joint Cartilage Degradation: Basic and Clinical Aspects*. Marcel Dekker Inc., New York, 1993, p1–36.
24. Mayne R. Structure and function of collagen. In: Koopman WJ (ed) *Arthritis and Allied Conditions*, 13th ed. Williams & Wilkins, Baltimore, 1997,1 (10):207–227
25. Diab M. The role of type IX collagen in osteoarthritis and rheumatoid arthritis. *Orthop Rev* 1993;**22**:165–170.
26. Lohmander LS. Markers of cartilage metabolism in arthrosis: a review. *Acta Orthop Scand* 1991;**62**:623–632.
27. Mankin HJ, Brandt KD. Pathogenesis of osteoarthritis. In: Kelly WN, Harris ED, Ruddy S, Sledge CB (eds) *Textbook of Rheumatology*, 5th ed. WB Saunders, Philadelphia, 1997, p1369.
28. Kuettner K, Thonar E, Aydelotte M. Articular cartilage – structure and chondrocyte metabolism. In: Muir H, Hirohata K, Shichikawa K (eds) *Mechanisms of Articular Cartilage Damage and Repair in Osteoarthritis*. Hogrefe & Huber, Toronto, 1990, p11.
29. Cohen NP, Foster RJ, Mow VC. Composition and dynamics of articular cartilage: structure, function, and maintaining healthy state. *J Orthop Sports Phys Ther* 1998;**28**:203–215.
30. Radin EL, Paul IL, Lowry M. A comparison of the dynamic force transmitting properties of subchondral bone and articular cartilage. *J Bone Joint Surg Am* 1970;**52**:444–456.
31. Radin EL, Paul IL. Does cartilage reduce skeletal impact loads? The relative force-attenuating properties of articular cartilage, synovial fluid, periarticular soft tissues and bone. *Arthritis Rheum* 1970;**13**:139–144.
32. Reimann I, Christensen SB. A histological demonstration of nerves in subchondral bone. *Acta Orthop Scand* 1977;**48**:345–352.
33. McDevitt C, Gilbertson E, Muir H. An experimental model of osteoarthritis: early morphological and biochemical changes. *J Bone Joint Surg Br* 1977;**59**:24–35.
34. Moskowitz RW, Goldberg VM. Studies of osteophyte pathogenesis in experimentally induced osteoarthritis. *J Rheumatol* 1987;**14**:311–320.
35. Gilbertson EM. Development of periarticular osteophytes in experimentally induced osteoarthritis in the dog. A study using microradiographic, microangiographic, and fluorescent bone-labelling techniques. *Ann Rheum Dis* 1975;**34**:12–25.
36. Mankin HJ, Radin EL. Structure and function of joints. In: Koopman WJ (ed) *Arthritis and Allied Conditions*, 13th ed. Williams & Wilkins, Baltimore, 1997,**1**(8) :175–191
37. Ralphs JR, Benjamin M. The joint capsule: structure, composition, ageing and disease. *J Anat* 1994;**184**:503–509.
38. Mine T, Kimura M, Sakka A, *et al*. Innervation of nociceptors in the menisci of the knee joint: an immunohistochemical study. *Arch Orthop Trauma Surg* 2000;**120**:201–204.
39. Simkin PA. Synovial physiology. In: Koopman WJ (ed) *Arthritis and Allied Conditions*, 13th ed. Williams & Wilkins, Baltimore, 1997, p193.
40. Simkin PA, Benedict RS. Iodide and albumin kinetics in normal canine wrists and knees. *Arthritis Rheum* 1990;**33**:73–79.
41. Brandt KD, Thonar EJM. Lack of association between serum keratan sulfate concentrations and cartilage changes of osteoarthritis after transection of the anterior cruciate ligament in the dog. *Arthritis Rheum* 1989;**32**:647–651.
42. Nakano T, Aherne FX, Thompson JR. Changes in swine knee articular cartilage during growth. *Can J Anim Sci* 1979;**59**:167–179.
43. Venn MF. Variation of chemical composition with age in human femoral head cartilage. *Ann Rheum Dis* 1978;**37**:168–174.
44. Roughley PJ. Changes in cartilage proteoglycan structure during ageing: origin and effects – a review. *Agents Actions Suppl* 1986;**18**:19–29.
45. Grieson HA, Summers BA, Lust G. Ultrastructure of the articular cartilage and synovium in the early stages of degenerative joint disease in canine hip joints. *Am J Vet Res* 1982;**43**:1963–1971.
46. Goldring MB. The role of the chondrocyte in osteoarthritis. *Arthritis Rheum* 2000;**43**:1916–1926.
47. Farahat MN. Cytokine expression in synovial membranes of patients with rheumatoid arthritis and osteoarthritis. *Ann Rheum Dis* 1993;**52**:870–875.
48. Venn G, Nietfeld JJ, Duits AJ, *et al*. Elevated synovial fluid levels of interleukin-6 and tumor necrosis factor associated with early experimental canine osteoarthritis. *Arthritis Rheum* 1993; **36**:819–826.
49. Bakker AC, van de Loo FA, van Beuningen HM, *et al*. Overexpression of active TGF-beta-1 in the murine knee joint: evidence for synovial-layer-dependent chondro-osteophyte formation. *Osteoarthritis Cartilage* 2001;**9**:128–136.

50. Blom AB, van Lent PL, Holthuysen AE, *et al.* Synovial lining macrophages mediate osteophyte formation during experimental osteoarthritis. Proceedings of the 49th Annual Meeting of the Orthopedic Research Society, 2003;353.
51. Walker ER, Body RD. Morphologic and morphometric changes in synovial membrane associated with mechanically induced osteoarthritis. *Arthritis Rheum* 1991;**34**:515–524.
52. Hough AJ. Pathology of osteoarthritis. In: Koopman WJ (ed.) *Arthritis and Allied Conditions: a Textbook of Rheumatology*, 14th ed. Lippincott Williams & Wilkins, Philadelphia, 2001, p2167–2194.
53. Haywood L, McWilliams DF, Pearson CI, *et al.* Inflammation and angiogenesis in osteoarthritis. *Arthritis Rheum* 2003;**48**:2173–2177.
54. Klocke NW, Snyder PW, Widmer WR, *et al.* Detection of synovial macrophages in the joint capsule of dogs with naturally occurring rupture of the cranial cruciate ligament. *Am J Vet Res* 2005;**66**:493–499.
55. Paulos CM, Turk MJ, Breur GJ, *et al.* Folate receptor-mediated targeting of therapeutic and imaging agents to activated macrophages in rheumatoid arthritis. *Adv Drug Deliv Rev* 2004;**56**:1205–1217.
56. Boniface RJ, Cain PR, Evans CH. Articular responses to purified cartilage proteoglycans. *Arthritis Rheum* 1988;**31**:258–266.
57. Carney SL, Billingham MEJ, Caterson B, *et al.* Changes in proteoglycan turnover in experimental canine osteoarthritic cartilage. *Matrix* 1992;**12**:137–147.
58. Broom N. Abnormal softening in articular cartilage. *Arthritis Rheum* 1982;**25**:1209–1216.
59. Hwang WS, Li B, Jin LH, Ngo K, *et al.* Collagen fibril structure of normal, aging, and osteoarthritic cartilage. *J Pathol* 1992;**167**:425–433.
60. Malemud CJ. Fundamental pathways in osteoarthritis: an overview. *Front Biosci* 1999;**4**:D659–661.
61. Dijkgraaf LC, De Bont LG, Boering G, *et al.* The structure, biochemistry, and metabolism of osteoarthritic cartilage: a review of the literature. *J Oral Maxillofac Surg* 1995;**53**:1182–1192.
62. Nagase H, Woessner JF. Role of endogenous proteinases in the degradation of cartilage matrix. In: Woessner JF, Howell DS (eds) *Joint Cartilage Degradation: Basic and Clinical Aspects*. Marcel Dekker, New York, 1993, p159.
63. Lotz M. Cytokines and their receptors. In: Koopman WJ (ed) *Arthritis and Allied Conditions*, 13th ed. Williams & Wilkins, Baltimore, 1997, p439.
64. Poole AR. An introduction to the pathophysiology of osteoarthritis. *Front Biosci* 1999;**4**:662–670.
65. Pelletier JP, Martel-Pelletier J, Howell DS. Etiopathogenesis of osteoarthritis. In: Koopman WJ (ed) *Arthritis and Allied Conditions*, 13th ed. Williams & Wilkins, Baltimore, 1997;2 : 1969–1984.
66. Johnston SA. Osteoarthritis: joint anatomy, physiology, and pathobiology. *Vet Clin North Am Small Anim Pract* 1997;**27**:699–723.
67. Burr DB, Radin EL. Trauma as a factor in the initiation of osteoarthritis. In: Brandt KD (ed) *Cartilage Changes in Osteoarthritis*. Indiana University School of Medicine, Indianapolis, 1990, p63.
68. Meyers SL, Brandt KD, O'Connor BL, *et al.* Synovitis and osteoarthritic changes in canine articular cartilage after anterior cruciate ligament transection: Effect of surgical hemostasis. *Arthritis Rheum* 1990;**33**:1406–1415.
69. Galloway RH, Lester SJ. Histopathological evaluation of canine stifle joint synovial membrane collected at the time of repair of cranial cruciate ligament rupture. *J Am Anim Hosp Assoc* 1995;**3**:289–294.
70. Lipowitz AJ, Wong PL, Stevens JB. Synovial membrane changes after experimental transaction of the cranial cruciate ligament in dogs. *Am J Vet Res* 1985;**46**:1166–1170.
71. Pelletier JP, Martel-Pelletier J, Ghandur-Mnaymneh L, *et al.* Role of synovial membrane inflammation in cartilage matrix breakdown in the Pond–Nuki dog model of osteoarthritis. *Arthritis Rheum* 1985;**28**:554–561.
72. Henderson B, Higgs GA. Synthesis of arachidonate oxidation products by synovial joint tissues during the development of chronic erosive arthritis. *Arthritis Rheum* 1987;**30**:1149–1156.
73. Schaible HGT, Grubb BD. Afferent and spinal mechanisms of joint pain. *Pain* 1993;**55**:5–54.
74. Ben-Av P, Crofford LJ, Wilder RL, *et al.* Induction of vascular endothelial growth factor expression in synovial fibroblasts by prostaglandin E and interleukin-1: a potential mechanism for inflammatory angiogenesis. *FEBS Lett* 1995;**372**:83–87.
75. Vignon E, Mathieu P, Louisot P, *et al.* Phospholipase A2 activity in human osteoarthritic cartilage. *J Rheumatol Suppl* 1989;**18**:35–38.
76. Sturge RA, Yates DB, Gordon D, *et al.* Prostaglandin production in arthritis. *Ann Rheum Dis* 1978;**37**:315–320.
77. Fulkerson JP, Laderbauer-Bellis IM, Chrisman OD. In vitro hexosamine depletion of intact articular cartilage by E-prostaglandins: prevention by chloroquine. *Arthritis Rheum* 1979;**22**:1117–1121.

78. Fox DB, Cook JL. Synovial fluid markers of osteoarthritis in dogs. *J Am Vet Med Assoc* 2001;**219**:756–761.
79. Bauer DC, Hunter DJ, Abramson SB, *et al.* Review: classification of osteoarthritis biomarkers: a proposed approach. *Osteoarthritis Cartilage* 2006;**14**:723–727.
80. Hadler N. Why does the patient with osteoarthritis hurt? In: Brandt KD, Doherty M, Lohmander LS (eds) *Osteoarthritis*. Oxford University Press, New York, 1998, p255–261.
81. Kellgren JH, Samuel EP. The sensitivity and innervation of the articular capsule. *J Bone Joint Surg* 1950;**4**:193–205.
82. Salo P. The role of joint innervation in the pathogenesis of arthritis. *Can J Surg* 1999;**42**:91–100.
83. Kellgren JH. Observations on referred pain arising from muscle. *Clin Sci* 1938;**3**:175–190.
84. Johannson H, Sjolander P, Sojka P. Receptors in the knee joint ligaments and their role in biomechanics of the joint. *CRC Crit Rev Biomed Engineering* 1991;**18**:341–368.
85. Mense S. Nociception from skeletal muscle in relation to clinical muscle pain. *Pain* 1993;**54**:241–289.
86. Wyke B. The neurology of joints. A review of general principles. *Clin Rheum Dis* 1981;**7**:223–239.
87. Caron JP. Neurogenic factors in joint pain and disease pathogenesis. In: Mcllwraith CW, Trotter GW (eds) *Joint Disease in the Horse*. WB Saunders, Philadelphia, 1996, p40–70.
88. Schmidt RF. The articular polymodal nocieceptor in health and disease. *Prog Brain Res* 1996;**113**:53–81.
89. Krauspe R, Schmidt M, Schaible H-G. Sensory innervation of the anterior cruciate ligament: an electrophysiological study of the response properties of single identified mechanoreceptors in the cat. *J Bone Joint Surg Am* 1992;**74**:390–397.
90. Schaible H-G, Schmidt RF. Time course of mechanosensitivity changes in articular afferents during a developing experimental arthritis. *J Neurophysiol* 1988;**60**:2180–2195.
91. Kanaka R, Schaible H-G, Schmidt RF. Activation of fine articular afferent units by bradykinin. *Brain Res* 1985;**327**:81–90.
92. Neugebauer V, Schaible H-G, Schmidt RF. Sensitization of articular afferents to mechanical stimuli by bradykinin. *Pflügers Archiv* 1989;**415**:330–335.
93. Birrell GM, McQueen DS, Iggo A, *et al.* Prostanoid-induced potentiation of the excitatory and sensitizing effects of bradykinin on articular mechanonociceptors in the rat ankle joint. *Neuroscience* 1993;**54**:537–544.
94. Schaible H-G, Schmidt RF. Excitation and sensitization of fine articular afferents from cat's knee joint by prostaglandin E2. *J Physiol* 1988;**403**:91–104.
95. Grubb BD, Birrell J, McQueen DS, *et al.* The role of PGE2 in the sensitization of mechanoreceptors in normal and inflamed ankle joints of the rat. *Exp Brain Res* 1991;**84**:383–392.
96. Schepelmann K, Messlinger K, Schaible H-G, *et al.* Inflammatory mediators and nociception in the joint: excitation and sensitization of slowly conducting afferent fibers of cat's knee by prostaglandin I2. *Neuroscience* 1992;**50**:237–247.
97. Birrell GM, McQueen DS, Iggo A, *et al.* PGI2-induced activation and sensitization of articular mechanoreceptors. *Neurosci Lett* 1991;**124**:5–8.
98. McQueen DS, Iggo A, Birrell GJ, *et al.* Effects of paracetamol and aspirin on neural activity of joint mechanonociceptors in adjuvant arthritis. *Br J Pharmacol* 1991;**104**:178–182.
99. Birrell GJ, McQueen DS, Iggo A, *et al.* The effects of 5-HT on articular sensory receptors in normal and arthritic rats. *Br J Pharmacol* 1990;**101**:715–721.
100. Herbert MK, Schmidt RF. Activation of normal and inflamed fine articular afferent units by serotonin. *Pain* 1992;**50**:79–88.
101. He X, Schepelmann K, Schaible H-G, *et al.* Capsaicin inhibits responses of fine afferents from the knee joint of the cat to mechanical and chemical stimuli. *Brain Res* 1990;**530**:147–150.
102. Gauldie SD, McQueen DS, Pertwee R, *et al.* Ananamide activates peripheral nociceptors in normal and arthritic rat knee joints. *Br J Pharmacol* 2001;**132**:617–621.
103. Kelly DC, Asghar AU, Marr CG, *et al.* Nitric oxide modulates articular sensory discharge and responsiveness to bradykinin in normal and arthritic rats in vivo. *Neuroreport* 2001;**12**:121–125.
104. Dowd E, McQueen DS, Chessell IP, *et al.* P2X receptor-mediated excitation of nociceptive afferents in the normal and arthritic rat knee joint. *Br J Pharmacol* 1998;**125**:341–346.
105. Dowd E, McQueen DS, Chessell IP, *et al.* Adenosine A1 receptor-mediated excitation of nociceptive afferents innervating the normal and arthritic rat knee joint. *Br J Pharmacol* 1998;**125**:1267–1271.
106. Heppelmann B, Pawlak M. Sensitisation of articular afferents in normal and inflamed knee joints by substance P in the rat. *Neurosci Lett* 1997;**223**:97–100.
107. Herbert MK, Schmidt RF. Sensitisation of group III articular afferents to mechanical stimuli by substance P. *Inflamm Res* 2001;**50**:275–282

108. Pawlak M, Schmidt RF, Nitz C, *et al.* The neurokinin-2 receptor is not involved in the sensitization of primary afferents of the rat knee joint. *Neurosci Lett* 2002;**326**:113–116.
109. Heppelmann B, Pawlak M. Inhibitory effects of somatostatin on the mechanosensitivity of articular afferents in normal and inflamed knee joints of the rat. *Pain* 1997;**73**:377–382.
110. Heppelmann B, Just S, Pawlak M. Galanin influences the mechanosensitivity of sensory endings in the rat knee joint. *Eur J Neurosci* 2000;**12**:1567–1572.
111. Just S, Heppelmann B. Neuropeptide Y changes the excitability of fine afferent units in the rat knee joint. *Br J Pharmacol* 2001;**132**:703–708.
112. McDougall JJ, Pawlak M, Hanesch U, *et al.* Peripheral modulation of rat knee joint afferent mechanosensitivity by nociceptin/orphanin FQ. *Neurosci Lett* 2000;**288**:123–126.
113. Mense S. Pathophysiologic basis of muscle pain syndromes. Myofascial pain – update in diagnosis and treatment. *Phys Med Rehabil Clin North Am* 1997;**8**:23–53.
114. Slemenda C, Brandt KD, Heilman DK, *et al.* Quadriceps weakness and osteoarthritis of the knee. *Ann Intern Med* 1997;**127**:97–104.
115. van Baar ME, Dekker J, Lemmens JAM, *et al.* Pain and disability in patients with osteoarthritis of hip or knee: the relationship with articular, kinesiological, and psychological characteristics. *J Rheumatol* 1998;**25**:125–133.
116. Arendt-Nielsen L, Laursen RJ, Drewes AM. Referred pain as an indicator for neural plasticity. In: Sandkuhler J, Bromm B, Beghart GF (eds) *Progress in Brain Research*. Elsevier, Amsterdam, 2000, p343–356.
117. Neugebauer V, Lücke T, Schaible H-G. N-methyl-D-aspartate (NMDA) and non-NMDA receptor antagonists block the hyperexcitability of dorsal horn neurons during development of acute arthritis in rat's knee joint. *J Neurophysiol* 1993;**70**: 1365–1377.
118. Schaible H-G, Freudenberger U, Neugebauer V, *et al.* Intraspinal release of immunoreactive calcitonin gene-related peptide during development of inflammation in the joint in vivo – a study with antibody microprobes in cat and rat. *Neuroscience* 1994;**62**:1293–1305.
119. Ebersberger A, Grubb BD, Willingale HL, *et al.* The intraspinal release of prostaglandin E2 in a model of acute arthritis is accompanied by an upregulation of cyclooxygenase-2 in the rat spinal cord. *Neuroscience* 1999;**93**:775–781.
120. Bendele AM. Progressive chronic osteoarthritis in femorotibial joints of partial medial meniscectomized guinea pigs. *Vet Pathol* 1987;**24**:444–448.
121. Bendele AM, White SL. Early histopathologic and ultrastructural alterations in femorotibial joints of partial medial meniscectomized guinea pigs. *Vet Pathol* 1987;**24**:436–443.
122. Kamekura S, Hoshi K, Shimoaka T, *et al.* Osteoarthritis development in novel experimental mouse models induced by knee joint instability. *Osteoarthritis Cartilage* 2005;**13**:632–641.
123. Bendele AM. Animal models of osteoarthritis. *J Musculoskel Neuron Interact* 2001;**1**:363–376.
124. Brandt KD, Braunstein EM, Visco DM, *et al.* Anterior (cranial) cruciate ligament transection in the dog: a bona fide model of osteoarthritis, mot merely of cartilage injury and repair. *J Rheumatol* 1991;**18**:436–446.
125. Oegema TR, Visco D. Animal models of osteoarthritis. In: An YH, Friedman RJ (eds) *Animal Models in Orthopaedic Research*. CRC Press, Boca Raton, 1999, p349–367.
126. Griffiths RJ, Schrier DJ. Advantages and limitations of animal models in the discovery and evaluation of novel disease-modifying osteoarthritis drugs (DMOADs). In: Brandt KD, Koherty M, Lohmander LS (eds) *Osteoarthritis*, 2nd ed. Oxford University Press, Oxford, 2003, p411–416.
127. Pritzker KP. Animal models for osteoarthritis: processes, problems and prospects. *Ann Rheum Dis* 1994;**53**:406–420.
128. Brandt KD, Myers SL, Burr D, *et al.* Osteoarthritic changes in canine articular cartilage, subchondral bone, and synovium fifty-four months after transection of the anterior cruciate ligament. *Arthritis Rheum* 1991;**34**:1560–1570.
129. Smith GN Jr, Myers SL, Brandt KD, *et al.* Diacerhein treatment reduces the severity of osteoarthritis in the canine cruciate-deficient model of osteoarthritis. *Arthritis Rheum* 1999;**42**:545–554.
130. Schawalder P, Gitterle E. Some methods for surgical reconstruction of ruptures of the anterior and posterior crucial ligaments. *Kleintiepraxis* 1989;**34**:323–330.
131. Cox JS, Nye CE, Schaefer WW, *et al.* The degenerative effects of partial and total resection of the medial meniscus in dogs' knees. *Clin Orthop Relat Res* 1975;178–183.
132. Frost-Christensen LN, Mastbergen SC, Vianen ME, *et al.* Degeneration, inflammation, regeneration, and pain/disability in dogs following destabilization or articular cartilage grooving of the stifle joint. *Osteoarthritis Cartilage* 2008;**16**:1327–1335.

133. Marijnissen ACA, van Roermund PM, TeKoppele JM, *et al.* The canine 'groove' model, compared with the ACLT model of osteoarthritis. *Osteoarthritis Cartilage* 2002;**10**:145–155.
134. Hulse DA, Butler DL, Kay MD, *et al.* Biomechanics of cranial cruciate ligament reconstruction in the dog. 1. In vitro laxity testing. *Vet Surg* 1983;**12**:109–112.
135. Kirby BM. Decision-making in cranial cruciate ligament ruptures. *Vet Clin North Am* 1993;**23**:797–819.
136. Lopez MJ, Kunz D, Wanderby R Jr, *et al.* A comparison of joint stability between anterior cruciate intact and deficient knees: a new canine model of anterior cruciate ligament disruption. *J Ortho Res* 2003;**21**:224–230.
137. Vasseur PB: Stifle joint. In: Slatter D (ed) *Textbook of Small Animal Surgery* 3rd Ed, Vol 2. WB Saunders, Philadelphia, 2003, p2090–2133.
138. Slocum B, Slocum TD. Tibial plateau leveling osteotomy for repair of cranial cruciate ligament rupture in the canine. *Vet Clin North Am Small Anim Pract* 1993;**23**:777–795.
139. Montavon PM, Damur DM, Tepic S. Advancement of the tibial tuberosity for the treatment of cranial cruciate deficient canine stifle. Proceedings of the 1st World Orthopaedic Veterinary Congress; Munich Germany, 2002;152.
140. Lafaver S, Miller NA, Stubbs WP, *et al.* Tibial tuberosity advancement for stabilization of the canine cranial cruciate ligament-deficient stifle joint: surgical technique, early results, and complications in 101 dogs. *Vet Surg* 2007;**36**:573–586.
141. Smith GK, Gregor TP, Rhodes WH, *et al.* Coxofemoral joint laxity from distraction radiography and its contemporaneous and prospective correlation with laxity, subjective score, and evidence of degenerative joint disease from conventional hip-extended radiography in dogs. *Am J Vet Res* 1993;**54**:1021–1042.
142. Smith GK, Popovitch CA, Gregor TP, *et al.* Evaluation of risk factors for degenerative joint disease associated with hip dysplasia in dogs. *J Am Vet Med Assoc* 1995;**206**:642–647.
143. Smith GK, Mayhew PD, Kapatkin AS, *et al.* Evaluation of risk factors for degenerative joint disease associated with hip dysplasia in German Shepherd Dogs, Golden Retrievers, Labrador Retrievers, and Rottweilers. *J Am Vet Med Assoc* 2001;**219**:1719–1724.
144. Samoy Y, Van Ryssen B, Gielen I, *et al.* Elbow incongruity in the dog: review of the literature. *Vet Comp Orthop Traumatol* 2006;**19**:1–8.
145. Evans RB, Gordon-Evans WJ, Conzemius MG. Comparison of three methods for the management of fragmented media coronoid process in the dog. A systematic review and meta-analysis. *Vet Comp Orthop Traumatol* 2008;**21**:106–109.
146. Morgan JP, Wind A. Osteochoondroses, hip dysplasia, elbow dysplasia. In: *Hereditary Bone and Joint Diseases in the Dog*. Schlütersche GmbH & Co., Hanover, 1999, p41–94.

CHAPTER 3

1. Vertosick FT. *Why we hurt: the natural history of pain*. Harcourt, Inc., New York, 2000.
2. Merskey H, Bogduk N (eds) *Classification of Chronic Pain*, 2nd ed. IASP Press, Seattle, 1994.
3. Ventafridda V, Caracen A. Cancer pain classification: a controversial issue. *Pain* 1991;**46**:1–2.
4. Caraceni A, Weinstein S. Classification of cancer pain syndromes. *Oncology (Williston Park)* 2001;**15**:1627–1640.
5. Twycross R. Cancer pain classification. *Acta Anaesthesiol Scand* 1997;**41**:141–145.
6. Verstappen C, Heimans J, Hoekman K, *et al.* Neurotoxic complications of chemotherapy in patients with cancer: clinical signs and optimal management. *Drugs* 2003;**63**:1549–1563.
7. Portenoy R. Cancer pain: pathophysiology and syndromes. *Lancet* 1992;**339**:1026–1031.
8. Stute P, Soukup J, Menzel M. Analysis and treatment of different types of neuropathic cancer pain. *J Pain Symptom Manage* 2003;**26**:1123–1131.
9. Portenoy R, Foley K, Intumisi C. The nature of opioid responsiveness and its implications for neuropathic pain: new hypotheses derived from studies of opioid infusions. *Pain* 1990;**43**:273–286.
10. Chong M, Bajwa Z. Diagnosis and treatment of neuropathic pain. *J Pain Symptom Manage* 2003;**25**:S4–S11.
11. Caraceni A, Zecca E, Martini C, *et al.* Gabapentin as an adjuvant to opioid analgesia for neuropathic cancer pain. *J Pain Symptom Manage* 1999;**17**:441–445.
12. Martin L, Hagen N. Neuropathic pain in cancer patients: mechanism, syndromes, and clinical controversies. *J Pain Symptom Manage* 1997;**14**:99–117.
13. Tasker R. The problem of deafferentation pain in the management of the patient with cancer. *J Palliat Care* 1987;**2**:8–12.
14. England J, Happel L, Kline D, *et al.* Sodium channel accumulation in humans with painful neuromas. *Neurology* 1996;**47**:272–276.

15. Ashby M, Fleming B, Brooksbank M, *et al.* Description of a mechanistic approach to pain management in advanced cancer. Preliminary report. *Pain* 1992;**51**:153–161.
16. World Health Organization. *Cancer Pain Relief.* World Health Organization, Geneva, 1986.
17. Dorn CR, Taylor DON, Frye FL, *et al.* Survey of animal neoplasms in Alameda and Contra Costa Counties, California. 1. Methodology and description of cases. *J Natl Cancer Inst* 1968;**40**:295–305.
18. Bronson RT. Variation in age at death of dogs of different sexes and breeds. *Am J Vet Res* 1982;**43**:2057–2059.
19. Reif JS. The epidemiology and incidence of cancer. In: Withrow SJ, Vail DM (eds) *Small Animal Clinical Oncology*. Saunders Elsevier, St Louis, Missouri, 2007.
20. Larue F, Colleau SM, Breasseur L, *et al.* Multicenter study of cancer pain and its treatment in France. *Br Med J* 1995;**310**:1034–1037.
21. Wagner G. Frequency of pain in patients with cancer. *Recent Results Cancer Res* 1984;**89**:64–71.
22. Capner CA, Lascelles BD, Waterman-Pearson AE. Current British veterinary attitudes to perioperative analgesia for dogs. *Vet Rec* 1999;**145**:95–99.
23. Dohoo SE, Dohoo IR. Postoperative use of analgesics in dogs and cats by Canadian veterinarians. *Can Vet J* 1996;**37**:546–551.
24. Portenoy RK, Lesage P. Management of cancer pain. *Lancet* 1999;**353**:1695–1700.
25. Lascelles BDX. Relief of chronic cancer pain. In: Dobson JM, Lascelles BDX (eds) *BSAVA Manual of Canine and Feline Oncology*. BSAVA, Quedgeley, Gloucester, 2003, p137–151.
26. Miguel RV. Initial approach to the patient with cancer pain. In: de Leon-Casasola OA (ed) *Cancer Pain: Pharmacology, Interventional and Palliative Care Approaches*. W.B. Saunders, Philadelphia, 2006, p26.
27. Yazbek KVB, Fantoni DT. Validity of a health-related quality-of-life scale for dogs with signs of pain secondary to cancer. *J Am Vet Med Assoc* 2005;**226**:1354–1358.
28. Conzemius MG, Hill CM, Sammarco JL, *et al.* Correlation between subjective and objective measures used to determine severity of postoperative pain in dogs. *J Am Vet Med Assoc* 1997;**210**:1619–1622.
29. Fox SM, Mellor DJ, Lawoko CRO, *et al.* Changes in plasma cortisol concentrations in bitches in response to different combinations of halothane and butorphanol, with or without ovariohysterectomy. *Res Vet Sci* 1998;**65**:125–133.
30. Fox SM, Mellor DJ, Stafford, KJ, *et al.* The effects of ovariohysterectomy plus different combinations of halothane anaesthesia and butorphanol analgesia on behaviour in the bitch. *Res Vet Sci* 2000;**68**:265–274.
31. Hardie EM, Hansen BD, Carroll GS. Behavior after ovariohysterectomy in the dog: what's normal? *Appl Anim Behav Sci* 1997;**51**:111–128.
32. Hunt SP, Mantyh PW. The molecular dynamics of pain control. *Nat Rev Neurosci* 2001;**2**:83–91.
33. Hunt SP, Pini A, Evan G. Induction of c-fos-like protein in spinal cord neurons following sensory stimulation. *Nature* 1987;**328**:632–634.
34. Dubois RN, Radhika A, Reddy BS, *et al.* Increased cyclooxygenase-2 levels in carcinogen-induced rat colonic tumors. *Gastroenterology* 1996;**110**:1259–1262.
35. Kundu N, Yang QY, Dorsey R, *et al.* Increased cyclooxygenase-2 (COX-2) expression and activity in a murine model of metastatic breast cancer. *Int J Cancer* 2001;**93**:681–686.
36. Masferrer JL, Leahy KM, Koki AT, *et al.* Antiangiogenic and antitumor activities of cyclooxygenase-2 inhibitors. *Cancer Res* 2000;**60**:1306–1311.
37. Moore BC, Simmons DL. COX-2 inhibition, apoptosis, and chemoprevention by non-steroidal anti-inflammatory drugs. *Curr Med Chem* 2000;**7**:1131–1144.
38. Dempke W, Rie C, Grothey A, *et al.* Cyclooxygenase-2: a novel target for cancer chemotherapy? *J Cancer Res Clin Oncol* 2001;**127**:411–417.
39. Khan KN, Knapp DW, Denicola DB, *et al.* Expression of cyclooxygenase-2 in transitional cell carcinoma of the urinary bladder in dogs. *Am J Vet Res* 2000;**61**:478–481.
40. Khan KN, Stanfield KM, Trajkovic D, *et al.* Expression of cyclooxygenase-2 in canine renal cell carcinoma. *Vet Pathol* 2001;**38**:116–119.
41. Pestili de Almeida EM, Piché C, Sirois J, *et al.* Expression of cyclo-oxygenase-2 in naturally occurring squamous cell carcinomas in dogs. *J Histochem Cytochem* 2001;**49**:867–875.
42. Tremblay C, Doré M, Bochsler PN, *et al.* Induction of prostaglandin G/H synthase-2 in a canine model of spontaneous prostatic adenocarcinoma. *J Natl Cancer Inst* 1999;**91**:1398–1403.
43. McEntee MF, Cates JM, Neilsen N. Cyclooxygenase-2 expression in spontaneous intestinal neoplasia of domestic dogs. *Vet Pathol* 2002;**39**:428–436.
44. Borzacchiello G, Paciello O, Papparella S. Expression of cyclooxygenase-1 and -2 in canine nasal carcinomas. *J Comp Path* 2004;**131**:70–76.

45. Mullins MN, Lana SE, Dernell WS, *et al.* Cyclooxygenase-2 expression in canine appendicular osteosarcoma. *J Vet Intern Med* 2004;**18**:859–865.
46. Heller DA, Clifford CA, Goldschmidt MH, *et al.* Cycloxygenase-2 expression is associated with histologic tumor type in canine mammary carcinoma. *Vet Pathol* 2005;**42**:776–780.
47. Mohammed SI, Khan KNM, Sellers RS, *et al.* Expression of cyclooxygenase-1 and 2 in naturally-occuring canine cancer. *Prostaglandins Leukot Essent Fatty Acids* 2004;**70**:479–483.
48. Beam SL, Rassnick KM, Moore AS, *et al.* An immunohistochemical study of cyclooxygenase-2 expression in various feline neoplasms. *Vet Pathol* 2003;**40**:496–500.
49. Pomonis JD, Rogers SD, Peters CM, *et al.* Expression and localization of endothelin receptors: Implications for the involvement of peripheral glia in nociception. *J Neurosci* 2001;**21**:999–1006.
50. Kurbel S, Kurbel B, Kovacic D, *et al.* Endothelin-secreting tumors and the idea of the pseudoectopic hormone secretion in tumors. *Med Hypotheses* 1999;**52**:329–333.
51. Nelson JB, Hedican SP, George DJ, *et al.* Identification of endothelin-1 in the pathophysiology of metastatic adenocarcinoma of the prostate. *Nat Med* 1995;**1**:944–999.
52. Julius D, Basbaum AL. Molecular mechanisms of nociception. *Nature* 2001;**413**:203–210.
53. Delaisse J-M, Vales G. Mechanism of mineral solubilization and matrix degradation in osteoclastic bone resorption. In: Rifkin BR, Gay CV (eds) *Biology and Physiology of the Osteoclast*. CRC, Ann Arbor, 1992.
54. Honore P, Menning PM, Rogers SD, *et al.* Neurochemical plasticity in persistent inflammatory pain. *Prog Brain Res* 2000;**129**:357–363.
55. Mannix K, Ahmedazai SH, Anderson H, *et al.* Using bisphosphonates to control the pain of bone metastases: evidence-based guidelines for palliative care. *Palliat Med* 2000;**14**:455–461.
56. Honore P, Rogers SD, Schwei MJ, *et al.* Murine models of inflammatory, neuropathic and cancer pain each generates a unique set of neurochemical changes in the spinal cord and sensory neurons. *Neuroscience* 2000;**98**:585–598.
57. Koltzenburg M. The changing sensitivity in the life of the nociceptor. *Pain* 1999;Suppl 6:S93–102.
58. Boucher TJ, McMahon SB. Neurotrophic factors and neuropathic pain. *Curr Opin Pharmacol* 2001;**1**:66–72.
59. Schwei MJ, Honore P, Rogers SD, *et al.* Neurochemical and cellular reorganization of the spinal cord in a murine model of bone cancer pain. *J Neurosci* 1999;**19**:10886–10897.
60. Ripamonti C, Dickerson ED. Strategies for the treatment of cancer pain in the new millennium. *Drugs* 2001;**61**:955–977.
61. Honore P, Schwei J, Rogers SD, *et al.* Cellular and neurochemical remodeling of the spinal cord in bone cancer pain. *Prog Brain Res* 2000;**129**:389–397.
62. Patrick DL, Ferketich SL, Frame PS, *et al.* National Institutes of Health State-of-the-Science Conference Statement: Symptom management in cancer: Pain, depression, and fatigue, July 15–17, 2002. *J Natl Cancer Inst* 2003;**95**:1110–1117.
63. Quasthoff S, Hartung H. Chemotherapy-induced peripheral neuropathy. *J Neurol* 2002;**249**:9–17.
64. Mangioni C, Bolis G, Pecorelli S, *et al.* Randomized trial in advanced ovarian cancer comparing cisplatin and carboplatin. *J Natl Cancer Inst* 1989;**81**: 1464–1471.
65. Rowinsky EK, Donehower RC. Paclitaxel (taxol). *N Engl J Med* 1995;**332**:1004–1014.
66. Verweij J, Clavel M, Chevalier B. Paclitaxel (Taxol™) and docetaxel (Taxotere™): not simply two of a kind. *Ann Oncol* 1994;**5**:495–505.
67. Harmers FPT, Gispen WH, Neijt JP. Neurotoxic side-effects of cisplatin. *Eur J Cancer* 1991;**27**:372–376.
68. Gurney H, Crowther D, Anderson H, *et al.* Five year follow-up and dose delivery analysis of cisplatin, iproplatin or carbopolatin in combination with cyclophosphamide in advanced ovarian carcinoma. *Ann Oncol* 1990;**1**:427–433.
69. Swenerton K, Jeffrey J, Stuart G, *et al.* Cisplatin-cyclophosphamide versus carboplatin-cyclophosphamide in advanced ovarian cancer: a randomized phase III study of the National Cancer Institute of Canada Clinical Trials Group. *J Clin Oncol* 1992;**10**:718–726.
70. Forman AD. Peripheral neuropathy in cancer patients: clinical types, etiology, and presentation. Part 2. *Oncology (Williston Park)* 1990;**4**:85–89.
71. Tuxen MK, Hansen SW. Neurotoxicity secondary to antineoplastic drugs. *Cancer Treat Rev* 1994;**20**:191–214.
72. McBride WH, Withers HR. Biological basis of radiation therapy. In: Perez CA (ed) *Principles and Practice of Radiation Oncology*. Lippincott, Philadelphia, 2002, p96–136.
73. Kerr JF, Winterford CM, Harmon BV. Apoptosis: Its significance in cancer and cancer therapy. *Cancer* 1994;**73**:2013–2026.

74. Azinovic I, Calvo FA, Puebla F, *et al.* Long-term normal tissue effects of intraoperative electron radiation therapy (IOERT): late sequelae, tumor recurrence, and second malignancies. *Int J Radiat Oncol Biol Phys* 2001;**49**:597–604.
75. Carsten RE, Hellyer PW, Bachand AM, *et al.* Correlations between acute radiation scores and pain scores in canine radiation patients with cancer of the forelimb. *Vet Anaesth Analg* 2008;**35**: 355–362.
76. Weil AB, Ko J, Inoue T. The use of lidocaine patches. *Compend Contin Educ Vet* 2007;**29**(4):208–215.
77. Robertson SA, Lascelles BDX, Taylor PM, *et al.* PK-PD modeling of buprenorphine in cats: intravenous and oral transmucosal administration. *J Vet Pharmacol Ther* 2005;**28**:453–460.
78. Carroll GL, Howe LB, Slater MR, *et al.* Evaluation of analgesia provided by postoperative administration of butorphanol to cats undergoing onychectomy. *J Am Vet Med Assoc* 1998;**213**:246–250.
79. Carroll GL, Howe, LB, Peterson KD. Analgesic efficacy of preoperative administration of meloxicam or butorphanol in onychectomized cats. *J Am Vet Med Assoc* 2005;**226**:913–919.
80. Franks JN, Boothe HW, Taylor L, *et al.* Evaluation of transdermal fentanyl patches for analgesia in cats undergoing onychectomy. *J Am Vet Med Assoc* 2000;**217**:1013–1020.
81. Glerum LE, Egger CM, Allen SW, *et al.* Analgesic effect of the transdermal fentanyl patch during and after feline ovariohysterectomy. *Vet Surg* 2001;**30**:351–358.
82. Lascelles BDX, Court MH, Hardie EM, *et al.* Nonsteroidal anti-inflammatory drugs in cats: a review. *Vet Anaesth Analg* 2007;**34**:228–250.
83. DeWys WD, Begg C, Lavin PT, *et al.* Prognostic effect of weight loss prior to chemotherapy in cancer patients. Eastern Cooperative Oncology Group. *Am J Med* 1980;**69**:491–497.
84. Langer CJ, Hoffman JP, Ottery FD. Clinical significance of weight loss in cancer patients: rationale for the use of anabolic agents in the treatment of cancer-related cachexia. *Nutrition* 2001;**17** (1 Suppl):S1–20.
85. Michel KE, Sorenmo K, Shofer FS. Evaluation of body condition and weight loss in dogs presented to a veterinary oncology service. *J Vet Intern Med* 2004;**18**:692–695.
86. Mauldin GE. Nutritional management of the cancer patient. In: Withrow SJ, Vail DM (eds) *Small Animal Clinical Oncology*, 4th ed. Saunders/Elsevier, St Louis, Missouri, 2007.
87. Lagoni L. Bond-centered cancer care: an applied approach to euthanasia and grief support for your clients, your staff, and yourself. In: Withrow SJ, Vail DM (eds) *Small Animal Clinical Oncology*, 4th ed. Saunders/Elsevier, St Louis, Missouri, 2007.

CHAPTER 4

1. Martin M, Matifas A, Maldonado R, *et al.* Acute antinociceptive responses in single and combinatorial opioid receptor knockout mice: distinct mu, delta and kappa tones. *Eur J Neurosci* 2003;**17**:701–708.
2. Pfeiffer A, Pasi A, Meraein P, *et al.* Opiate receptor binding sites in human brain. *Brain Res* 1982;**248**:87–96.
3. Dourish CT, Hawley D, Iversen SD. Enhancement of morphine analgesia and prevention of morphine tolerance in the rat by cholecystokinin antagonist L-364, 718. *Eur J Pharmacol* 1988;**147**:469–472.
4. Jordan B, Devi LA. Molecular mechanisms of opioid receptor signal transduction. *Br J Anaesth* 1998;**81**:12–19.
5. Jadad AR, Carroll D, Glynn CJ, *et al.* Morphine responsiveness of chronic pain: double-blind randomized crossover study with patient controlled analgesia. *Lancet* 1992;**339**:1367–1371.
6. Robertson SA, Hauptan JG, Nachreiner RF, *et al.* Effects of acetylpromazine or morphine on urine production in halothane-anesthetized dogs. *Am J Vet Res* 2001;**62**:1922–1927.
7. Chu LF, Clark DJ, Angst MS. Opioid tolerance and hyperalgesia in chronic pain patients after one month of oral morphine therapy: a preliminary prospective study. *J Pain* 2006;**7**:43–48.
8. Mercadante S, Ferrera P, Villari P, *et al.* Hyperalgesia: an emerging iatrogenic syndrome. *J Pain Symptom Manage* 3003;**26**:769–775.
9. Gardell LR, Wang R, Burgess SE, *et al.* Sustained morphine exposure induces a spinal dynorphin-dependent enhancement of excitatory transmitter release from primary afferent fibers. *J Neurosci* 2002;**22**:6747–6755.
10. Ossipov MH, Lai J, King T, *et al.* Antinociceptive and nociceptive actions of opioids. *J Neurobiol* 2004;**61**:126–148.
11. King T, Vardanyan A, Majuta L, *et al.* Morphine treatment accelerates sarcoma-induced bone pain, bone loss, and spontaneous fracture in a murine model of bone cancer. *Pain* 2007;**132**:154–168.
12. Kukanich B, Lascelles BD, Aman AM, *et al.* The effects of inhibiting cytochrome P450 3A, p-glycoprotein, and gastric acid secretion on the oral

bioavailability of methadone in dogs. *J Vet Pharmacol Ther* 2005;**28**:461–466.
13. Kukanich B, Lascelles BD, Papich MG. Pharmacokinetics of morphine and plasma concentrations of morphine-6-glucuronide following morphine administration to dogs. *J Vet Pharmacol Ther* 2005;**28**:371–376.
14. Hansen B. How to prevent and relieve patient pain. *Vet Forum* 1996;**8**:34–39.
15. Barnhart MD, Hubbell JAE, Muir WW, *et al.* Pharmacokinetics, pharmacodynamics, and analgesic effects of morphine after rectal, intramuscular, and intravenous administration in dogs. *Am J Vet Res* 2000;**61**:24–28.
16. Egger CM, Duke T, Archer J, *et al.* Comparison of plasma fentanyl concentrations by using three transdermal fentanyl patch sizes in dogs. *Vet Surg* 1998;**27**(2):159–166.
17. Kyles AE, Papich M, Hardie EM. Disposition of transdermally administered fentanyl in dogs. *Am J Vet Res* 1996;**57**:715–719.
18. Scherk-Nixon M. A study of the use of a transdermal fentanyl patch in cats. *J Am Anim Hosp Assoc* 1996;**32**:19–24.
19. Lee DD, Papich MG, Hardie EM. Pharmacokinetics of intravenously and transdermally administered fentanyl in cats (abstr). In Proceedings of the ACVS Symposium 1998:15.
20. Boden BP, Fassler S, Cooper S, *et al.* Analgesic effect of intraarticular morphine, bupivacaine, and morphine/bupivacine after arthroscopic knee surgery. *Arthroscopy* 1994;**10**:104–107.
21. Raffa RB, Friderichs E, Reimann W, *et al.* Opioid and nonopioid components independently contribute to the mechanism of action of tramadol, an 'atypical' opioid analgesic. *J Pharmacol Exp Ther* 1992;**260**:275–285.
22. Bianchi M, Broggini M, Balzarini P, *et al.* Effects of tramadol on synovial fluid concentrations of substance P and interleukin-6 in patients with knee osteoarthritis: comparison with paracetamol. *Int Immunopharmacol* 2003;**3**:1901–1908.
23. Wu WN, McKown LA, Gauthler AD, *et al.* Metabolism of the analgesic drug, tramadol hydrochloride, in rat and dog. *Xenobiotica* 2001;**31**:423–441.
24. Kukanich B, Papich MG. Pharmacokinetics of tramadol and the metabolite O-desmethyltramadol in dogs. *J Vet Pharmacol Ther* 2004;**27**:239–246.
25. Pypendop BH, Ilkiw JE. Pharmacokinetics of tramadol and O-desmethyltramadol in cats. *J Vet Pharmacol Ther* 2007;**31**:52–59.
26. Armstrong PJ, Bersten A. Normeperidine toxicity. *Anesth Analg* 1986;**65**(5):536–538.
27. Robertson SA, Lascelles BDX, Taylor PM, *et al.* PK-PD modeling of buprenorphine in cats: intravenous and oral transmucosal administration. *J Vet Pharmacol Ther* 2005;**28**:453–460.
28. Caraco Y, Sheller J, Wood AJ. Pharmacogenetic determination of the effects of codeine and prediction of drug interactions. *J Pharmacol Exp Ther* 1996;**278**(3):1165–1174.
29. Webb, AR, Leong S, Myles PS, *et al.* The addition of a tramadol infusion to morphine patient-controlled analgesia after abdominal surgery: a double-blinded, placebo-controlled randomized trial. *Anesth Analg* 2002;**95**:1713–1718.
30. Tuncer S, Pirbudak L, Balat O, *et al.* Adding ketoprofen to intravenous patient-controlled analgesia with tramadol after major gynecological cancer surgery: a double-blinded, randomized, placebo-controlled clinical trial. *Eur J Gynaecol Oncol* 2003;**24**:181–184.
31. Sindrup SH, Andersen G, Madsen C, *et al.* Tramadol relieves pain and allodynia in polyneuropathy: a randomized, double-blind, controlled trial. *Pain* 1999;**83**(1):85–90.
32. Virtanen R. Pharmacologic profiles of medetomidine and its antagonist, antipamezole. *Acta Vet Scand* (Suppl) 1989;**85**:29–37.
33. Duke T, Cox AM, Remedios AM, *et al.* The cardiopulmonary effects of placing fentanyl or medetomidine in the lumbosacral epidural space of isoflurane-anesthetized cats. *Vet Surg* 1994;**23**:149–155.
34. Pan H-L, Chen S-R, Eisenach JC. Intrathecal clonidine alleviates allodynia in neuropathic rats: interaction with spinal muscarinic and nicotinic receptors. *Anesthesiology* 1999;**90**:509–514.
35. Schwinn DA. Adrenoceptors as models for G protein-coupled receptors: structure, function and regulation. *Br J Anaesth* 1993;**71**:77–85.
36. Aantaa R, Marjamäki A, Scheinin M. Molecular pharmacology of 2-adrenoceptor subtypes. *Ann Med* 1995;**27**:439–449.
37. Grimm IKA, Lemke KA. Preanesthetics and anesthetic adjuncts. In: Thurman JC, Tranquilli WJ (eds) *Lumb & Jones' Veterinary Anesthesia and Analgesia*, 4th ed. Blackwell Publishing, Ames, 2007.
38. Dworkin RH, Backonja M, Rowbotham MC, *et al.* Advances in neuropathic pain: diagnosis, mechanisms, and treatment recommendations. *Arch Neurol* 2003;**60**:1524–1534.

39. Devor M, Wall PD, Catalan N. Systemic lidocaine silences ectopic neuroma and DRG discharge without blocking nerve conduction. *Pain* 1992;**48**:261–268.
40. Biella G, Sotgiu ML. Central effects of systemic lidocaine mediated by glycine spinal receptors: an iontophoretic study in the rat spinal cord. *Brain Res* 1993;**603**:201–206.
41. Chabal C, Jacobson L, Mariano A, *et al.* The use of oral mexiletine for the treatment of pain after peripheral nerve injury. *Anesthesiology* 1992;**76**:513–517.
42. Koppert W, Weigand M, Neumann F, *et al.* Perioperative intravenous lidocaine has preventive effects on postoperative pain and morphine consumption after major abdominal surgery. *Anesth Analg* 2004;**98**:1050–1055.
43. Insler SR, O'Conner RM, Samonte AF, *et al.* Lidocaine and the inhibition of postoperative pain in coronary artery bypass patients. *J Cardiothorac Vasc Anesth* 1995;**9**:541–546.
44. Birch K, Jørgensen J, Chraemmer-Jørgensen B, *et al.* Effect of i.v. lignocaine on pain and the endocrine metabolic responses after surgery. *Br J Anaesth* 1987;**59**:721–724.
45. Cassuto J, Wallin G, Högstr M S, *et al.* Inhibition of postoperative pain by continuous low-dose intravenous infusion of lidocaine. *Anesth Analg* 1985;**64**:971–974.
46. Sjøgren P, Banning AM, Hebsgaard K, *et al.* [Intravenous lidocaine in the treatment of chronic pain caused by bone metastases.] *Ugeskr Laeger* 1989;**151**:2144–2146.
47. Elleman K, Sjögren P, Banning AM, *et al.* Trial of intravenous lidocaine on painful neuropathy in cancer patients. *Clin J Pain* 1989;**5**:291–294.
48. Nagaro T, Shimizu C, Inoue H, *et al.* [The efficacy of intravenous lidocaine on various types of neuropathic pain.] *Masui* 1995;**44**:862–867.
49. Tanelian DL, Brose WG. Neuropathic pain can be relieved by drugs that are use-dependent sodium channel blockers: lidocaine, carbamazepine, and mexiletine. *Anesthesiology* 1991;**74**:949–951.
50. Ferrante FM, Paggioli J, Cherukuri S, *et al.* The analgesic response to intravenous lidocaine in the treatment of neuropathic pain. *Anesth Analg* 1996;**82**:91–97.
51. Wallace MS, Dyck JB, Rossi SS, *et al.* Computer-controlled lidocaine infusion for the evaluation of neuropathic pain after peripheral nerve injury. *Pain* 1996;**66**:69–77.
52. Galer BS, Miller KV, Rowbotham MC. Response to intravenous lidocaine infusion differs based on clinical diagnosis and site of nervous system injury. *Neurology* 1993;**43**:1233–1235.
53. Edmondson SA, Simpson RK Jr, Stubler DK, *et al.* Systemic lidocaine therapy for poststroke pain. *South Med J* 1993;**86**:1093–1096.
54. Rowbotham MC, Reisner-Keller LA, Fields HL. Both intravenous lidocaine and morphine reduce the pain of postherpetic neuralgia. *Neurology* 1991;**41**:1024–1028.
55. Sörensen J, Bengtsson A, Bäckman E, *et al.* Pain analysis in patients with fibromyalgia. Effects of intravenous morphine, lidocaine, and ketamine. *Scand J Rheumatol* 1995;**24**:360–365.
56. Bach FW, Jensen TS, Kastrup J, *et al.* The effect of intravenous lidocaine on nociceptive processing in diabetic neuropathy. *Pain* 1990;**40**:29–34.
57. Ackerman WE 3rd, Colclough GW, Juneja MM, *et al.* The management of oral mexiletine and intravenous lidocaine to treat chronic painful symmetrical distal diabetic neuropathy. *J Ky Med Assoc* 1991;**89**:500–501.
58. McGeeney BE. Anticonvulsants. In: de Leon-Casasola OA (ed) *Cancer Pain: Pharmacological, Interventional and Palliative Care Approaches.* Saunders Elsevier, Philadelphia, 2006.
59. Raymond SA, Steffensen SC, Gugino LD, *et al.* The role of length of nerve exposed to local anesthetics in impulse blocking action. *Anesth Analg* 1989;**68**:563–570.
60. Campoy L, Martin-Flores M, Looney AL, *et al.* Distribution of a lidocaine-methylene blue solution staining in brachial plexus, lumbar plexus and sciatic nerve blocks in the dog. *Vet Anaesth Analg* 2008;**35**:348–354.
61. Chabal C, Russell LC, Burchiel K. The effect of intravenous lidocaine, tocainide, and mexiletine on spontaneously active fibers arising in rat sciatic nerve neuromas. *Pain* 1989;**38**:333–338.
62. Devers A, Galer BS. Topical lidocaine patch relieves a variety of neuropathic pain conditions: an open label study. *Clin J Pain* 2000;**16**:205–208.
63. Paoli F, Darcourt G, Cossa P. Note preliminaire sur l'action de l'imipramine dans les états douloureux. *Rev Neurol (Paris)* 1960;**102**:503–504.
64. Hansson PT, Fields HL, Hill RG, *et al.* *Neuropathic Pain: Pathophysiology and Treatment.* IASP Press, Seattle, 2001, p169–183.
65. Hall H, Ögren S-O. Effects of antidepressant drugs on different receptors in the brain. *Eur J Pharmacol* 1981;**70**:393–407.
66. Nelson KA, Park KM, Robinovitz E, *et al.* High-dose oral dextromethorphan versus placebo in painful

diabetic neuropathy and postherpetic neuralgia. *Neurology* 1997;**48**:1212–1218.

67. Sato J, Perl ER. Adrenergic excitation of cutaneous pain receptors induced by peripheral nerve injury. *Science* 1991;**251**:1608–1611.
68. Pancrazio JJ, Kamatchi GL, Roscoe AK, *et al.* Inhibition of neuronal Na^+ channels by antidepressant drugs. *J Pharmacol Exp Ther* 1998;**284**:208–214.
69. Sindrup SH, Jensen TS. Efficacy of pharmacological treatments of neuropathic pain: an update and effect related to mechanism of drug action. *Pain* 1999;**83**:389–400.
70. Sindrup SH, Brosen K, Gram LF. The mechanism of action of antidepressants in pain treatment: controlled cross-over studies in diabetic neuropathy. *Clinical Neuropharmacology* 1992;**15**(suppl 1 part A):380A-381A.
71. Max M, Culnane M, Schafer S, et. al. Amitriptyline relieves diabetic neuropathy pain in patients with normal or depressed mood. *Neurology* 1987;**37**:589-596
72. Sudoh Y, Cahoon EE, Gerner P, et. al. Tricyclic antidepressants as long-acting local anesthetics. *Pain* 2003;**103**:49-55
73. Lesch KP, Wolozin BL, Murphy DL, et. al. Primary structure of the human platelet serotonin uptake site: identity with the brain serotonin transporter. *J Neurochem* 1993;**60**:2319-2322.
74. Skop BP, Brown TM. Potential vascular and bleeding complications of treatment with selective serotonin reuptake inhibitors. *Psychosomatics* 1996;**37**:12-16.
75. De Abajo FJ, Montero D, Garcia Rodriguez LA, et. al. Antidepressants and risk of upper gastrointestinal bleeding. *Basic & Clinical Pharmacology & Toxicology* 2006;**98**:304-310.
76. Martesson B, Wagner A, Beck O, et. al. Effects of clomipramine treatment on cerebrospinal fluid monoamine metabolites and platelet 3H-imipramine binding and serotonin uptake and concentration in major depressive disorder. *Acta psychiat scand 1991*;**83**:125-133.
77. White HS. Comparative anticonvulsant and mechanistic profile of the established and newer antiepileptic drugs. *Epilepsia* 1999;**40**(Suppl 5):S2–10.
78. Tremont-Lukats IW, Megeff C, Backonja MM. Anticonvulsants for neuropathic pain syndromes: mechanisms of action and place in therapy. *Drugs* 2001;**60**:1029–1052.
79. Fields HL, Rowbotham MC, Devor M. Excitability blockers: anticonvulsants and low concentration local anesthetics in the treatment of chronic pain. In: Dickenson AH, Besson JM (eds) *Handbook of Experimental Pharmacology*. Springer-Verlag, Berlin, 1997.
80. Taylor CP, Gee NS, Su TZ, *et al.* A summary of mechanistic hypotheses of gabapentin pharmacology. *Epilepsy Res* 1998;**29**:233–249.
81. Rock DM, Kelly KM, Macdonald RL. Gabapentin actions on ligand- and voltage-gated responses in cultured rodent neurons. *Epilepsy Res* 1993;**16**: 89–98.
82. Shimoyama N, Shimoyama M, Davis AM, *et al.* Spinal gabapentin is antinociceptive in the rat formalin test. *Neurosci Lett* 1997;**222**:65–67.
83. Field MJ, Oles RJ, Lewis AS, *et al.* Gabapentin (Neurontin) and S-(+)-3-isobutylgaba represent a novel class of selective antihyperalgesic agents. *Br J Pharmacol* 1997;**121**:1513–1522.
84. Houghton AK, Lu Y, Westlund KN. S-(+)-3-Isobutylgaba and its stereoisomer reduces the amount of inflammation and hyperalgesia in an acute arthritis model in the rat. *J Pharmacol Exp Ther* 1988;**285**: 533–538.
85. Lu L, Westlund KN. Gabapentin attenuates nociceptive behaviors in an acute arthritis model in rats. *J Pharm Exp Ther* 1999;**290**:214–219.
86. Woolf CJ, Thompson SWN. The induction and maintenance of central sensitization is dependent on N-methyl-D-aspartic acid receptor activation; implications for the treatment of post-injury pain hypersensitivity states. *Pain* 1991;**44**:293–299.
87. Dambisya YM, Lee TL. Antinociceptive effects of ketamine-opioid combinations in the mouse tail flick test. *Methods Find Exp Clin Pharmacol* 1994;**16**:179–184.
88. Field MJ, Holloman EF, McCleary S, *et al.* Evaluation of gabapentin and S-(+)-isobutylgaba in a rat model of postoperative pain. *J Pharmacol Exp Ther* 1997;**282**: 1242–1246.
89. Hanesch U, Pawlak M, McDougall JJ. Gabapentin reduces the mechanosensitivity of fine afferent nerve fibres in normal and inflamed rat knee joints. *Pain* 2003;**104**:363–366.
90. Ivanavicius SP, Ball AD, Heapy CG, *et al.* Structural pathology in a rodent model of osteoarthritis is associated with neuropathic pain: Increased expression of ATF-3 and pharmacological characterization. *Pain* 2007;**128**:272–282.
91. Maneuf YP, Hughes J, McKnight AT. Gabapentin inhibits the substance P-facilitated K(+)-evoked release of [(3)H]glutamate from rat caudal trigeminal nucleus slices. *Pain* 2001;**93**:191–196.

92. Boileau C, Martel-Pelletier J, Brunet J, *et al.* Oral treatment with PD-0200347, an alpha2delta ligand, reduces the development of experimental osteoarthritis by inhibiting metalloproteinases and inducible nitric oxide synthase gene expression and synthesis in cartilage chondrocytes. *Arthritis Rheum* 2005;**52**:488–500.
93. Boel A, Fransson KE, Peck JK, *et al.* Transdermal absorption of a liposome encapsulated formulation of lidocaine following topical administration in cats. *Am J Vet Res* 2002;**63**(9):1309–1312.
94. Beydoun A, Uthman BM, Sackellares C. Gabapentin: pharmacokinetics, efficacy and safety. *Clin Neuropharmacol* 1995;**18**:469–481.
95. Mather LE, Edwards SR. Chirality in anaesthesia – ropivacaine, ketamine and thiopentone. *Curr Opin Anaesthesiol* 1998;**11**:383–390.
96. Scheller M, Bufler J, Hertle I, *et al.* Ketamine blocks currents through mammalian nicotinic acetylcholine receptor channels by interaction with both the open and the closed state. *Anesth Analg* 1996;**83**:830–836.
97. Hirota K, Lambert DG. Ketamine: its mechanism(s) of action and unusual clinical uses. *Br J Anaesth* 1996;**77**:441–444.
98. Tverskoy M, Yuval O, Isakson A, *et al.* Preemptive effect of fentanyl and ketamine on postoperative pain and wound hyperalgesia. *Anaesth Analg* 1994;**78**:1–5.
99. Slingsby LS, Waterman-Pearson AE. The post-operative analgesic effects of ketamine after canine ovariohysterectomy – a comparison between pre- or post-operative administration. *Res Vet Sci* 2000;**69**:147–152.
100. Van Pragg H. The role of glutamate in opiate descending inhibition of nociceptive spinal reflexes. *Brain Res* 1990;**524**:101–105.
101. Backonja M, Arndt G, Gombar KA, *et al.* Response of chronic neuropathic pain syndromes to ketamine: a preliminary study. *Pain* 1994;**56**:51–57.
102. Eide PK, Stubhaug A, Øye I, *et al.* Continuous subcutaneous administration of the N-methyl-D-aspartic acid (NMDA) receptor antagonist ketamine in the treatment of post-herpetic neuralgia. *Pain* 1995;**61**:221–228.
103. Hoffmann V, Copperjans H, Vercauteren M, *et al.* Successful treatment of postherpetic neuralgia with oral ketamine. *Clin J Pain* 1994;**10**:240–242.
104. Eisenberg E, Pud D. Can patients with chronic neuropathic pain be cured by acute administration of the NMDA receptor antagonist amantadine? *Pain* 1998;**74**:337–339.
105. Pud D, Eisenberg E, Spitzer A, *et al.* The NMDA receptor antagonist amantadine reduces surgical neuropathic pain in cancer patients: a double blind, randomized, placebo controlled trial. *Pain* 1998;**75**:349–354.
106. Kleinbohl D, Gortelmeyer R, Bender HJ, *et al.* Amantadine sulfate reduces experimental sensitization and pain in chronic back pain patients. *Anesth Analg* 2006;**102**:840–847.
107. Lascelles BDX, Gaynor JS, Smith SC, *et al.* Amantadine in a multimodal analgesic regimen for alleviation of refractory osteoarthritis pain in dogs. *J Vet Intern Med* 2008;**22**:53–59.
108. Lascelles BDX, Gaynor JS. Cancer Patients. In: Tranquilli WJ, Thurmon JC, Grimm KA (eds) *Lumb & Jones Veterinary Anesthesia and Analgesia*, 4th ed. Blackwell Publishing, Ames, 2007.
109. Enarson MC, Hays H, Woodroffe MA. Clinical experience with oral ketamine. *J Pain Symptom Manage* 1999;**17**:384–386.
110. Kukanich B, Papich MG. Plasma profile and pharmacokinetics of dextromethorphan after intravenous and oral administration in healthy dogs. *J Vet Pharmacol Therap* 2004;**27**:337–341.

CHAPTER 5

1. Wallace JL, Keenan CM, Gale D, *et al.* Exacerbation of experimental colitis by nonsteroidal anti-inflammatory drugs is not related to elevated leukotriene B4 synthesis. *Gastroenterology* 1992;**102**(1):18–27.
2. Martel-Pelletier J, Mineau F, Fahmi H, *et al.* Regulation of the expression of 5-lipoxygenase-activating protein/5-lipoxygenase and the synthesis of leukotrienes B_4 in osteoarthritic chondrocytes. *Arthritis Rheum* 2004;**50**: 3925-3933.
3. Lascelles BDX, Blikslager AT, Fox SM, *et al.* Gastrointestinal tract perforations in dogs treated with a selective cyclooxygenase-2 inhibitor: 29 cases (2002–2003). *J Am Vet Med Assoc* 2005;**227**(7):1112–1117.
4. Dow SW, Rosychuk RA, McChesney AE, *et al.* Effects of flunixin and flunixin plus prednisone on the gastrointestinal tract of dogs. *Am J Vet Res* 1990;**51**:1131–1138.
5. Boston SE, Moens NM, Kruth SA, *et al.* Endoscopic evaluation of the gastroduodenal mucosa to determine the safety of short-term concurrent administration of meloxicam and dexamethasone in healthy dogs. *Am J Vet Res* 2003;**64**:1369–1375.
6. De Leon-Casasola OA (ed) *Cancer Pain. Pharmacologic, Interventional, and Palliative Approaches.* W. B. Saunders, Philadelphia, 2006, p284.
7. Hemler M, Lands WE. Purification of the cyclooxygenase that forms prostaglandins.

Demonstration of two forms of iron in the holoenzyme. *J Biol Chem* 1976;**251**:5575–5579.

8. Vane JR, Botting RM. A better understanding of anti-inflammatory drugs based on isoforms of cyclooxygenase (COX-1 and COX-2). *Adv Prostaglandin Thromboxane Leukot Res* 1995;**23**:41–48.
9. Warner TD, Mitchell JA. Cyclooxygenases: new forms, new inhibitors, and lessons from the clinic. *FASEB J* 2004;**18**:790–804.
10. Kay-Mungerford P, Benn SJ, LaMarre J, *et al.* In vitro effects of nonsteroidal anti-inflammatory drugs on cyclooxygenase activity in dogs. *Am J Vet Res* 2000;**61**:802–810.
11. Brideau C, Van Staden C, Chan CC. In vitro effects of cyclooxygenase inhibitors in whole blood of horses, dogs, and cats. *Am J Vet Res* 2001;**62**: 1755–1760.
12. Streppa HK, Jones CJ, Budsberg SC. Cyclooxygenase selectivity of nonsteroidal anti-inflammatory drugs in canine blood. *Am J Vet Res* 2002;**63**:91–94.
13. Li J, Lynch MP, Demello KL, *et al.* In vitro and in vivo profile of 2-(3-di-fluoromethyl-5-phenylpyrazol-1-yl)-5-methanesulfonylpyridine, a potent, selective, and orally active canine COX-2 inhibitor. *Bioorg Med Chem* 2005;**13**:1805–1809.
14. Warner TD, Mitchell JA. Cyclooxygenase-3 (COX-3): filling in the gaps toward a COX continuum? *Proc Natl Acad Sci USA* 2002;**99**:13371–13373.
15. Singh G, Fort JG Goldstein JL, *et al.* Celecoxib versus naproxen and diclofenac in osteoarthritis patients: SUCCESS-I Study. *Am J Med* 2006;**119**:255–266.
16. Liu SK, Tilley LP, Tappe JP, *et al.* Clinical and pathologic findings in dogs with atherosclerosis: 21 cases (1970–1983). *J Am Vet Med Assoc* 1986;**189**(2):227–232.
17. Trepanier LA. Idiosyncratic toxicity associated with potentiated sulfonamides in the dog. *J Vet Pharmacol Ther* 2004;**27**:129–138.
18. Tegeder I, Pfeilschifter J, Geisslinger G. Cyclooxygenase-independent actions of cyclooxygenase inhibitors. *FASEB J* 2001;**15**:2057–2072.
19. Kopp E, Ghosh S. Inhibition of NF-kappa B by sodium salicylate and aspirin. *Science* 1994;**265**:956–959.
20. Zingarelli B, Sheehan M, Wong HR. Nuclear factor-kappaB as a therapeutic target in critical care medicine. *Crit Care Med* 2003;**31**(Suppl):S105–S111.
21. Almawi WY, Melemedjian OK. Negative regulation of nuclear factor-kappaB activation and function by glucocorticoids. *J Mol Endocrinol* 2002;**28**:69–78.
22. Heidrich JE, *et al.* Unpublished, 2008.
23. Hampshire VA, Doddy FM, Post LO, *et al.* Adverse drug event reports at the United States Food and Drug Administration Center for Veterinary Medicine. *J Am Vet Med Assoc* 2004;**225**:533–536.
24. Menguy R, Masters YF. Effect of cortisone on mucoprotein secretion by gastric antrum of dogs: pathogenesis of steroid ulcer. *Surgery* 1963;**54**:19–28.
25. Sessions JK, Reynolds LR, Budsberg SC. In vivo effects of carprofen, deracoxib, and etodolac on prostanoid production in blood, gastric mucosa, and synovial fluid in dogs with chronic osteoarthritis. *Am J Vet Res* 2005;**66**:812–817.
26. Jones CJ, Streppa Hk, Harmon BG, *et al.* In vivo effects of meloxicam and aspirin on blood, gastric mucosal, and synovial fluid prostanoid synthesis in dogs. *Am J Vet Res* 2002;**63**:1527–1531.
27. Agnello KA, Reynolods LR, Budsberg SC. In vivo effects of tepoxalin, an inhibitor of cyclooxygenase and lipoxygenase, on prostanoid and leukotriene production in dogs with chronic osteoarthritis. *Am J Vet Res* 2005;**66**:966–972.
28. Wooten JG, Blikslager AT, Ryan KA, *et al.* Cyclooxygenase expression and prostanoid production in pyloric and duodenal mucosae in dogs after administration of nonsteroidal anti-inflammatory drugs. *Am J Vet Res* 2008;**69**:457–464.
29. Brainard BM, Meredith CP, Callan MB, et al. Changes in platelet function, hemostasis, and prostaglandin expression after treatment with nonsteroidal anti-inflammatory drugs with various cyclooxygenase selectivities in dogs. *AJVR* 2007; **68(3)**: 251–257
30. Blikslager AT, Zimmel DN, Young KM, *et al.* Recovery of ischaemic injured porcine ileum: evidence for a contributory role of COX-1 and COX-2. *Gut* 2002;50:615–623.
31. Punke JP, Reynolds LR, Speas AL, *et al.* Early in vivo effects of firocoxib, tepoxalin and meloxicam on blood and gastric and duodenal prostaglandin synthesis in dogs with osteoarthritis. (Poster presentation). ACVS Annual Meeting 2007, Chicago.
32. Deracoxib: 3 Year Adverse Drug Event Report. Data on file: Novartis Animal Health US.
33. Cheng HF, Harris RC. Renal effects of non-steroidal anti-inflammatory drugs and selective cyclooxygenase-2 inhibitors. *Curr Pharm Des* 2005;**11**:1795–1804.
34. Cohen HJ, Marsh DJ, Kayser B. Autoregulation in vasa recta of the rat kidney. *Am J Physiol* 1983;**245**:F32–F40.
35. Nantel F, Meadows E, Denis D, *et al.* Immunolocalization of cyclooxygenase-2 in the macula densa of human elderly. *FEBS Lett* 1999;**457**:474–477.

36. Schnermann J, Briggs P. The macula densa is worth its salt. *J Clin Invest* 1999;**104**:1007–1009.
37. Pages JP. Nephropathies dues aux anti-inflammatores non steroidiens (AINS) chez le Chat: 21 observations (1993–2001). *Prat Med Chir Anim Comp* 2005;**40**:177–181.
38. Harvey JW, Kaneko JJ. Oxidation of human and animal haemoglogins with ascorbate, acetylphenylhydrazine, nitrite, and hydrogen peroxide. *Br J Haematol* 1976;**32**:193–203.
39. Fox SM, Gorman MP. New study findings and clinical experiences enhance understanding of Rimadyl (carprofen). Pfizer Animal Health Technical Bulletin, August 1998.
40. Boelsterli UA, Zimmerman HJ, Kretz-Rommel A. Idiosyncratic liver toxicity of nonsteroidal antiinflammatory drugs: molecular mechanisms and pathology. *Crit Rev Toxicol* 1995;**25**:207–235.
41. Boelsterli UA. Xenobiotic acyl glucuronides and acyl CoA thioesters as protein-reactive metabolites with the potential to cause idiosyncratic drug reactions. *Curr Drug Metab* 2002;**3**:439–450.
42. Bailey MJ, Dickinson RG. Acyl glucuronide reactivity in perspective: biological consequences. *Chem Biol Interact* 2003;**145**:117–137.
43. Dahl G, Dahlinger L, Ekenved G, *et al.* The effect of buffering of acetylsalicylic acid on dissolution, absorption, gastric pH and faecal blood loss. *Int J Pharm* 1982;**10**:143–151.
44. Phillips BM. Aspirin-induced gastrointestinal microbleeding in dogs. *Toxicol Appl Pharmacol* 1973;**24**:182–189.
45. Singh G, Triadafilopoulos G. Epidemiology of NSAID-induced GI complications. *J Rheumatol* 1999;**26**(Suppl):18–24.
46. Morton DJ, Knottenbelt DC. Pharmacokinetics of aspirin and its application in canine veterinary medicine. *J S Afr Vet Assoc* 1989;**60**(4):191–194.
47. Price AH, Fletcher M. Mechanisms of NSAID-induced gastroenteropathy. *Drugs* 1990;**40**(Suppl 5):1–11.
48. Christoni A, Lapressa F. Richerche farmalologiche sull asspirinia. *Arch Farmarol* 1909;**8**:63. Cited by Ghross M, Greenburg LA. *The Salicylates.* Hillhouse Press, New Haven, CT, 1948.
49. Boulay JP, Lipowitz AJ, Klausner JS. The effect of cimetidine on aspirin-induced gastric hemorrhage in dogs. *Am J Vet Res* 1986;**47**:1744–1746.
50. Hurley JW, Crandall LA. The effects of salicylates upon the stomachs of dogs. *Gastroenterology* 1964;**46**:36–43.
51. Taylor LA, Crawford LM. Aspirin-induced gastrointestinal lesions in dogs. *J Am Vet Med Assoc* 1968;**152**(6):617–619.
52. Lipowitz AJ, Boulay JP, Klausner JS. Serum salicylate concentrations and endosopic evaluation of the gastric mucosa in dogs after oral administration of aspirin-containing products. *Am J Vet Res* 1986;**47**(7):1586–1589.
53. Nap RC, Breen DJ, Lam TJGM, *et al.* Gastric retention of enteric-coated aspirin tablets in beagle dogs. *J Vet Pharmacol Ther* 1990;**13**:148–153.
54. Kotob F, Lema MJ. Nonopioid Analgesics. In: de Leon-Casasola OA (ed) *Cancer Pain: Pharmacological, Interventional and Palliative Care Approaches.* Saunders / Elsevier, Philadelphia, 2006, p284.
55. Wallace JL, Fiorucci S. A magic bullet for mucosal protection...and aspirin is the trigger! *Trends Pharmacol Sci* 2003;**24**(7):323–326.
56. Dowers KL, Uhrig SR, Mama KR, *et al.* Effect of short-term sequential administration of nonsteroidal anti-inflammatory drugs on the stomach and proximal portion of the duodenum in healthy dogs. *Am J Vet Res* 2006;**67**(10):1794–1801.
57. Williams JT. The painless synergism of aspirin and opium. *Nature* 1997;**390**:557–559.
58. Lee A, Cooper MC, Craig JC, *et al.* Effects of nonsteroidal anti-inflammatory drugs on postoperative renal function in adults with normal renal function. *Cochrane Database Syst Rev* (2):CD002765, 2004.
59. Radi ZA, Khan NK. Review: effects of cyclooxygenase inhibition on bone, tendon, and ligament healing. *Inflamm Res* 2005;**54**:358–366.
60. Clark TP, Chieffo C, Huhn JC, *et al.* The steady-stage pharmacokinetics and bioequivalence of carprofen administered orally and subcutaneously in dogs. *J Vet Pharmacol Ther* 2003;**26**:187–192.
61. Quinn MM, Keuler NS, Lu Y, *et al.* Evaluation of agreement between numerical rating scales, visual analogue scoring scales, and force plate gait analysis in dogs. *Vet Surg* 2007;**36**:360–367.
62. Millis DL. A Multimodal approach to treating osteoarthritis. 2006 Western Veterinary Conference Symposium Proceedings.
63. Franks JN, Boothe HW, Taylor L, *et al.* Evaluation of transdermal fentanyl patches for analgesia in cats undergoing onychectomy. *J Am Vet Med Assoc* 2000;**217**:1013–1020.
64. Lascelles BDX, Hansen BD, Thomson A, *et al.* Evaluation of a digitally integrated accelerometer-based activity monitor for the measurement of activity in cats. *Vet Anaesth Analg* 2008;**35**:173–183.
65. Trepanier LA. Potential interactions between non-steroidal anti-inflammatory drugs and other drugs. *J Vet Emerg Crit Care* 2005;**15**(4):248–253.

66. Goodman L, Trepanier L. Potential drug interactions with dietary supplements. *Compendium (SAP)* 2005;October:780–789.
67. Rostom A, Dube C, Lewin G, *et al.* Nonsteroidal anti-inflammatory drugs and cyclooxygenase-2 inhibitors for primary prevention of colorectal cancer: a systematic review prepared for the US Preventive Services Task Force. *Ann Intern Med* 2007;**146**:376–389.
68. Page GG, Blakely WP, Ben-Eliyahu S. Evidence that postoperative pain is a mediator of the tumor-promoting effects of surgery in rats. *Pain* 2001;**90**(1–2):191–199.
69. Zweifel BS, Davis TW, Ornberg RL, *et al.* Direct evidence for a role of cyclooxygenase-2-derived prostaglandin E2 in human head and neck xenograft tumors. *Cancer Res* 2002;**62**:6706–6711.
70. Rüegg C, Dormond O. Suppression of tumor angiogenesis by nonsteroidal anti-inflammatory drugs: a new function for old drugs. *ScientificWorldJournal* 2001;**1**:808–811.
71. Ohno R, Yoshinaga K, Fujita T, *et al.* Depth of invasion parallels increased cyclooxygenase-2 levels in patients with gastric carcinoma. *Cancer* 2001;**91**:1876–1881.
72. Boria PA, Biolsi SA, Greenberg CB, *et al.* Preliminary evaluation of deracoxib in canine transitional cell carcinoma of the urinary bladder. *Vet Cancer Soc Proc* 2003;17.
73. Wise JK, Heathcott BL, Gonzales ML. Results of the AVMA survey on companion animal ownership in US pet-owning households. *J Am Vet Med Assoc* 2002;**221**:1572–1573.
74. Lascelles BDX, Court MH, Hardie EM, *et al.* Nonsteroidal anti-inflammatory drugs in cats: a review. *Vet Anaesth Analg* 2007;**34**:228–250.
75. Hardie EM, Roe SC, Martin FR. Radiographic evidence of degenerative joint disease in geriatric cats: 100 cases (1994–1997). *J Am Vet Med Assoc* 2002;**220**:628–632.
76. Court MH, Greenblatt DJ. Molecular genetic basis for deficient acetaminophen glucuronidation by cats: UGT1A6 is a pseudogene, and evidence for reduced diversity of expressed hepatic UGT1A isoforms. *Pharmacogenetics* 2000;**10**:355–369.
77. Savides M, Oehme F, Nash S, *et al.* The toxicity and biotransformation of single doses of acetaminophen in dogs and cats. *Toxicol Appl Pharmacol* 1984;**74**:26–34.
78. Dittert LW, Caldwell HC, Ellison T, *et al.* Carbonate ester prodrugs of salicylic acid. Synthesis, solubility characteristics, in vitro enzymatic hydrolysis rates, and blood levels of total salicylate following oral administration to dogs. *J Pharm Sci* 1968;**57**:828–831.
79. Parton K, Balmer TV, Boyle J, *et al.* The pharmacokinetics and effects of intravenously administered carprofen and salicylate on gastrointestinal mucosa and selected biochemical measurements in healthy cats. *J Vet Pharmacol Ther* 2000;**23**:73–79.
80. Davis LE, Westfall BA. Species differences in biotransformation and excretion of salicylate. *Am J Vet Res* 1972;**33**:1253–1262.
81. Clark TP, Chieffo C, Huhn JC, *et al.* The steady-state pharmacokinetics and bioequivalence of carprofen administered orally and subcutaneously in dogs. *J Vet Pharmacol Ther* 2003;**26**:187–192.
82. Taylor PM, Delatour P, Landoni FM, *et al.* Pharmacodynamics and enantioselectivity pharmacokinetics of carprofen in the cat. *Res Vet Sci* 1996;**60**:144–151.
83. Hardie EM, Hardee GE, Rawlings CA. Pharmacokinetics of flunixin meglumine in dogs. *Am J Vet Res* 1985;**46**:235–237.
84. Lees P, Taylor PM. Pharmacodynamics and pharmacokinetics of flunixin in the cat. *Br Vet J* 1991;**147**:298–305.
85. Horii Y, Ikenaga M, Shimoda M, *et al.* Pharmacokinetics of flunixin in the cat: enterohepatic circulation and active transport mechanism in the liver. *J Vet Pharmacol Ther* 2004;**27**:65–69.
86. Montoya L, Ambros L, Kreil V, *et al.* A pharmacokinetic comparison of meloxicam and ketoprofen following oral administration to healthy dogs. *Vet Res Commun* 2004;**28**:415–428.
87. Lees P, Taylor PM, Landoni FM, *et al.* Ketoprofen in the cat: pharmacodynamics and chiral pharmacokinetics. *Vet J* 2003;**165**:21-35.
88. Castro E, Soraci A, Fogel F, *et al.* Chiral inversion of R(–) fenoprofen and ketoprofen enantiomers in cats. *J Vet Pharmacol Ther* 2000;**23**:265–271.
89. Busch U, Schmid J, Heinzel G, *et al.* Pharmacokinetics of meloxicam in animals and the relevance to humans. *Drug Metab Dispos* 1998;**26**:576–584.
90. Galbraith EA, McKellar QA. Pharmacokinetics and pharmacodynamics of piroxicam in dogs. *Vet Rec* 1991;**128**:561–565.
91. Heeb HL, Chun R, Koch DE, *et al.* Single dose pharmacokinetics of piroxicam in cats. *J Vet Pharmacol Ther* 2003;**26**:259–263.

CHAPTER 6

1. Animal Pharm Report. Nutraceuticals for companion animals. October (2005); www.animalpharmreports.com
2. Consumer Reports January 2002: p18.
3. Diplock AT, Charleux JL, Crozier-Willi G, *et al.* Functional food science and defence against reactive oxidative species. *Br J Nutr* 1998;**80**(Suppl 1):S77–S112.
4. Lascelles BDX, Blikslager AT, Fox SM, *et al.* Gastrointestinal tract perforations in dogs treated with a selective cyclooxygenase-2 inhibitor: 29 cases (2002–2003). *J Am Vet Med Assoc* 2005;**227**(7):1112–1117.
5. Dingle JT. The effect of nonsteroidal anti-inflammatory drugs on human articular cartilage glycosaminoglycan synthesis. *Osteoarthritis Cartilage* 1999;**7**:313–314.
6. Goldring MB. The role of the chondrocyte in osteoarthritis. *Arthritis Rheum* 2000;**43**:1916–1926.
7. Billinghurst RC, Dahlberg L, Ionescu M, *et al.* Enhanced cleavage of type II collagen by collagenases in osteoarthritic articular cartilage. *J Clin Invest* 1997;**99**:1534–1545.
8. Mengshol JA, Mix KS, Brinckerhoff CE. Matrix metalloproteinases as therapeutic targets in arthritic diseases: bull's-eye or missing the mark? *Arthritis Rheum* 2002;**46**:13–20.
9. Reboul P, Pelletier JP, Tardif G, *et al.* The new collagenase, collagenase 3, is expressed and synthesized by human chondrocytes but not by synovial fibroblasts: a role in osteoarthritis. *J Clin Invest* 1996;**97**:2011–2019.
10. Sandy JD, Verscharen C. Analysis of aggrecan in human knee cartilage and synovial fluid indicates that aggrecanase (ADAMTS) activity is responsible for the catabolic turnover and loss of whole aggrecan whereas other protease activity is required for C-terminal processing in vivo. *Biochem J* 2001;**358**:615–626.
11. Pelletier JP, McCollum R, Cloutier JM, *et al.* Synthesis of metalloproteases and interleukin 6 (IL-6) in human osteoarthritic synovial membrane is an IL-1 mediated process. *J Rheumatol Suppl* 1995;**43**:109–114.
12. Pelletier JP, DiBattista JA, Roughley P, *et al.* Cytokines and inflammation in cartilage degradation. *Rheum Dis Clin North Am* 1993;**19**:545–568.
13. Neil KM, Caron JP, Orth MW. The role of gulcosamine and chondroitin sulfate in treatment for and prevention of osteoarthritis in animals. *J Am Vet Med Assoc* 2005;**226**:1079–1088.
14. Bassleer C, Rovati L, Franchimont P. Stimulation of proteoglycan production by glucosamine sulfate in chondrocytes isolated from human osteoarthritis articular cartilage in vitro. *Osteoarthritis Cartilage* 1998;**6**:427–434.
15. Ronca F, Palmieri L, Panicucci P, *et al.* Anti-inflammatory activity of chondroitin sulfate. *Osteoarthritis Cartilage* 1998;**6**(suppl A):14–21.
16. Adebowale AO, Cox DS, Liang Z, *et al.* Analysis of glucosamine and chondroitin sulfate content in marketed products and the Caco-2 permeability of chondroitin sulfate raw materials. *J Am Nutraceutical Assoc* 2000;**3**:33–44.
17. Volpi N. Oral absorption and bioavailability of ichthyic origin chondroitin sulfate in healthy male volunteers. *Osteoarthritis Cartilage* 2003;**11**:433–441.
18. Volpi N. Oral bioavailability of chondroitin sulfate (Chondrosulf) and its constituents in healthy male volunteers. *Osteoarthritis Cartilage* 2002;**10**:768–777.
19. Liau YH, Horowitz MI. Desulfation and depolymerization of chondroitin-4-sulfate and its degradation products by rat stomach, liver and small intestine. *Proc Soc Exp Biol Med* 1974;**146**:1037–1043.
20. King M. Equine joint treatments and applications. *Vet Prac News* 2007;July:38.
21. Dobenecker B, Beetz Y, Kienzle E. A placebo-controlled double-blind study on the effect of nutraceuticals (chondroitin sulfate and mussel extract) in dogs with joint diseases as perceived by their owners. *J Nutr* 2002;**132**:1690S–1691S.
22. Largo R, Alverez-Soria MA, Diez-Ortego I, *et al.* Glucosamine inhibits IL-1-induced NFB activation in human osteoarthritic chondrocytes. *Osteoarthritis Cartilage* 2003;**11**:290–298.
23. Platt D. The role of oral disease-modifying agents glucosamine and chondroitin sulphate in the management of equine degenerative joint disease. *Equine Vet Educ* 2001;**3**:262–272.
24. Fenton JI, Chlebek-Brown KA, Peters TL, *et al.* The effects of glucosamine derivatives on equine articular cartilage degradation in explant culture. *Osteoarthritis Cartilage* 2000;**8**:444–451.
25. Hoffer LJ, Kaplan LN, Hamadeh MT, *et al.* Sulfate could mediate the therapeutic effect of glucosamine sulfate. *Metabolism* 2001;**50**:767–770.
26. Dodge GR, Hawkins JF, Jimenez SA. Modulation of aggrecan, MMP1 and MMP3 productions by glucosamine sulfate in cultured human osteoarthritis articular chondrocytes. *Arthritis Rheum* 1999;**42S**:253.
27. Basleer C, Rovati L, Franchimont P. Stimulation of proteoglycan production by glucosamine sulfate in chondrocytes isolated from human osteoarthritis articular cartilage in vitro. *Osteoarthritis Cartilage* 1998;**6**:427–434.

28. Abelda SM, Buck CA. Integrins and other cell adhesion molecules. *FASEB J* 1990;**4**:2868–2880.
29. Piperno M, Reboul P, Hellio Le Graverand MP, *et al.* Glucosamine sulfate modulates dysregulated activities of human osteoarthritis chondrodytes in vitro. *Osteoarthritis Cartilage* 2000;**8**:207–212.
30. Rovati LC. Clinical development of glucosamine sulfate as selective drug in osteoarthritis. *Rheumatol Europe* 1997;**26**:70.
31. Houpt JB, McMillan R, Wein C, *et al.* Effect of glucosamine hydrochloride in the treatment of pain of osteoarthritis of the knee. *J Rheumatol* 1999;**26**:2413–2430.
32. Russell AS, Aghazadeh-Habashi A, Jamali F. Active ingredient consistency of commercially available glucosamine sulfate products. *J Rheumatol* 2001;**29**:2407–2409.
33. Persiani S, Rotini R, Trisolino G, *et al.* Synovial and plasma glucosamine concentrations in osteoarthritic patients following oral crystalline glucosamine sulphate at therapeutic dose. *Osteoarthritis Cartilage* 2007;**15**:764–772.
34. Cordoba F, Nimni ME. Chondroitin sulfate and other sulfate containing chondroprotective agents may exhibit their effects by overcoming a deficiency of sulphur amino acids. *Osteoarthritis Cartilage* 2003;**11**:228–230.
35. Piepoli T, Zanelli T, Letari O, *et al.* Glucosamine sulfate inhibits IL1β-stimulated gene expression at concentrations found in humans after oral intake (Abstract). *Arthritis Rheum* 2005;**52**(9 Suppl):1326.
36. Largo R, Alvarez-Soria MA, Díez-Ortego I, *et al.* Glucosamine inhibits IL-1 beta-induced NFkappaB activation in human osteoarthritic chondrocytes. *Osteoarthritis Cartilage* 2003;**11**:290–298.
37. Bond M, Baker AH, Newby AC. Nuclear factor kappaB activity is essential for matrix metalloproteinase-1 and -3 upregulation in rabbit dermal fibroblasts. *Biochem Biophys Res Commun* 1999;**264**:561–567.
38. Kuroki K, Cook JL, Stoker AM. Evaluation of chondroprotective nutriceuticals in an *in vitro* osteoarthritis model. Poster. 51st Annual Meeting of the Orthopaedic Research Society, 2005.
39. Ramey DW. Skeptical of treatment with glucosamine and chondroitin sulfate. (editorial) *J Am Vet Med Assoc* 2005;**226**:1797–1799.
40. Adebowale A, Du J, Liang Z, *et al.* The bioavailability and pharmacokinetics of glucosamine hydrochloride and low molecular weight chondroitin sulfate after single and multiple doses to beagle dogs. *Biopharm Drug Dispos* 2002;**23**:217–225.
41. McAlindon T. Why are clinical trials of glucosamine no longer uniformly positive? *Rheum Dis Clin North Am* 2003;**29**:789–801.
42. Clegg DO, Reda DJ, Harris CL, *et al.* Glucosamine, chondroitin sulfate, and the two in combination for painful knee osteoarthritis. *New Engl J Med* 2006;**354**:795–808.
43. Hochberg MC. Nutritional supplements for knee osteoarthritis – still no resolution (editorial). *New Engl J Med* 2006;**354**:858–860.
44. Hazewinkel HAW, Frost-Christensen LFN. Disease-modifying drugs in canine osteoarthritis. 13th ESVOT Congress, Munich, 7–10 September 2006:5054.
45. Aragon CL, Hofmeister EH, Budsberg SC. Systematic review of clinical trials of treatments for osteoarthritis in dogs. *J Am Vet Med Assoc* 2007;**230**:514–521.
46. Horstman J. *The Arthritis Foundation's Guide to Alternative Therapies*. The Arthritis Foundation, Atlanta, GA, 1999, p179–180.
47. Henrotin YE, Labasse AH, Jaspar JM, *et al.* Effects of three avocado/soybean unsaponifiable mixtures on metalloproteinases, cytokines and prostaglandin E2 production by human articular chondrocytes. *Clin Rheumatol* 1998;**17**:31–39.
48. Maheu E, Mazieres B, Valat JP, *et al.* Symptomatic efficacy of avacado/soybean unsaponifiables in the treatment of osteoarthritis of the knee and hip. A prospective randomized, double-blind, placebo-controlled multicenter clinical trial with six-month treatment period and a two-month follow-up demonstrating a persistent effect. *Arthritis Rheum* 1998;**41**:81–91.
49. Henrotin YE, Sanchez C, Deberg MA, *et al.* Avocado/soybean unsaponifiables increase aggrecan synthesis and reduce catabolic and proinflammatory mediator production by human osteoarthritic chondrocytes. *J Rheumatol* 2003;**30**:1825–1834.
50. Hilal G, Martel-Pelletier J, Pelletier JP, *et al.* Osteoblast-like cells from human subchondral osteoarthritic bone demonstrate an altered phenotype in vitro: possible role in subchondral bone sclerosis. *Arthritis Rheum* 1998;**41**:891–899.
51. Hilal G, Massicotte F, Martel-Pelletier J, *et al.* Endogenous prostaglandin E2 and insulin-like growth factor 1 can modulate the levels of parathyroid hormone receptor in human osteoarthritic osteoblasts. *J Bone Miner Res* 2001;**16**:713–721.
52. Imhof H, Breitenseher M, Kainberger F, *et al.* Importance of subchondral bone to articular cartilage in health and disease. *Top Magn Reson Imaging* 1999;**10**:180–192.

53. Henrotin YE, Deberg MA, Crielaard J, *et al.* Avocado/soybean unsaponifiables prevent the inhibitory effect of osteoarthritic subchondral osteoblasts on aggrecan and type II collagen synthesis by chondrocytes. *J Rheumatol* 2006;**33**:1668–1678.
54. Kawcak CE, Frisbie DD, McIlwraith W, *et al.* Evaluation of avocado and soybean unsaponifiable extracts for treatment of horses with experimentally induced osteoarthritis. *Am J Vet Res* 2007;**68**:598–604.
55. Altinel L, Saritas ZK, Kose KC, *et al.* Treatment with unsaponifiable extracts of avocado and soybean increases TGF-beta1 and TGF-beta2 levels in canine joint fluid. *Tohoku J Exp Med* 2007;**211**:181–186.
56. Grimaud E, Heymann D, Rédini F. Recent advances in TGF-beta effects on chondrocyte metabolism. Potential therapeutic roles of TGF-beta in cartilage disorders. *Cytokine Growth Factor Rev* 2002;**13**:241–257.
57. Reddy CM, Bhat VB, Kiranmai G, *et al.* Selective inhibition of cyclooxygenase-2 by C-phycocyanin, a biliprotein from *Spirulina platensis. Biochem Biophys Res Comm* 2000;**277**:599–603.
58. Romay C, Ledón N, Gonzalez R. Further studies on anti-inflammatory activity of phycocyanin in some animal models of inflammation. *Inflamm Res* 1998;**47**:334–338.
59. Cherng S, Cheng S, Tarn A, *et al.* Anti-inflammatory activity of c-phycocyanin in lipopolysaccharide-stimulated RAW 264.7 macrophages. *Life Sci* 2007;**81**:1431–1435.
60. Caterson B. Cartilage physiology: unique aspects of canine cartilage. In: Proceedings of the Symposium on Nutritional Management of Chronic Canine Osteoarthritis. North American Veterinary Conference, Orlando FL, 2005.
61. Caterson B, *et al.* The modulation of canine articular cartilage degradation by omega-3 (n-3) polyunsaturated fatty acids. In: Proceedings of the 77th Western Veterinary Conference, Las Vegas, NV, 2005.
62. Wang CT, Lin J, Chang CJ, *et al.* Therapeutic effects of hyaluronic acid on osteoarthritis of the knee. A meta-analysis of randomized controlled trials. *J Bone Joint Surg Am* 2004;**86-A**(3):538–545.
63. Frizziero L, Govoni E, Bacchini P. Intra-articular hyaluronic acid in the treatment of osteoarthritis of the knee: clinical and morphological study. *Clin Exp Rheumatol* 1998;**16**:441–449.
64. Smith MM, Ghosh P. The synthesis of hyaluronic acid by human synovial fibroblasts is influenced by the nature of the hyaluronate in the extracellular environment. *Rheumatol Int* 1987;**7**:113–122.
65. Creamer P, Sharif M, George E, *et al.* Intra-articular hyaluronic acid in osteoarthritis of the knee: an investigation into mechanisms of action. *Osteoarthritis Cartilage* 1994;**2**:133–140.
66. Marshall KW. Intra-articular hyaluronan therapy. *Curr Opin Rheumatol* 2000;**12**:468–474.
67. Takahashi K, Hashimoto S, Kubo T, *et al.* Hyaluronan suppressed nitric oxide production in the meniscus and synovium of rabbit osteoarthritis model. *J Orthop Res* 2001;**19**:500–503.
68. Yasui T, Akatsuka M, Tobetto K, *et al.* The effect of hyaluronan on interleukin-1-alpha in induced prostaglandin E2 production in human osteoarthritic synovial cells. *Agents Actions* 1992;**37**:155–156.
69. DeVane CL. Substance P: a new era, a new role. *Pharmacotherapy* 2001;**21**:1061–1069.
70. Moore AR, Willoughby DA. Hyaluronan as a drug delivery system for diclofenac: a hypothesis for mode of action. *Int J Tissue React* 1995;**17**:153–156.
71. Pozo MA, Balazs EA, Belmonte C. Reduction of sensory responses to passive movements of inflamed knee joints by hylan, a hyaluronan derivative. *Exp Brain Res* 1997;**116**:3–9.
72. Soeken KL, Lee WL, Bausell RB, *et al.* Safety and efficacy of S-adenosylmethionine (SAMe) for osteoarthritis. *J Fam Pract* 2002;**51**:425–430.
73. Konig B. A long-term (two years) clinical trial with S-adenosinemethionine for the treatment of osteoarthritis. *Am J Med* 1987;**83**:78–80.
74. Center SA. S-adenosylmethionine (SAMe): an antioxidant and anti-inflammatory nutraceutical. Proceedings of the 18th American College of Veterinary Internal Medicine Conference. Seattle, WA, 2000, p549–552.
75. Steinmeyer J, Burton-Wurster N. Effects of three antiarthritic drugs on fibronectin and keratin sulfate synthesis by cultured canine articular cartilage chondrocytes. *Am J Vet Res* 1992;**53**:2077–2083.
76. Harmand MF, Jana JV, Maloche E, *et al.* Effects of S-adenosylmethionine on human articular chondrocyte differentiation. *Am J Med* 1987;**83**:48–54.
77. Lippiello L, Prudhomme A. Advantageous use of glucosamine combined with S-adenosylmethionine in veterinary medicine: preservation of articular cartilage in joint disorders. *Int J Appl Res Vet Med* 2005;**3**:6–12.
78. Innes JF, Caterson B, Little CB, *et al.* Effect of omega-3 fatty acids on canine cartilage: using an in vitro model to investigate therapeutic mechanisms. In: Proceedings of the 13th ESVOT Congress, Munich, 7–10 September, 2006.

CHAPTER 7

1. Kehlet H, Dahl JB. The value of 'multimodal' or 'balanced analgesia' in postoperative pain treatment. *Anesth Analg* 1993;77:1048–1056.
2. Penning JP, Yaksh TL. Interaction of intrathecal morphine with bupivacaine and lidocaine in the rat. *Anesthesiology* 1992;77:1186–1200.
3. Grimm KA, Tranquilli WJ, Thurmon JC, *et al.* Duration of nonresponse to noxious stimulation after intramuscular administration of butorphanol, medetomidine, or a butorphanol–medetomidine combination during isoflurane administration in dogs. *Am J Vet Res* 2000;**61**(1):42–47.
4. Skinner HB. Multimodal acute pain management. *Am J Orthop* 2004;**33**:5–9.
5. Rockemann MG, Seeling W, Bischof C, *et al.* Prophylactic use of epidural mepivacaine/morphine, systemic diclofenac, and metamizole reduces postoperative morphine consumption after major abdominal surgery. *Anesthesiology* 1996;**84**:1027–1034.
6. American Pain Society. *Guideline for the management of pain in osteoarthritis, rheumatoid arthritis, and juvenile chronic arthritis. Clin Pract Guide*, 2002, p2.
7. Muir WW, Woolf CJ. Mechanisms of pain and their therapeutic implications. *J Am Vet Med Assoc* 2001;**219**:1346–1356.
8. *An Animated Guide to the Multimodal Management of Canine Osteoarthritis*. Novartis Animal Health USA, Inc., 2007.
9. McQuay HJ, Moore A. NSAIDS and Coxibs: clinical use In: McMahon SB, Koltzenburg M. (eds) *Wall and Melzack's Textbook of Pain*, 5th ed. Elsevier, London, 2006, p474.
10. Kukanich B, Papich MG. Plasma profile and pharmacokinetics of dextromethorphan after intravenous and oral administration in healthy dogs. *J Vet Pharmacol Ther* 2004;**27**:337–341.
11. Skarda RT, Tranquilli WJ. Local Anesthetics. In: Tranquilli WJ, Thurmon JC, Grimm KA, (eds) *Lumb and Jones' Veterinary Anesthesia and Analgesia*, 4th ed. Blackwell, Ames, 2007, p395–419.
12. Feldman HS, Arthur GR, Covino BG. Comparative systemic toxicity of convulsant and supraconvulsant doses of intravenous ropivacaine, bupivacaine, and lidocaine in the conscious dog. *Anesth Analg* 1989;**69**:794–801.
13. Liu PL, Feldman HS, Giasi R, *et al.* Comparative CNS toxicity of lidocaine, etidocaine, bupivacaine, and tetracaine in awake dogs following rapid intravenous administration. *Anesth Analg* 1983;**62**:375–379.
14. Patronek GJ. Assessment of claims of short- and long-term complications associated with onychectomy in cats. *J Am Vet Med Assoc* 2001;**219**:932–937.
15. Cambridge AJ, Tobias KM, Newberry RC, *et al.* Subjective and objective measurements of postoperative pain in cats. *J Am Vet Med Assoc* 2000;**217**:685–690.
16. Tranquilli WJ, Grimm KA, Lamont LA. *Pain Management for the Small Animal Practitioner*, 2nd ed. Teton NewMedia, Jackson, WY, 2004.
17. Curcio K, Bidwell LA, Boohart GV, *et al.* Evaluation of signs of postoperative pain and complications after forelimb onychectomy in cats receiving buprenorphine alone or with bupivacaine administered as a four-point regional nerve block. *J Am Vet Med Assoc* 2006;**228**:65–68.
18. Conzemius MG, Brockman DJ, King LG, *et al.* Analgesia in dogs after intercostal thoracotomy: A clinical trial comparing intravenous buprenorphine and interpleural bupivacaine. *Vet Surg* 1994;**23**:291–298.
19. Dhokarikar P, Caywood DD, Stobie D, *et al.* Effects of intramuscular or interpleural administration of morphine and interpleural administration of bupivacaine on pulmonary function in dogs that have undergone median sternotomy. *Am J Vet Res* 1996;**57**:375–380.
20. Lemke KA, Dawson SD. Local and regional anesthesia. *Vet Clin North Am Small Anim Pract* 2000;**30**(4):839–857.
21. Carpenter RE, Wilson DV, Evans AT. Evaluation of intraperitoneal and incisional lidocaine or bupivacaine for analgesia following ovariohysterectomy in the dog. *Vet Anaesth Analg* 2004;**31**:46–52.
22. Møiniche S, Mikkelsen S, Wetterslev J, *et al.* A systematic review of intra-articular local anesthesia for postoperative pain relief after arthroscopic knee surgery. *Reg Anesth Pain Med* 1999;**24**:430–437.
23. Sammarco JL, Conzemius MG, Perkowski SZ, *et al.* Postoperative analgesia for stifle surgery: a comparison of intra-articular bupivacaine, morphine, or saline. *Vet Surg* 1996;**25**:59–69.
24. Barber FA, Herbert MA. The effectiveness of an anesthetic continuous-infusion device on postoperative pain control. *Arthroscopy* 2002;**18**:76–81.
25. Wolfe TM, Bateman SW, Cole LK. Evaluation of a local anesthetic delivery system for the postoperative analgesic management of canine total ear canal ablation – a randomized, controlled, double-blinded study. *Vet Anaesth Analg* 2006;**33**:328–339.

26. Radlinsky MG, Mason DE, Roush JK, *et al.* Use of a continuous, local infusion of bupivacaine for postoperative analgesia in dogs undergoing total ear canal ablation. *J Am Vet Med Assoc* 2005;**227**:414–419.
27. Davis KM, Hardie EM, Martin FR, *et al.* Correlation between perioperative factors and successful outcome in fibrosarcoma resection in cats. *Vet Rec* 2007;**161**:199–200.
28. Yaksh TL, Rudy TA. Analgesia mediated by a direct spinal action of narcotics. *Science* 1976;**192**:1357–1358.
29. Valverde A, Dyson DH, McDonell WN. Epidural morphine reduces halothane MAC in the dog. *Can J Anaesth* 1989;**36**:629–632.
30. Wetmore LA, Glowaski MM. Epidural analgesia in veterinary critical care. *Clin Tech Small Anim Pract* 2000;**15**:177–188.
31. Robertson SA, Lascelles BDX, Taylor PM, *et al.* Pk-Pd modeling of buprenorphine in cats: intravenous and oral transmucosal administration. *J Vet Pharmacol Ther* 2005;**28**:453–460.
32. World Health Organization. *WHO Traditional Medicine Strategy 2002–2005*. Geneva, World Health Organization, 2002.
33. Bache F. Cases illustrative of the remedial effects of acupuncture. *North Am Med Surg J* 1826;**1**: 311–321.
34. Skarda RT, Glowaski M. Acupuncture. In: Tranquilli WJ, Thurman JC, Grimm KA (eds) *Lumb and Jones' Veterinary Anesthesia and Analgesia*, 4th ed. Blackwell, Ames, 2007, p683–697.
35. Ma Y, Ma M, Cho ZH. *Biomedical Acupuncture for Pain Management: An Integrative Approach*. Elsevier, St. Louis, 2005.
36. Helms JM. *Acupuncture Energetics: A Clinical Approach for Physicians*. Medical Acupuncture Publishers, Berkeley, 1997.
37. Poneranz B, Chiu D. Naloxone blockade of acupuncture analgesia; endorphin implicated. *Life Sci* 1976;**19**:1757–1762.
38. Lee A, Done ML. The use of nonpharmacologic techniques to prevent postoperative nausea and vomiting. A meta-analysis. *Anesth Analg* 1999;**88**:1362–1369.
39. American Cancer Society. *American Cancer Society's Guide to Complementary and Alternative Cancer Methods*. American Cancer Society, Atlanta, 2000.

CHAPTER 8

1. Grimm KA, Tranquilli WJ, Thurmon JC, *et al.* Duration of nonresponse to noxious stimulation after intramuscular administration of butorphanol, medetomidine, or a butorphanol–medetomidine combination during isoflurane administration in dogs. *Am J Vet Res* 2000;**61**(1):42–47.
2. Williams JT. The painless synergism of aspirin and opium. *Nature* 1997;**390**:557–558.
3. Aragon CL, Hofmeister EH, Budsberg SC. Systematic review of clinical trials of treatments for osteoarthritis in dogs. *J Am Vet Med Assoc* 2007;**230**:514–521.
4. Impellizeri JA, Tetrick MA, Muir P. Effect of weight reduction on clinical signs of lameness in dogs with hip osteoarthritis. *J Am Vet Med Assoc* 2000;**216**(7):1089–1091.
5. Kealy RD, Lawler DF, Ballam JM, *et al.* Five-year longitudinal study on limited food consumption and development of osteoarthritis in coxofemoral joints of dogs. *J Am Vet Med Assoc* 1997;**210**(2):222–225.
6. Kealy RD, Lawler DF, Ballam JM, *et al.* Evaluation of the effect of limited food consumption on radiographic evidence of osteoarthritis in dogs. *J Am Vet Med Assoc* 2000;**217**(11):1678–1680.
7. Johnston SA. Osteoarthritis. Joint anatomy, physiology, and pathobiology. *Vet Clin North Am Small Anim Pract* 1997;**27**(4):699–723.
8. Hayek MG, Lepine AJ, Martinez SA, *et al.* Articular Cartilage and Joint Health. Proceedings from a Symposium on March 7, 2000 at the Veterinary Orthopedic Society 27th Annual Conference, Val d' Isere, France.
9. Clinician's update™, Supplement to NAVC Clinician's Brief®. April 2005.
10. Solomon L. Clinical features of osteoarthritis. In: Kelley WN, Ruddy S, Harris EDJ, Sledge C (eds) *Textbook of Rheumatology*, Vol 2. WB Saunders, Philadelphia, 1997, p1383–1408.
11. 1999 Rimadyl A&U Study – USA: 039 DRIM 197. Pfizer Animal Health USA.
12. Lascelles BDX, Blikslager AT, Fox SM, *et al.* Gastrointestinal tract perforations in dogs treated with a selective cyclooxygenase-2 inhibitor: 29 cases (2002–2003). *J Am Vet Med Assoc* 2002;**227**(7):1112–1117.
13. 3-Year Deramaxx Update. Novartis Animal Health USA, Inc. 2007:DER 060058A 35618.
14. Mamdani M, Rochon PA, Juurlink DN, *et al.* Observational study of upper gastrointestinal haemorrhage in elderly patients given selective cyclo-oxygenase-2 inhibitors or conventional

non-steroidal anti-inflammatory drugs. *BMJ* 2002;**325**:624.

15. Liu S, Tilley LP, Tappe JP, Fox PR. Clinical and pathologic findings in dogs with atherosclerosis: 21 cases (1970–1983). *J Am Vet Med Assoc* 1986;**189**(2):227–232.
16. Pharmacovigilance summary: clinical experience with Deramaxx (deracoxib) since its US Launch. Advisor for the Practicing Veterinarian. 2004 (DER 030103A).
17. Lascelles BDX, McFarland JM. *Guidelines for safe and effective use of non-steroidal anti-inflammatory drugs in dogs*. Technical Bulletin, Pfizer Animal Health. November 2004.
18. Dowers KL, Uhrig SR, Mama KR, *et al*. Effect of short-term sequential administration of nonsteroidal anti-inflammatory drugs on the stomach and proximal portion of the duodenum in healthy dogs. *Am J Vet Res* 2006;**67**(10):1794–1801.
19. Henrotin Y. Nutraceuticals in the management of osteoarthritis: an overview. *J Vet Pharmacol Ther* 2006;**29**(Suppl 1):201–210.
20. Henrotin YE, Deberg MA, Crielaard JM, *et al*. Avocado/soybean unsaponifiables prevent the inhibitory effect of osteoarthritic subchondral osteoblasts on aggrecan and Type II collagen synthesis by chondrocytes. *J Rheumatol* 2006;**33**:1668–1678.
21. *Consumer Reports*, January 2002, p19.
22. Animal Pharm Report October 2005 www.animalpharmreports.com.
23. McAlindon TE, La Valley MP, Gulin JP, *et al*. Glucosamine and chondroitin for treatment of osteoarthritis: a systematic quality assessment and meta-analysis. *J Am Med Assoc* 2000;**283**:1469–1475.
24. Clegg DO, Reda DJ, Harris CL, *et al*. Glucosamine, chondroitin sulfate, and the two in combination for painful knee osteoarthritis. *New Engl J Med* 2006;**354**(8):795–808.
25. Adebowale AO, Cox DS, Liang Z, *et al*. Analysis of glucosamine and chondroitin sulfate content in marketed products and the Caco-2 permeability of chondroitin sulfate raw materials. *J Am Nutraceutical Assoc* 2000;**3**:37–44.
26. Russell AS, Aghazadeh-Habashi A, Jamali F. Active ingredient consistency of commercially available glucosamine sulfate products. *J Rheumatol* 2002;**29**:2407–2409.
27. FDA. Available at: www.fda.gov//ohrms/dockets/dailys/04/oct04/101304/04p-0060/pdn0001-yoc.htm as accessed 27 April 2005.
28. Rovati LC. Clinical development of glucosamine sulfate as selective drug in osteoarthritis. *Rheumatol Eur* 1997;**26**:70.
29. Dodge GR, Hawkins JF, Jimenez SA. Modulation of aggrecan, MMP1 and MMP3 productions by glucosamine sulfate in cultured human osteoarthritis articular chondrocytes. *Arthritis Rheum* 1999;**42S**:253.
30. Piperno M, Reboul P, Hellio Le Graverand MP, *et al*. Glucosamine sulfate modulates dysregulated activities of human osteoarthritis chondrocytes in vitro. *Osteoarthritis Cartilage* 2000;**8**:207–212.
31. Neil KM, Caron JP, Orth MW. The role of glucosamine and chondroitin sulfate in treatment for and prevention of osteoarthritis in animals. *J Am Vet Med Assoc* 2006;**226**(7):1079–1088.
32. Cook JL, Anderson CC, Kreeger JM, *et al*. Effects of human recombinant interleukin-1 beta on canine articular chondrocytes in three-dimensional culture. *Am J Vet Res* 2000;**61**:766–770.
33. Tung JT, Fenton JI, Arnold C, *et al*. Recombinant equine interleukin-1 beta induces putative mediators of articular cartilage degradation in equine chondrocytes. *Can J Vet Res* 2002;**66**:19–25.
34. Morris EA, Treadwell BV. Effect of interleukin 1 on articular cartilage from young and aged horses and comparison with metabolism of osteoarthritic cartilage. *Am J Vet Res* 1994;**55**:138–146.
35. Richardson DW, Dodge GR. Effects of interleukin-1 beta and tumor necrosis factor-alpha on expression of matrix-related genes by cultured equine articular chondrocytes. *Am J Vet Res* 2000;**61**:624–630.
36. MacDonald MH, Stover SM, Willits NH, *et al*. Regulation of matrix metabolism in equine cartilage explant cultures by interleukin 1. *Am J Vet Res* 1992;**53**:2278–2285.
37. Platt D, Bayliss MT. An investigation of the proteoglycan metabolism of mature equine articular cartilage and its regulation by interleukin-1. *Equine Vet J* 1994;**26**:297–303.
38. Fenton JL, Chlebek-Brown KA, Caron JP, *et al*. Effect of glucosamine on interleukin-1-conditioned articular cartilage. *Equine Vet J Suppl* 2002;**34**:219–223.
39. Largo R, Alvarez-Soria MA, Diez-Ortego I, *et al*. Glucosamine inhibits IL-1 beta-induced NFkappaB activation in human osteoarthritic chondrocytes. *Osteoarthritis Cartilage* 2003;**11**:290–298.
40. Fenton JL, Chlebek-Brown KA, Peters TL, *et al*. Glucosamine HCl reduces equine articular cartilage degradation in explant culture. *Osteoarthritis Cartilage* 2000;**8**:258–265.
41. Byron CR, Orth MW, Venta PJ, *et al*. Influence of glucosamine on matrix metalloproteinase expression and activity in lipopolysaccharide-stimulated equine chondrocytes. *Am J Vet Res* 2003;**64**:666–671.

42. Sandy JD, Gamett D, Thompson V, *et al.* Chondrocyte-mediated catabolism of aggrecan: aggrecanase-dependent cleavage induced by interleukin-1 or retinoic acid can be inhibited by glucosamine. *Biochem J* 1998;**335**:59–66.
43. Shikhman AR, Kuhn K, Alaaeddine N, *et al.* N-acetylglucosamine prevents IL-1 beta-mediated activation of human chondrocytes. *J Immuol* 2001;**166**:5155–5160.
44. Bassleer C, Rovati L, Franchimont P. Stimulation of proteoglycan production by glucosamine sulfate in chondrocytes isolated from human osteoarthritic articular chartilage in vitro. *Osteoartitis Cartilage* 1998;**6**:427–434.
45. Dodge CR, Jimenez SA. Glucosamine sulfate modulates the levels of aggrecan and matrix metalloproteinase-3 synthesized by cultured human osteoarthritis articular chondrocytes. *Osteoarthritis Cartilage* 2003;**11**:424–432.
46. Gouze JN, Bianchi A, Becuwe P, *et al.* Glucosamine modulates IL-1-induced activation of rat chondrocytes at a receptor level, and by inhibiting the NF-kappa B pathway. *FEBS Lett* 2002;**510**:166–170.
47. Orth MW, Peters TL, Hawkins JN. Inhibition of articular cartilage degradation by glucosamine-HCl and chondroitin sulphate. *Equine Vet J Suppl* 2002;**3**:224–229.
48. Bassleer C, Henrotin Y, Franchimont P. In-vitro evaluation of drugs proposed as chondroprotective agents. *Int J Tissue React* 1992;**14**:231–241.
49. Dechant JE, Baxter GM, Frisbie DD, *et al.* Effects of glucosamine hydrochloride and chondroitin sulphate, alone and in combination, on normal and interleukin-1 conditioned equine articular cartilage explant metabolism. *Equine Vet J* 2005;**37**:227–231.
50. Uebelhart D, Thonar DJ, Delmas PD, *et al.* Effects of oral chondroitin sulfate on the progression of knee osteoarthritis: a pilot study. *Ostoarthritis Cartilage* 1998;**6**(suppl A):37–38.
51. Adebowale A, Du J, Liang Z, *et al.* The bioavailability and pharmacokinetics of glucosamine hydrochloride and low molecular weight chondroitin sulfate after single and multiple doses to beagle dogs. *Biopharm Drug Dispos* 2002;**23**:217–225.
52. Setnikar I, Palumbo R, Canali S, *et al.* Pharmacokinetics of glucosamine in man. *Arzneimittelforschung* 1993;**43**:1109–1113.
53. McAlindon T. Why are clinical trials of glucosamine no longer uniformly positive? *Rheum Dis Clin North Am* 2003;**29**:789–801.
54. Burkhardt D, Ghosh P. Laboratory evaluation of antiarthritic drugs as potential chondroprotective agents. *Semin Arthritis Rheum* 1987;**17**(2 Suppl 1):3–34.
55. Baici A, Salgram P, Fehr K, *et al.* Inhibition of human elastase from polymorphonuclear leukocytes by a glycosaminoglycan polysulfate (Arteparon). *Biochem Pharmacol* 1980;**29**:1723–1727.
56. Stephens RW, Walton EA, Ghosh P, *et al.* A radioassay for proteolytic cleavage of isolated cartilage proteoglycan. 2. Inhibition of human leukocyte elastase and cathepsin G by anti-inflammatory drugs. *Arzneimittelforschung* 1980;**30**:2108–2112.
57. Stanciková M, Trnavsky K, Keilová H. The effect of antirheumatic drugs on collagenolytic activity of cathepsin B1. *Biochem Pharmacol* 1977;**26**:2121–2124.
58. Egg D. Effects of glycosaminoglycan-polysulfate and two nonsteroidal anti-inflammatory drugs on prostaglandin E2 synthesis in Chinese hamster ovary cell cultures. *Pharmacol Res Commun* 1983;**15**:709–717.
59. Nishikawa H, Mori I, Umemoto J. Influences of sulfated glycosaminoglycans on biosynthesis of hyaluronic acid in rabbit knee synovial membrane. *Arch Biochem Biophys* 1985;**240**:146–153.
60. Bianchi M, Broggini M, Balzarini P, *et al.* Effects of tramadol on synovial fluid concentrations of substance P and interleukiin-6 in patients with knee osteoarthritis: comparison with paracetamol. *Int Immunopharmacol* 2003;**3**(13–14):1901–1908.
61. American College of Rheumatology Subcommittee on Osteoarthritis. Recommendations for the medical management of osteoarthriis of the hip and knee. *Arthritis Rheum* 2000;**43**:1905–1915.
62. American Medical Directors Association. *Chronic pain management in the long-term care setting: clinical practice guideline.* American Medical Directors Association, Baltimore, 1999, p1–32.
63. Millis DL. Nonsteroidal anti-inflammatory drugs, disease-modifying drugs, and osteoarthritis. A multimodal approach to treating osteoarthritis: symposium proceedings. Western Veterinary Conference, 2006, Las Vegas.
64. Millis DL, Weigel JP, Moyers T, *et al.* Effect of deracoxib, a new COX-2 inhibitor, on the prevention of lameness induced by chemical synovitis in dogs. *Vet Ther* 2002;**24**:7–18.
65. Vasseur PB, Johnson AL, Budsberg SC, *et al.* Randomized, controlled trial of the efficacy of carprofen, a nonsteroidal anti-inflammatory drug, in the treatment of osteoarthritis in dogs. *J Am Vet Med Assoc* 1995;**206**:807–811.
66. Peterson KD, Keef TJ. Effects of meloxicam on severity of lameness and other clinical signs of osteoarthritis in dogs. *J Am Vet Med Assoc* 2004;**225**:1056–1060.

67. Lust G, Williams AJ, Burton-Wurster N, *et al.* Effects of intramuscular administration of glycosaminoglycan polysulfates on signs of incipient hip dysplasia in growing pups. *Am J Vet Res* 1992;**53**:1836–1843.
68. De Haan JJ, Goring RL, Beale BS. Evaluation of polysulfated glycosaminoglycan for the treatment of hip dysplasia in dogs. *Vet Surg* 1994;**23**:177–181.
69. Sevalla K, Todhunter RJ, Vernier-Singer M, *et al.* Effect of polysulfated glycosaminoglycan on DNA content and proteoglycan metabolism in normal and osteoarthritic canine articular cartilage explants. *Vet Surg* 2000;**29**:407–414.
70. Millis DL, Korvick D, Dean D, *et al.* Proceedings of the 45th Meeting of the Orthopaedic Research Society, 1999, p792.
71. Kukanich B, Papich MG. Pharmacokinetics of tramadol and the metabolite O-desmethyltramadol in dogs. *J Vet Pharmacol Ther* 2004;**27**:239–246.
72. Emkey R, Rosenthal N, Wu SC, *et al.* Efficacy and safety of tramadol/acetaminophen tablets (Ultracet) as add-on therapy for osteoarthritis in subjects receiving a COX-2 nonsteroidal antiinflammatory drug: a multicenter, randomized, double-blind, placebo-controlled trial. *J Rheumatol* 2004;**31**:150–156.
73. Bennett GJ. Update on the neurophysiology of pain transmission and modulation: focus on the NMDA-receptor. *J Pain Symptom Manage* 2000;**19**(1 Suppl):S2–S6.
74. www.hosppract.com 2000 (discontinued).
75. Kealy RD, Lawler DF, Ballam JM, *et al.* Effects of diet restriction on life span and age-related changes in dogs. *J Am Vet Med Assoc* 2002;**220**:1315–1320.
76. Kealy RD, Olsson SE, Monti KL, *et al.* Effects of limited food consumption on the incidence of hip dysplasia in growing dogs. *J Am Vet Med Assoc* 1992;**201**:857–863.
77. Burkholder WJ, Taylor L, Hulse DA. Weight loss to optimal body condition increases ground reaction forces in dogs with osteoarthritis. Purina Research Report, 2000.
78. Johnston SA, Budsberg SC, Marcellin-Little D, *et al.* *Canine Osteoarthritis: Overview, Therapies, & Nutrition*. NAVC Clinician's Brief, April 2005; Supplement.
79. Waldron M. The role of fatty acids in the management of osteoarthritis. *Nestlé Purina Clinical Edge*, October 2004, p14–16.
80. Nutrition plays a key role in joint health. Study finds that proactive nutrition can minimize use of NSAIDs. *Iams Partners for Health*, July 2003;V1, No.3.
81. Laflamme DP. *Fatty Acids in Health and Disease.* Nestlé Purina Research Report 2006;10(2).
82. Bauer JE. Responses of dogs to dietary omega-3 fatty acids. *J Am Vet Med Assoc* 2007;**231**:1657–1661.
83. Innes JF, Caterson B, Little CB, *et al.* Effect of omega-3 fatty acids on canine cartilage: using an in vitro model to investigate therapeutic mechanisms. 13th ESVOT Congress, 2006, Munich.
84. Levine D, Millis DL, Marcellin-Little DM. Introduction to veterinary physical rehabilitation. *Vet Clin North Am Small Anim Pract* 2005;**35**(6):1247–1254, vii.
85. Millis DL, Levine D, Brumlow M, *et al.* A preliminary study of early physical therapy following surgery for cranial cruciate ligament rupture in dogs. Proceedings of the 24th Annual Conference of the Veterinary Orthopaedic Society, 1997, p39.
86. Marcellin-Little D. Multimodal management of osteoarthritis in dogs. Symposium: a multimodal approach to treating osteoarthritis. Western Veterinary Conference, 2007, Las Vegas.
87. Millis DL, Levine D, Taylor RA. *Canine Rehabilitation & Physical Therapy*. WB Saunders, Philadelphia, 2004.

CHAPTER 9

1. Miller N. *Sensory Innervation of the Eye and Orbit*, 4th ed. Williams and Wilkins, Baltimore, 1985.
2. Barrett PM, Scagliotti RH, Merideth RE, *et al.* Absolute corneal sensitivity and corneal trigeminal nerve anatomy in normal dogs. *Vet Comp Ophthalmol* 1991;**1**:245–254.
3. Marfurt CF, Murphy CJ, Florczak JL. Morphology and neurochemistry of canine corneal innervation. *Invest Ophthalmol Vis Sci* 2001;**42**:2242–2251.
4. Moreira LB, Kasetsuwan N, Sanchez D, *et al.* Toxicity of topical anesthetic agents to human keratocytes *in vivo*. *J Cataract Refract Surg* 1999;**25**:975–980.
5. Williamson CH. Topical anesthesia using lidocaine. In: Fine IH, Fichman RA, Grabow HB, (eds) *Clear-Corneal Cataract Surgery and Topical Anesthesia.* Slack, Thorofare, NJ, 1993, p121–128.
6. Maurice DM, Singh T. The absence of corneal toxicity with low-level topical anesthesia. *Am J Ophthalmol* 1985;**99**:691–696.
7. Liu JC, Steinemann TL, McDonald MB, *et al.* Topical bupivacaine and proparacaine: a comparison of toxicity, onset of action, and duration of action. *Cornea* 1993;**12**:228–232.
8. Sun R, Hamilton RC, Gimbel HV. Comparison of 4 topical anesthetic agents for effect and corneal toxicity in rabbits. *J Cataract Refract Surg* 1999;**25**:1232–1236.

9. DiFazio CA, Carron H, Grosslight KR, *et al.* Comparison of pH-adjusted lidocaine solutions for epidural anesthesia. *Anesth Analg* 1986;**65**:760–764.
10. Galindo A. pH-adjusted local anesthetics: clinical experience (abstract). *Reg Anesth* 1983;**8**:35–36.
11. Zagelbaum BM, Tostanoski JR, Hochman MA, *et al.* Topical lidocaine and proparacaine abuse. *Am J Emerg Med* 1994;**12**:96–97.
12. Smith LJ, Bentley E, Shih A, *et al.* Systemic lidocaine infusion as an analgesic for intraocular surgery in dogs: a pilot study. *Vet Anaesth Analg* 2004;**31**:53–63.
13. Boneham GC, Collin HB. Steroid inhibition of limbal blood and lymphatic vascular cell growth. *Curr Eye Res* 1995;**14**:1–10.
14. Musson DG, Bidgood AM, Olejnik O. An in vitro comparison of the permeability of prednisolone, prednisolone sodium phosphate and prenisolone acetate across the NZW rabbit cornea. *J Ocul Pharmacol* 1992;**8**:139–150.
15. Kalina PH, Erie JC, Rosenbaum L. Biochemical quantification of triamcinolone in subconjunctival depots. *Arch Ophthalmol* 1995;**113**:867–869.
16. Spandau UHM, Derse M, Schmitz-Valckenberg P, *et al.* Dosage dependency of intravitreal triamcinolone acetonide as treatment for diabetic macular oedema. *Br J Ophthalmol* 2005;**89**:999–1003.
17. Regnier A. Clinical pharmacology and therapeutics. Part 2: antimicrobials, anti-inflammatory agents, and antiglaucoma drugs. In: Gelatt KN (ed) *Veterinary Ophthalmology*, 4th ed. Blackwell, Ames, IA, 2007, p300.
18. Zhan G-L, Miranda OC, Bito LZ. Steroid glaucoma: Corticosteroid-induced ocular hypertension in cats. *Exp Eye Res* 1992;**54**:211–218.
19. Gelatt KN, Mackay EO. The ocular hypertensive effects of topical 0.1% dexamethasone in beagles with inherited glaucoma. *J Ocul Pharmacol Ther* 1998;**14**:57–66.
20. Millichamp NJ, Dziezyc J. Mediators of ocular inflammation. *Prog Vet Comp Ophthalmol* 1991;**1**:41–58.
21. Sawa M, Masuda K. Topical indomethacin in soft cataract aspiration. *Jpn Ophthalmol* 1976;**20**:514–519.
22. Miyake K. Prevention of cystoid macular edema after lens extraction by topical indomethacin (II): a control study in bilateral extraction. *Jpn Ophthalmol* 1978;**22**:80–94.
23. Keates RH, McGowan KA. The effect of topical indomethacin ophthalmic solution in maintaining mydriasis during cataract surgery. *Ann Ophthalmol* 1984;**16**:1116–1121.
24. Arshinoff S, D'Addario D, Sadler C, *et al.* Use of topical nonsteroidal anti-inflammatory drugs in excimer laser photorefractive keratectomy. *J Cataract Refract Surg* 1994;**20**(Suppl):216–222.
25. Koay P. The emerging roles of non-steroidal anti-inflammatory agents in ophthalmology. *Br J Ophthalmol* 1996;**80**:480–485.
26. Gaynes BI, Fiscella R. Topical non-steroidal anti-inflammatory drugs for ophthalmic use: a safety review. *Drug Saf* 2002;**25**:233–250.
27. Samiy N, Foster CS. The role of non-steroidal anti-inflammatory drugs in ocular inflammation. *Int Ophthalmol Clin* 1996;**36**:195–206.
28. Ward DA. Comparative efficacy of topically applied flurbiprofen, diclofenac, tolmetin, and suprofen for the treatment of experimentally induced blood–aqueous barrier disruption in dogs. *Am J Vet Res* 1996;**57**:875–878.
29. Regnier AM, Dossin O, Cutzach EE, *et al.* Comparative effects of two formulations of indomethacin eyedrops on the paracentesis-induced inflammatory response in the canine eye. *Vet Comp Ophthalmol* 1995;**5**:242–246.
30. Spiess BM, Mathis GA, Franson KL, *et al.* Kinetics of uptake and effects of topical indomethacin application on protein concentration in the aqueous humor of dogs. *Am J Vet Res* 1991;**52**:1159–1163.
31 Gilmour MA, Lehenhauer TW. Comparison of tepoxalin, carprofen, and meloxicam for reducing intraocular inflammation in dogs. *AJVR* 2009; **70**(7):902–907.
32. O'Brien TP, Li QJ, Sauerburger F, *et al.* The role of matrix metalloproteinases in ulcerative keratolysis associated with perioperative diclofenac use. *Ophthalmalogy* 2001;**108**:656–659.
33. Flach AJ. Misuse and abuse of topically applied nonsteroidal anti-inflammatory drugs. (Letter to the Editor.) *Cornea* 2006;**25**:1265–1266.
34. Stiles J, Honda CN, Krohne SG, *et al.* Effect of topical administration of 1% morphine sulfate solution on signs of pain and corneal wound healing in dogs. *Am J Vet Res* 2003;**64**:813–818.
35. Whitley RD, Gilger BC. Diseases of the canine cornea and sclera. In: Gelatt KN (ed) *Veterinary Ophthalmology*, 3rd ed. Lippincott Williams & Wilkins, Baltimore, 1999, p635–673.
36. Szucs PA, Nashed AH, Allegra JR, *et al.* Safety and efficacy of diclofenac ophthalmic solution in the treatment of corneal abrasions. *Ann Emerg Med* 2000;**35**:131–137.
37. Alberti MM, Bouat CG, Allaire CM, *et al.* Combined indomethacin/gentamicin eyedrops to reduce pain after

traumatic corneal abrasion. *Eur J Ophthalmol* 2001;**11**:233–239.
38. Peyman GA, Rahimy MH, Fernandes ML. Effects of morphine on corneal sensitivity and epithelial wound healing: implications for topical ophthalmic analgesia. *Br J Ophthal* 1994;**78**:138–141.
39. Gelatt KN, Brooks DE. The canine glaucomas. In: Gelatt KN (ed) *Veterinary Ophthalmology*, 3rd edn. Lippincott Williams & Wilkins, Baltimore, 1999, p701–754.
40. Foster PJ, Buhrmann R, Quigley HA, *et al.* The definition and classification of glaucoma in prevalence surveys. *Br J Opthalmol* 2002;**86**:238–242.
41. Kavalieratos C, Dimou T. Gabapentin therapy for painful, blind glaucomatous eye: case report. *Pain Med* 2008;**9**:377–378.
42. Nepp J, Jandrasits K, Schauersberger J, *et al.* Is acupuncture a useful tool for pain-treatment in ophthalmology? *Acupunct Electrother Res* 2002;**27**:171–182.
43. Grönlund MA, Stenevi U, Lundeberg T. Acupuncture treatment in patients with keratoconjunctivitis sicca: a pilot study. *Acta Ophthalmol Scand* 2004;**82**:283–290.
44. Gotthelf LN. Primary causes of ear disease. In: Gotthelf LN (ed) *Small Animal Ear Diseases. An Illustrated Guide*, 2nd edn. Elsevier Saunders, St. Louis, 2000, p24.
45. Little CJL, Lane JG, Pearson GR. Inflammatory middle ear disease of the dog: the pathology of otitis media. *Vet Rec* 1991;**128**:293–296.
46. Wolfe TM, Bateman SW, Cole LK, *et al.* Evaluation of a local anesthetic delivery system for the postoperative analgesic management of canine total ear canal ablation – a randomized, controlled, double-blinded study. *Vet Anaesth Analg* 2006;**33**:328–339.
47. Beebe DE, Holmstrom SE. *Complications of Periodontal Therapy*. NAVC Clinician's Brief, 2007 (October), 63–66.
48. Salvi GE, Lang NP. The effects of non-steroidal anti-inflammatory drugs (selective and non-selective) on the treatment of periodontal diseases. *Curr Pharm Des* 2005;**11**:1757–1769.

CASE REPORTS

1. Lascelles BDX, Robertson SA, Gaynor JS. Can chronic pain in cats be managed? Yes! In: *Managing Pain in Cats, Dogs, Small Mammals and Birds*. Proceedings of a symposium held at the North American Veterinary Conference and the American Animal Hospital Association Annual Meeting, 2003.
2. Hardie EM, Lascelles BDX, Gaynor JS. Managing chronic pain in dogs: the next level. In: *Managing Pain in Cats, Dogs, Small Mammals and Birds.* Proceedings of a symposium held at the North American Veterinary Conference and the American Animal Hospital Association Annual Meeting, 2003.

GLOSSARY

1. Cervero F, Laird JM. Mechanism of touch-evoked pain (allodynia): a new model. *Pain* 1996;**68**:13–23.
2. McMahon S, Koltzenburg M. The changing role of primary afferent neurons in pain. *Pain* 1990;**43**:269–272.

GLOSSARY

Aβ fiber afferents: nociceptors can be activated by mechanical stress resulting from direct pressure, tissue deformation or changes in osmolarity. Based upon sensory modality and electrical response, mammalian mechanosensory neurons can be classified into four groups:

- Aα fibers are proprioceptors that detect muscle tension or joint position.
- Aβ fibers include touch receptors that are activated by low pressure.
- Aδ and C fibers are nociceptors that respond to strong mechanical, thermal, electrical or chemical stimulation.

Action potential: the means by which information signals are transmitted in nerves–abrupt pulse-like changes in the membrane potential. An action potential can be elicited in a nerve fiber by almost any factor that suddenly increases the permeability of the membrane to sodium ions, such as electrical stimulation, mechanical compression of the fiber, application of chemicals to the membrane, or almost any other event that disturbs the normal resting state of the membrane.

Adenosine: an endogenous nucleotide that generally serves inhibitory functions and it acts as a depressant in the CNS. It can be progressively phosphorylated to generate the high-energy molecules of adenosine mono-, di-, and triphosphate (AMP, ADP, and ATP), and from ATP, may be further modified to generate the intracellular second-messenger cyclic-AMP (cAMP).

Adjunct: refers to a drug, agent, or therapy that is added to a 'baseline' protocol, e.g. addition of tramadol to an NSAID protocol, or acupuncture added to a drug therapy.

Afferent: incoming, or conducted toward the CNS.

Aggrecan: major proteoglycan of articular cartilage, consisting of the proteoglycan monomer that aggregates with hyaluronan.

Aggrecanase: enzyme that degrades aggrecan.

Agonist (opioid): binds to one or more receptor types and causes certain effects.

Agonist–antagonist (opioid): simultaneously binds to more than one type of receptor, causing an effect at one receptor, but no or a lesser effect at another receptor.

Allodynia: pain due to a stimulus which does not normally provoke pain. A mechanism of touch-evoked pain[1] places the emphasis of a mechanistic model on presynaptic interactions between A and C fibers, with enhancement of the inflammatory response resultant from release of vasoactive peptides (sP and CGRP) from the terminal endings of afferent Aδ and C fibers by antidromic action potentials (neurogenic inflammation or axon reflexes).

Analgesia: absence of pain sensation.

Angiogenesis: the development of blood vessels, e.g. the induction of blood vessel growth from surrounding tissue into a tumor by a diffusible chemical factor released by the tumor cells.

Antagonist (opioid): binds to one or more receptor types, but causes no effect at those receptors–by competitive displacement, reverses the effect of an agonist.

Apoptosis: a process including coagulative necrosis and shrinkage. Programmed cell death as signaled by the nuclei in normally functioning human and animal cells when age or state of cell health and condition dictates. Cells that die by apoptosis do not usually elicit the inflammatory responses that are associated with necrosis, though the reasons are not clear. Cancerous cells, however, are unable to experience the normal cell transduction or apoptosis-driven natural cell death process.

Arachidonic acid pathway: metabolic pathway giving rise to a variety of eicosanoids including prostaglandins from cyclo-oxygenase (COX) and leukotrienes via lipoxygenase (LOX).

Aspirin triggered lipoxin (ATL): 15(R)-epi-LXA_4

- Under normal circumstances PGs produced by COX-1 and COX-2 contribute to many aspects of mucosal defense.
- Aspirin suppresses PG synthesis via both COX-1 and COX-2, thereby impairing mucosal defense and leading to hemorrhagic erosion formation. Aspirin also triggers generation of ATL, which partially counteracts the detrimental effects of PG suppression. ATL is produced via COX-2, but not via COX-1.
- Inhibition of COX-2 activity by any NSAID removes the formation of ATL by aspirin. In the absence of the protective effects of ATL, the extent of gastric damage is likely increased.
- Therefore, the combined use of aspirin together with any other NSAID may accentuate the gastric damage of aspirin.

ASU: avocado/soybean unsaponifiables–a nutraceutical compound.

Biomarkers: specific biochemicals in the body with a well defined molecular feature that makes them useful for diagnosing a disease, measuring the progress of a disease, or determining the effects of a treatment.

Blotting: general term for the transfer of protein, RNA or DNA molecules from a relatively thick acrylamide or agarose gel or to a paper-like membrane (usually nylon or nitrocellulose) by capillarity or an electric field, preserving the spatial arrangement. Once on the membrane, the molecules are immobilized, typically by baking or by ultraviolet irradiation and can then be detected at high sensitivity by hybridization (in the case of DNA and RNA) or antibody labeling (in the case of protein). Northern blot is a technique to study gene expression by detection of RNA (or isolated mRNA); Western blots detect specific proteins; Southern blots detect specific DNA sequences.

Calcium channels: activated by relatively strong membrane depolarization, they permit calcium ion influx in response to action potentials. Consequential secondary actions include neurotransmitter release. These channels thus provide a major link between neuronal excitability and synaptic transmission.

Calcitonin gene related peptide: CGRP is found in a number of tissues including nervous tissue. It is a vasodilator that may participate in the cutaneous triple response. Co-localizes with substance P in neurons. It occurs as a result of alternative processing of mRNA from the calcitonin gene. The neuropeptide is widely distributed in neural tissue of the brain, gut, perivascular nerves, and other tissue. The peptide produces multiple biological effects and has both circulatory and neurotransmitter actions. In particular, it is a potent endogenous vasodilator. Intracerebral administration leads to a rise in noradrenergic sympathetic outflow, a rise in blood pressure and a fall in gastric secretion.

Capsaicin: trans-8-methyl-n-vanillyl-6-nonenamide. Cytotoxic alkaloid from various species of capsicum (pepper, paprika), of the solanaceae; causes pain, irritation, and inflammation, due to substance P depletion from sensory (afferent) nerve fibers; used mainly to study the physiology of pain and in the form of capsicum as a counterirritant and gastrointestinal stimulant.

Cartesian model: refers to Rene Descartes' theory of the early 1600s–a fixed relationship between the magnitude of stimulus and subsequent sensation.

Central sensitization: denotes augmentation of responsiveness of central pain-signaling neurons to input from low-threshold mechanoreceptors; playing a major role in secondary hyperalgesia.

C-*fos*: a proto-oncogene that encodes nuclear proteins that act as transcriptional regulators of target genes. C-*fos* is considered an immediate-early gene (IEG), a class of genes which respond to a variety of stimuli by rapid but transient expression. The nomenclature originates in virology where viral genes are defined as 'early' or 'late', depending on whether their expression occurs before or after replication of the viral genome. Further, a set of viral genes is expressed rapidly or 'immediately' after infection of a cell, even in the presence of protein synthesis inhibitors. Thus, the term 'viral immediate-early gene' (e.g. *v-fos*) was adopted and modified to 'cellular immediate-early gene' (e.g. *c-fos*) for cellular genes which are rapidly induced in the presence of protein synthesis inhibition. C-*fos* is activated in the brain and spinal cord under various conditions including seizures and noxious stimulation, and C-*fos* expression may be a marker for neuroaxis excitation.

Chondrocyte: the only cellular element of articular cartilage.

Chondroprotectant: an agent that 'spares' cartilage degradation.

Chronic pain: results from sustained noxious stimuli such as ongoing inflammation or may be independent of the inciting cause. It extends beyond the period of tissue healing and/or with low levels of identified pathology that are insufficient to explain the presence and/or extent of pain. It is maladaptive and offers no useful biological function or survival advantage. Accordingly, chronic pain may be considered a disease *per se*.

Convergence: where somatic and visceral afferents come together on the same dorsal horn neuron within the spinal cord, as a result 'referred' pain is sensed in a given soma although the stimulus is from the viscera.

Coxib-class NSAIDs: nonsteroidal anti-inflammatory drugs designed to suppress cyclo-oxygenase-2 mediated eicosanoids only and spare cyclo-oxygenase-1 mediated eicosanoids.

Cytokines: a heterogeneous group of polypeptides that activate the immune system and mediate inflammatory responses, acting on a variety of tissues, including the PNS and CNS. Cytokines act at hormonal concentrations, but in contrast to circulating endocrine hormones, they exert their effects on nearby cells over short extracellular distances at low concentrations, and thus serum levels may not reliably reflect local activation. Models of painful nerve injury reveal changes in cytokine expression in the injured nerve itself, in the DRG, in the spinal cord dorsal horn, and in the CNS.

Dorsal root ganglion (DRG): collection of neuronal cell bodies that send their afferent fibers into the spinal dorsal horn: may become a source for ectopic or spontaneous electrical signal generation following axonal injury.

Dysethesia: spontaneous pain.

Eburnation: a late stage of OA, where all cartilage is eroded and the exposed subchondral bone takes on a 'polished ivory' appearance.

Ectopic discharge: can arise from the DRG following peripheral axotomy. A direct relationship exists between ectopic afferent firing and allodynia in neuropathic pain.

Efferent: outgoing; conducted away from the CNS.

Eicosanoid: generic term for compounds derived from arachidonic acid. Includes leukotrienes, prostacyclin, prostaglandins and thromboxanes. Eicosanoid activity is tissue dependent.

Eicosapentaenoic acid (EPA): a precursor for the synthesis of eicosanoids, derived from α-linolenic acid and/or docosahexaenoic acid. Eicosanoids produced from EPA appear to be less inflammatory than those formed from the more common precursor, arachidonic acid.

ELISA: the enzyme-linked immunoabsorbent assay is a serological test used as a general screening tool for the detection of antibodies. Reported as positive or negative. Since false positive tests do occur (for example recent flu shot), positives may require further evaluation using the Western blot. ELISA technology links a measurable enzyme to either an antigen or an antibody. In this way, it can then measure the presence of an antibody or an antigen in the bloodstream.

Enantiomer: a pair of chiral isomers (stereoisomers) that are direct, nonsuperimposable mirror images of each other.

Endbulb: a terminal swelling at the proximal stump when an axon is severed.

Enthesiophytes: bony proliferations found at the insertion of ligaments, tendons, and joint capsule to bone.

Ephatic cross-talk: excitatory interactions among neighboring neurons, amplifying sensory signals and causing sensation spread.

Epitope: that part of an antigenic molecule to which the T-cell receptor responds, a site on a large molecule against which an antibody will be produced and to which it will bind.

Evidence-based: the conscientious, explicit, and judicious use of current best evidence in making decisions.

Excitability: refers to the translation of the generator potential into an impulse train, where sodium and potassium channels play a major role. If excitability is suppressed, the cell loses its ability to respond to all stimuli.

Excitation: refers to the transduction process, the ability of a stimulus to depolarize a sensory neuron, creating a generator potential.

Fibrillation: seen in the early stages of OA, where the superficial layer of the hyaline cartilage begins 'flaking' and is lost.

Force plate platform: a device for objective measurement of ground reaction forces; frequently used to compare efficacy of different treatment protocols.

GABA: is the most abundant inhibitory neurotransmitter in the CNS and plays a role in the control of the pathways that transmit sensory events, including nociception. GABAergic interneurons can be found in nearly all layers of the spinal cord, with the highest concentrations in laminae I–III. A decrease in GABAergic tone in the spinal cord may underlie the state of allodynia.

Gate theory: proposed by Melzack and Wall in 1965, suggesting that the CNS controls nociception: activity in large (non-nociceptive) fibers can inhibit the perception of activity in small (nociceptive) fibers and that descending activity from the brain also can inhibit that perception, i.e. encoding of high-intensity afferent input to the CNS was subject to modulation.

Glasgow Pain Scale: a multidimensional scheme for assessing pain. It takes into account the sensory and affective qualities of pain in addition to its intensity.

Glial cells: astrocytes, oligodendrocytes, and microglia. Microglia are resident tissue macrophages of the CNS, and when activated, can release chemical mediators that can act on neurons to alter their function.

Glycosaminoglycans (GAGs): hydrophilic 'bristles' attached to the hyaluronan backbone, thereby forming the 'bottle brush' appearance of the cartilage aggrecan.

Glutamate: the predominant neurotransmitter used by all primary afferent fibers.

Hyperalgesia: an increased response to a stimulus which is normally painful.

IC_{50}: the concentration of drug needed to inhibit the activity of an enzyme by 50%. (IC_{80} is sometimes referenced.)

Idiosyncratic: cause/etiology is unknown.

Incisional pain (postoperative): a specific form of acute pain, routinely lasting 2 (mechanical stimulus) to 7 (heat stimulus) days.

Kinematic gait analysis (motion analysis): measures changes in joint angles with gait, the velocity and acceleration of changes in joint angles, stride length, as well as gait swing and stance times. Often used in conjunction with force platform gait analysis, providing a powerful method of detecting musculoskeletal abnormalities and response to therapy.

Ligand: any molecule that binds to another, in normal usage a soluble molecule such as a hormone or neurotransmitter, that binds to a receptor. The decision as to which is the ligand and which the receptor is often a little arbitrary when the broader sense of receptor is used (where there is no implication of transduction of signal). In these cases it is probably a good rule to consider the ligand to be the smaller of the two.

Matrix metalloproteinase (MMP): a family of enzymes involved in the degradation of cartilage matrix.

Membrane remodeling: inappropriate distribution of membrane proteins such as ion channels, transducer molecules, and receptors synthesized in the cell soma and transported into the cell membrane of endbulbs and sprouts by vesicle exocytosis following injury to afferent neurons. This leads to altered axonal excitability.

Meta-analysis: a quantitative method of combining the results of independent studies (usually drawn from the published literature) and synthesizing summaries and conclusions which may be used to evaluate therapeutic effectiveness or to plan new studies, with application chiefly in the areas of research and medicine. It is often an overview of clinical trials. It is usually called a meta-analysis by the author or sponsoring body and should be differentiated from reviews of the literature.

Modulation: alterations of ascending signals initially in the dorsal horn and continuing throughout the CNS.

Multimodal analgesia: the administration of a combination of different drugs from different pharmacological classes, as well as different delivery forms, and techniques.

Nerve fiber: refers to the combination of the axon and Schwann cell as a functional unit.

Neurogenic inflammation: driven by events in the CNS and not dependent on granulocytes or lymphocytes as the classic inflammatory response to tissue trauma or immune-mediated cell damage. Dendrite release of inflammatory mediators causes action potentials to fire backwards down nociceptors, potentiating transmission of nociceptive signals from the periphery.

Neuroma: formed by failed efforts of injured peripheral nerve sprouts to re-establish normal functional contact, that can become ectopic generators of neural activity.

Neuropathic pain: arises from injury to or sensitization of the PNS or CNS.

Neurotransmitter: any of a group of endogenous substances that are released on excitation from the axon terminal of a presynaptic neuron of the CNS or PNS and travel across the synaptic cleft to either excite or inhibit the target cell. Among the many substances that have the properties of a neurotransmitter are acetylcholine, norepinephrine, glutamate, epinephrine, dopamine, glycine, gamma-aminobutyrate, glutamic acid, substance P, enkephalins, endorphins, and serotonin.

NMDA (N-methyl-D-aspartate) receptor: has been implicated in the phenomenon of windup and in related changes such as spinal hyperexcitability, that enhance and prolong sensory transmission. Persistent injury states such as neuropathy may produce a prolonged activation of the NMDA receptor subsequent to a sustained afferent input that causes a relatively small, but continuous increase in the levels of glutamate and enhances the evoked release of the amino acid. NMDA receptors are not functional unless there has been a persistent or large-scale release of glutamate. Ketamine, memantine, and amantadine are common NMDA antagonists.

Nitric oxide synthase (NOS): synthesizes nitric oxide (NO) from L-arginine; three isoforms are known to exist: endothelian NOS (eNOS), neuronal NOS (nNOS), and inducible NOS (iNOS).

Nociception: the physiological activity of transduction, transmission, and modulation of noxious stimuli; may or may not include perception, depending on the conscious state of the animal, i.e. the result of nociception in the conscious animal is pain.

Nociceptive pain (physiological pain): everyday acute pain, purposeful, short-acting, and relatively easy to treat.

Nuclear factor kappa B (NF-κB): a transcription factor that regulates gene expression of many cellular mediators influencing the immune and inflammatory response.

Number needed to treat (NNT): an estimate of the number of patients that would need to be given a treatment for one of them to achieve a desired outcome, e.g. the number of patients that must be treated, after correction for placebo responders, to obtain one patient with at least 50% pain relief. In a similar manner, number needed to harm (NNH) is a calculation of adverse effects.

Nutraceutical: a nondrug, food additive that is given orally to benefit the wellbeing of the recipient.

OP3: opioid mu receptor.

OP2: opioid kappa receptor.

OP1: opioid delta receptor.

Osteoarthritis (OA): (degenerative joint disease (DJD)) disorder of the total movable joints characterized by deterioration of articular cartilage; osteophyte formation and bone remodeling; pathology of periarticular tissues including synovium, subchondral bone, muscle, tendon, and ligament; and a low-grade, nonpurulent inflammation of variable degree. Pain is the hallmark clinical sign.

Osteophytes: a central core of bone frequently found at the junction of the synovium, perichondrium, and periosteum of arthritic joints.

Paresthesias: dysesthesia, and hyperpathia refer to odd, unnatural sensations like 'pins-and needles', sudden jabs, or electric-shock-like sensations. These occur when nerves are partially blocked (e.g. 'my leg went to sleep') or when there is nerve damage.

Partial agonist (opioid): binds at a given receptor causing an effect less pronounced than that of a pure agonist.

Pathological pain (inflammatory pain, neuropathic pain): implies tissue damage, nontransient, and may be associated with significant tissue inflammation and nerve injury.

Perception: receipt and cognitive appreciation of signals arriving at higher CNS structures, thereby allowing the interpretation as pain.

P2X: ionotropic receptors for ATP.

Phenotype: the total characteristics displayed by an organism under a particular set of environmental factors, regardless of the actual genotype of the organism. Results from interaction between the genotype and the environment.

Peripheral nervous system (PNS): cranial nerves, spinal nerves with their roots and rami, peripheral components of the autonomic nervous system, and peripheral nerves whose primary sensory neurons are located in the associated dorsal root ganglion.

Postherpetic neuralgia: PHN is commonly used as a model for neuropathic pain. PHN is a consequence of herpes zoster, where pain will continue long after the rash has resolved, causing a great deal of suffering and disability. Herpes zoster results from activation of the varicella-zoster virus, which has remained latent in the dorsal root ganglion since the first infection (usually chickenpox). The varicella-zoster virus has a vary narrow host range, and natural infection occurs only in humans and other primates.

Physical rehabilitation: activities involved in the goal to restore, maintain, and promote optimal function, optimal fitness, wellness, and quality of life as they relate to movement disorders and health.

Plasticity: refers to neuronal information processing which can change in a manner dependent on levels of neuronal excitability and synaptic strength, diversifying for short periods (seconds) or prolonged periods (days), or perhaps indefinitely.

Pre-emptive analgesia: presurgical blockade of nociception intended to prevent or lessen postsurgical pain or pain hypersensitivity. Best clinical application is actually 'perioperative', where analgesia is administered long enough to last throughout surgery and even into the postoperative period.

Primary hyperalgesia: hyperalgesia at the site of injury, while hyperalgesia in the uninjured skin surrounding the injury is termed secondary hyperalgesia.

Qi: a tenet of traditional Chinese medicine holding that Qi is a fundamental and vital substance of the universe, with all phenomena being produced by its changes. Traditional Chinese medicine suggests that a balanced flow of Qi throughout the system is required for good health, and acupuncture stimulation can correct imbalances.

Referred pain: a pain sensation felt at an anatomical location different from its origin; most often associated with visceral pain where the CNS is sensing a somatic input rather than visceral nociception.

Reversal of GABA/glycinergic inhibition: a microglial activity occurring only following neuropathic injury but not peripheral inflammation, where reversing the direction of anionic flux in lamina I neurons reverses the effect of GABA and glycine, changing inhibition to excitation.

Schwann cell: plays a major role in nerve regeneration and axonal maintenance. Some cells produce myelin, a lipid-rich insulating covering.

Secondary hyperalgesia: hyperalgesia in the uninjured skin surrounding the injury, including two different components: (1) a change in the modality of the sensation evoked by low-threshold mechanoreceptors, from touch to pain, and (2) an increase in the magnitude of the pain sensations evoked by mechanically sensitive nociceptors.

Sensitization: a leftward shift of the stimulus–response function that relates magnitude of the neural response to stimulus intensity.

Silent afferents (sleeping nociceptors, mechanically insensitive nociceptors): these afferents are ubiquitous and have been found in skin, joint, and viscera in rat, cat, and monkey:[2] 20–40% of C fibers in skin, 30–40% in muscle, 50–75% in joint, and possibly more than 90% of C fibers to colon and bladder fail to respond to acute noxious stimuli. In joints that have been artificially inflamed, these previously silent afferents develop an ongoing discharge and fire vigorously during ordinary movement.

Sodium channels: voltage-dependent sodium channels produce the inward transmembrane current that depolarizes the cell membrane, and thus are critically important contributors to action potential electrogenesis. Compelling evidence indicates that sodium channels participate substantially in the hyperexcitability of sensory neurons that contributes to neuropathic pain.

Subchondral bone: a thin layer of bone that joins hyaline cartilage with cancellous bone supporting the bony plate. Compliance of subchondral bone to applied joint forces allows congruity of joint surfaces for increasing the contact area of load distribution, i.e. a shock absorber, thereby reducing peak loading and potentially damaging effects on cartilage.

Substance P (sP): a vasoactive peptide found in the brain, spinal ganglia and intestine of vertebrates. Induces vasodilatation, salivation and increases capillary permeability. A tachykinin, released only after intense, constant peripheral stimuli. sP, acting at NK_1 receptors, plays an important role in nociception and emesis. 'Phylogenetic switch' is a term given to myelinated axons that normally do not make sP, but become capable of manufacturing sP after a prolonged inflammatory stimulus.

Synergism: a response greater than the additive response, e.g. the effect of opioids combined with alpha-2 adrenoceptor agonists is greater than the additive effect of each class of drug individually.

Synovial fluid: a dialysate of plasma containing electrolyes and small molecules in similar proportions as in plasma.

Synovial intima: lining of the joint capsule, containing synoviocytes A and B.

Synovitis: inflammation of the synovial intima.

Tetrodotoxin (TTX): a toxin derived from puffer fish, sensitivity to which is useful for classifying sodium currents (sensitive or resistant).

Tidemark: the upper limit of the calcified cartilage layer (zone 4) of articular cartilage.

Transcutaneous electrical nerve stimulation (TENS): a method of producing electroanalgesia through current applied to electrodes placed in the skin.

Transduction: conversion of energy from a noxious stimulus into nerve impulses by sensory receptors.

Transmission: transference of neural signals from the site of transduction (periphery) to the CNS.

Transmucosal (transbuccal): not to be confused with oral administration, refers to placement of a drug for absorption across the mucous membranes (as by placement in the guttural pouch). This route of absorption avoids hepatic first-pass elimination, because venous drainage is systemic.

TRPV (vanilloid or capsaicin) receptor: a detector of noxious heat.

Viscosupplementation: intra-articular injection of a chondroprotectant intended to increase the viscoelastic properties of the synovial fluid.

Voltage-gated sodium and calcium channel: voltage-gated sodium channels (VGSCs) are complex, transmembrane proteins that have a role in governing electrical activity in excitable tissues. The channel is activated in response to depolarization of the cell membrane that causes a voltage-dependent conformational change in the channel from a resting, closed conformation to an active conformation which increases membrane permeability. Gabapentin is thought to work via a voltage-dependent calcium channel (VDCC).

Wallerian degeneration: a form of degeneration occurring in nerve fibers as a result of their division; so called from Dr. Waller, who published an account of it in 1850.

Washout: refers to the time interval between different NSAID administrations presumed to reduce the risk for contributing to adverse drug reactions. Empirically, recommendations range from 1–7 days in healthy dogs.

WHO cancer pain ladder: the World Health Organization's analgesic ladder provides clinical guidance from a severity-based pain classification system.

Windup: a form of activity-dependent plasticity characterized by a progressive increase in action potential output from dorsal horn neurons elicited during the course of a train of repeated low-frequency C fiber or nociceptor stimuli. Resultant cumulative depolarization is boosted by recruitment of NMDA receptor current through inhibition of magnesium channel suppression.

Ω-conotoxin: found in the venoms of predatory marine snails that blocks depolarization-induced calcium influx through voltage-sensitive calcium channels.

INDEX

Note: Page references in *italic* refer to tables in the text